The Design and Statistical Analysis of Animal Experiments

Written specifically for animal researchers, this is the first book to provide a comprehensive guide to the design and statistical analysis of animal experiments. It has long been recognised that the proper implementation of these techniques can help to optimise the number of animals used in an experiment. By using real-life examples to make them more accessible, this book explains the statistical tools that are routinely employed by practitioners.

A wide range of design types are considered in detail, including block, factorial, nested, crossover, dose-escalation and repeated measures. Alongside each design, techniques are introduced to analyse the experimental data generated. Each analysis approach is described in non-mathematical terms, helping readers without a statistical background to understand key techniques such as: *t*-tests, ANOVA, repeated measures, analysis of covariance, multiple comparison tests, non-parametric methods and survival analysis.

This is also the first text to describe technical aspects of InVivoStat, a powerful open-source software package developed by the authors to enable animal researchers to analyse their data and obtain informative results. InVivoStat can be downloaded at www.invivostat.co.uk.

Simon T. Bate is a Principal Statistician at GlaxoSmithKline, supporting pre-clinical research. He has spent over 12 years supporting the design and statistical analysis of animal experiments, including drug discovery research, toxicology studies and safety assessment. He presents many statistics courses around Europe, including the statistics module of the British Association for Psychopharmacology's Pre-Clinical Certificate.

Robin A. Clark is a Senior Analyst Programmer at Huntingdon Life Sciences, Alconbury. Originally qualified as a marine ecologist, he is now a software architect producing data collection and statistical applications for the pharmaceutical industry. Robin produced the user interface and designed the system architecture for InVivoStat.

The Design and Statistical Analysis of Animal Experiments

Simon T. Bate

GlaxoSmithKline, UK

and

Robin A. Clark

Huntingdon Life Sciences, UK

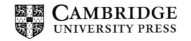

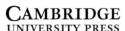

University Printing House, Cambridge CB2 8BS, United Kingdom

Published in the United States of America by Cambridge University Press, New York

Cambridge University Press is part of the University of Cambridge.

It furthers the University's mission by disseminating knowledge in the pursuit of
education, learning and research at the highest international levels of excellence.

www.cambridge.org
Information on this title: www.cambridge.org/9781107030787

First published 2014

Printed in the United Kingdom by Clays, St Ives plc

A catalogue record for this publication is available from the British Library

Library of Congress Cataloguing in Publication data
Bate, Simon T., 1975–
The design and statistical analysis of animal experiments / Simon Bate, GlaxoSmithKline, UK,
Robin Clark, Huntingdon Life Sciences, UK.
    pages   cm.
Includes bibliographical references and index.
ISBN 978-1-107-03078-7 (hardback) – ISBN 978-1-107-69094-3 (paperback)
1. Animal experimentation–Statistical methods.   2. Experimental design.   I. Clark, Robin A.,
software developer.   II. Title. HV4930.D47 2002
590.72′4–dc23
2013033851

ISBN 978-1-107-03078-7 Hardback
ISBN 978-1-107-69094-3 Paperback

Additional resources for this publication at www.cambridge.org/9781107030787

To

RB, NRB, MTB, EC, EJC, ZMC

Contents

Preface

This book is aimed at practitioners who do not have a statistics degree and yet wish to apply statistics to help them arrive at valid and reliable conclusions while minimising the animal numbers required. Descriptions of the mathematical methods underpinning the topics covered in the book are purposefully kept to a minimum. If readers wish to gain a better understanding of the mathematics behind experimental design and statistical analysis then reading a more advanced textbook would help further their understanding.

The solutions to practical problems encountered when conducting animal experiments are explained using non-technical approaches. We believe that in many situations advanced statistical ideas can be employed successfully by researchers with no statistical qualification, using a combination of common sense and modern statistical analysis software packages. In our experience statistical ideas are often introduced to scientists using mathematical terminology. This can be off-putting to non-mathematicians and can leave researchers with, at best, only rudimentary statistical tools and at worst a fear of statistics.

To keep the descriptions of the statistical tools covered in this book as simple as possible, we shall occasionally give pragmatic explanations. While such explanations may not apply in all cases and in all scientific disciplines, this approach does allow us to introduce methods in a clear and concise way. By allowing ourselves the freedom to simplify the problems pragmatically, we aim to make statistical tools more accessible. The reader is invited, once they have familiarised themselves with (and hopefully found the benefit of using) the tools described in this book, to read more advanced texts on the subject.

This book is divided into seven chapters which loosely correspond to the procedure a researcher should take when planning the experimental design, running the experiment and evaluating the data generated. Following an introductory chapter and a second describing certain statistical concepts, the third chapter covers different types of designs. Designs are outlined, where possible, in simple non-technical language. This is followed by a chapter describing the randomisation of the experimental material. The fifth chapter discusses the statistical analysis of animal experiments and this is followed by a chapter describing how these methods can be applied within the statistical software package InVivoStat. The final chapter draws some conclusions about the ideas contained within the text.

A scientist can apply all of the methodology described in this book. Certain topics covered are more advanced than others and while we aim to make all subjects accessible, the reader should be aware that the help of a professional statistician may be advisable when first implementing some of the more advanced tools. However, once the readers have familiarised themselves with the ideas contained within this book, we hope they will have a fuller appreciation of the help statistics can offer to improve the conclusions that can be made when running animal experiments.

Acknowledgments

We would like to thank all our colleagues, both past and present, for providing so much inspiration for this book. We hope this text reflects the discussions, consultations and the range of examples that we have worked on together. There are simply too many scientists to mention, but you know who you are! We hope the wide variety of interesting practical problems we have faced together is reflected throughout this book.

Special thanks also to the statisticians who have advised us over the years and shaped our views on this subject matter. Simon would especially like to thank Philip Overend and Andrew Lloyd for their input and encouragement and Janet and Ed Godolphin for their help and support over the years.

We would like to give an extra special thanks to Gillian Amphlett, Gill Fleetwood, David Willé, Clare Stanford and Nathalie Percie du Sert for giving up their time to review sections of the book, and providing ideas, advice and feedback. Their input has been most helpful and improved the text considerably.

Finally we would like to thank our friends and family for putting up with the long unsociable hours we spent writing this book.

Introduction

Many researchers, either directly or indirectly, rely on statistical ideas when carrying out animal experiments. While some statistical tools are well known and are applied routinely, other tools are less well understood and so are less well used. The overall aim of this book is to discuss statistical methodologies that can be applied throughout the many stages of the experimental process. Researchers should be able to carry out most of the techniques described, although the advice of a professional statistician is advisable for some of the more advanced topics. Making use of these techniques will ensure that experiments are conducted in a logical and efficient way, which should result in reliable and reproducible decisions.

The particular types of study addressed in this book, as the title suggests, are studies involving animals. We attempt to cover all of the statistical tools that the animal researcher should use to run successful studies. Of course many of the problems faced by the animal researcher are common to other disciplines, and hence the ideas contained within this book can be applied to other areas. It should be noted that certain topics described in the text have been simplified to allow non-statisticians to apply the ideas without professional statistical support. Such pragmatic descriptions, while simplifying the technical details, are not universal and will not be applicable in all scientific disciplines.

There has been much interest in the use of statistics in animal research, in particular in the application of the 3Rs, replacement, reduction and refinement, as described by Russell and Burch (1959):

Every time any particle of statistical method is properly used, fewer animals are employed than would otherwise have been necessary.

Many authors have since highlighted how important the use of good experimental design is when conducting animal experiments; see Festing (1994, 2003a, 2003b) and the references contained within. Some of the more practical, as well as statistical, aspects of experimental design and statistics when applying the 3Rs are described in the book by Festing *et al.* (2002). There have also been surveys into the use of statistics in refereed journals; see McCance (1995) and more recently Kilkenny *et al.* (2009). The latter draws attention to some of the mistakes that can be made by researchers when designing and analysing animal experiments. The reliability of the reporting of animal experiments has been considered in, for example, Macleod *et al.* (2009) and Rooke *et al.* (2011). These articles highlight that papers describing experiments that do not employ suitable randomisation techniques and/or blinding may contain biased results.

The main goal of this text is to demonstrate how statistics can aid the reduction and refinement of animal studies. The efficient use of statistics, both in terms of complex experimental design and powerful statistical analysis, can reduce the number of animals required. Statistics can also help the researcher understand the processes that underpin the animal model and help identify factors that are influencing the experimental results. Such an understanding will inevitably lead to a refinement in the experimental process and a reduction in the total number of animals used.

Statistics, as a discipline, provides researchers with tools to help them arrive at valid conclusions. However, statistics, along with the application of some common sense, can also increase the understanding of the animal model through the application of graphical and mathematical techniques. For example, graphical tools play an important role in helping the researcher understand the effect of the features of the experimental design and also uncover overall patterns present in the data. The application of a formal statistical test, without first investigating the data graphically, can lead to the researcher drawing incorrect conclusions from the data. Consider the following real-life case study, which used graphical, as well as statistical, tools. If a conventional statistical analysis had been carried out, without first investigating all of the information gathered within the experiment, then the conclusions would have been misleading.

Example 1.1: Reducing blood cholesterol levels in mice

A scientist wanted to test the hypothesis that a novel compound had a beneficial effect on reducing high-density lipoprotein (HDL) cholesterol levels in a transgenic C57Bl/6J strain of mice. A blood sample was taken pre-treatment and the baseline cholesterol level for each animal measured. The mice were then randomised to either the drug treatment group or the control group and dosed with either the drug treatment or vehicle twice daily for two weeks. At the end of this period, a terminal blood sample was taken and the HDL cholesterol level measured.

As the scientist wanted to make use of the baseline information in the statistical analysis, it was decided that the percentage change from baseline would be a suitable response to investigate. This would, the scientist hoped, effectively remove the animal-to-animal differences by normalising to the baseline level. While there was evidence of a decrease in HDL cholesterol level in the group of animals administered the drug treatment (a 20% decrease from baseline in the drug treatment group compared to a 10% decrease in the control group) this was not deemed statistically significant using an unpaired t-test (p = 0.191). A means with standard errors of the mean (SEMs) plot of the data (see Section 5.3.5) is presented in Figure 1.1.

As a follow-up the scientist also analysed the terminal HDL cholesterol level. From this analysis it appeared that there was a statistically significant increase in cholesterol level in the drug-treated group compared to the control. A plot of the means with SEMs of the terminal HDL cholesterol level is presented in Figure 1.2.

Based on the results of this experiment, should we conclude the drug increases cholesterol levels? And why did the two analyses give such different conclusions? These questions can be answered

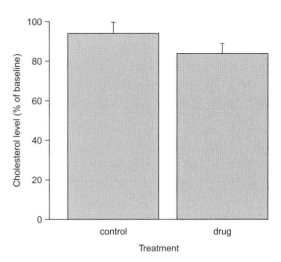

Figure 1.1. Plot of treatment means with standard errors for the percentage of baseline cholesterol response for Example 1.1.

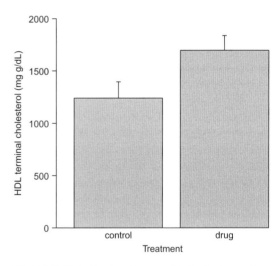

Figure 1.2. Plot of treatment means with standard errors for the terminal HDL cholesterol for Example 1.1.

by a simple scatterplot of the measured HDL cholesterol levels. If we plot terminal vs. baseline HDL cholesterol levels, an underlying problem with the experiment becomes clear. The scatterplot is presented in Figure 1.3.

From Figure 1.3 it can be seen that there are two distinct groupings along the X-axis. The plot reveals that, in terms of the HDL baseline cholesterol level, the animals belong to one of two

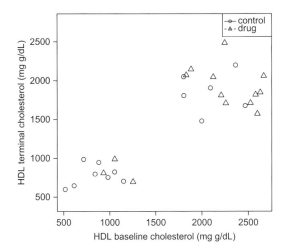

Figure 1.3. Scatterplot of terminal HDL cholesterol vs. baseline HDL cholesterol, categorised by treatment for Example 1.1.

sub-populations. Unless we are careful how these baseline differences are accounted for, we could draw incorrect conclusions from the analysis. Given that there appears to be a correlation between baseline and terminal cholesterol levels, this baseline difference is probably the most important feature of the experiment that influences the conclusion – perhaps more so than the treatment effect itself. The treatment effect observed in the experiment will be influenced by the allocation of the mice (within each sub-population) to the treatment groups. In this case most of the mice that were allocated to the novel drug group were from the sub-population with the high baseline level. So it is not surprising that, when analysing the terminal HDL cholesterol level, it appears that the terminal cholesterol level is higher in the treatment group. Obviously the researcher was unlucky that the randomisation of the mice to the treatment groups produced such an allocation.

The solution is twofold. Firstly, and most importantly, the researcher should try to identify what is causing the baseline differences. We can then account for this effect in the experimental design. However, if we fail to identify what is causing the baseline differences, then the randomisation should be carried out so that the treatment replication is equal in both sub-populations. This will, of course, depend on whether the baseline information is available when allocating the mice to the treatment groups.

If the researcher produces the scatterplot shown in Figure 1.3, then it will become apparent that the treatment effects may be due to baseline cholesterol levels. However, without such a graphical investigation of the data the problem may not have been identified. It is important at this stage of the book to note that a valid statistical investigation of a dataset is more about understanding the information contained within the data. It does not just involve the

calculation of *p*-values. Graphs can be the best and simplest way to achieve this and should always be considered first, ideally by plotting the individual data points.

In reality the treatment allocation observed in this example is quite extreme and perhaps indicates a biased selection process. It should be noted, however, that there is always a chance, however small, that the randomisation will generate a significant treatment effect due to differences at baseline. This will occasionally happen, even when the allocation process is valid. As long as the randomisation is performed correctly, then we should not be too concerned that effects present at the baseline will influence the treatment comparisons.

1.1 Structure of this book

The majority of the remainder of this text is split up into three main chapters. In Chapter 3 we describe families of experimental designs that can be employed when conducting animal research. The chapter consists of a description of each design and practical examples of their use. Also given is an explanation of when and where to apply each design. The section attempts to introduce each experimental design, without overuse of mathematical terminology.

In Chapter 4 some general issues involving randomisation are discussed. We consider why the experimental material should be randomised and describe the influence this has on the statistical analysis. Techniques that can be employed to perform the randomisation are also given.

When conducting a statistical analysis, one of the first steps in the process is to define the statistical model that will be used to explain the observed data. There are several ways to justify the choice of statistical model. Given that the animal researcher has control over the experimental design, it seems sensible to make use of the design when deciding which statistical model to apply. One way of linking the experimental design to the statistical analysis is by considering the randomisation applied to the experimental material. Most analyses, and certainly those considered in this book, make assumptions about the allocation of animals to treatment groups. For a valid statistical analysis of a designed experiment, a suitable randomisation should have been carried out.

Chapter 5 describes the statistical analysis techniques that the researcher should employ when analysing data generated using the designs discussed in Chapter 3. We approach the subject in a practical way, without the use of mathematical formulae. We assume the researcher has access to an advanced statistical package, such as InVivoStat, to compute all numerical results. The tools described in this book are flexible enough to cope with most experimental situations. Any assumptions made during the statistical analysis are also discussed. When these assumptions do not hold alternative approaches are given.

In Chapter 6 we describe how the researcher can perform the analyses discussed in Chapter 5 using the InVivoStat statistical software package. For each InVivoStat module the analysis procedure is described, including input and output options, and a worked example given. Where appropriate, a technical description of the implementation of the analysis methodology is also presented.

This text contains many ideas that the researcher may need to employ during the course of the experimental process. Some of the techniques will be applied frequently during routine work and hence will be of interest to all readers. Other sections describe techniques that are more advanced and would only be used occasionally, for example when setting up a new animal model.

1.1.1 Introductory sections

The following sections should be read by the casual reader who wishes to get a simple overview of the ideas contained within this text. These sections provide a flavour of some of the more advanced sections.

Sections 2.1 and 2.3 – Statistical concepts

Readers should familiarise themselves with these sections as they provide the framework for all following sections on experimental design and statistical analysis.

Section 3.1 – Why design experiments?

This section is an introduction into why we should be designing animal experiments and some information

on the benefits that can be gained from an understanding of experimental design.

Section 3.3 – Summary of design types

This section introduces the types of experimental design that are available to the researcher. Information is given on when and why they should be used.

Section 3.7.2 – Sample size and power

This section discusses the factors that influence sample size and gives information on how to calculate suitable sample sizes in animal experiments.

Sections 4.2 and 4.4 – Randomisation

These sections describe why we need to randomise our experimental material and give practical examples of how to carry out the randomisation.

Section 5.1 – Introduction into statistical analysis

This section is a description, including a worked example, of our preferred analysis procedure using the InVivoStat software package.

Section 5.4 – Parametric analysis

This section describes the types of parametric analysis, some of their properties and gives information on when to use them.

1.1.2 Approaches to consider when setting up a new animal model

When setting up a new animal model, or perhaps trying to replicate a model described in the literature, there may be many factors that influence the animals' responses which will need to be quantified. Perhaps the researcher needs to decide which sex to use, how old the animals need to be, how long to dose the animals prior to testing... the list goes on. A common approach taken by researchers is to investigate each of these factors one at a time. However, there are better and more efficient (not to say more informative) ways to conduct these investigations. Use:

- Large factorial designs (Section 3.5.4) to assess factors and factor interactions and to maximise the window of opportunity;
- Nested designs (Section 3.7) to decide on the replication required within the experiment;
- Power analysis to select sample sizes (Section 3.7.2);
- Parametric analysis tools, such as ANOVA (Section 5.4.2), repeated measures analysis (Section 5.4.4) or graphical tools (Section 5.3) to investigate how the factors relate to each other.

1.1.3 Approaches to consider when generating hypotheses

Once the animal model has been set up, the researcher might wish to start generating hypotheses. Consider using:
- Small factorial designs (Section 3.5.3) to assess interactions between factors of interest;
- Block designs to reduce variability and allow the researcher to manage experiments more efficiently (Section 3.4);
- Parametric analysis tools, such as ANOVA (Section 5.4.3), repeated measures analysis (Section 5.4.4) or graphical tools (Section 5.3) to investigate how the factors relate to each other.

1.1.4 Approaches to consider when testing hypotheses

When testing specific hypotheses, the researcher should be stricter (in the analysis) to avoid generating false positive results. Consider using:
- Block designs to reduce variability and manage the experiments more efficiently (Section 3.4);
- Parametric analysis tools, such as ANOVA (Section 5.4.3) or repeated measures analysis (Section 5.4.4);
- Planned comparisons or other suitable multiple comparison procedures to compare individual group means (Section 5.4.8).

1.2 Statistical problems faced by animal researchers

From a statistical point of view the animal researcher faces two major issues. The first problem is that there will usually be substantial animal-to-animal variability. If two animals are given the same treatment regime, then they will respond in subtly different ways. This, combined with the ethical imperative to use as few animals as possible, will cause many problems for the researcher.

The level of animal-to-animal variability varies between different animal models, disease areas, species and even batches of animals. This has, perhaps, been reduced by the advent of inbred isogenic strains, which has meant that the animals themselves are less phenotypically variable (Festing *et al.*, 2002, pp. 17–26). However, it is probably correct to assume that this source of variability will still be large in most animal experiments. The researcher should aim to quantify the size of the animal-to-animal variability but also try to discover any other sources of variability within the experiment that will increase this.

Once all the sources of variability have been identified and quantified, another problem is determining the sample size required for the experiment. Sadly, many assume the advice of a statistician will be to increase sample size, regardless of the practical implications! While there are benefits to be gained from increasing sample size (for purely statistical reasons) there may be other techniques that statistics can offer, other than simply increasing animal numbers, which will improve the reliability and reproducibility of the experimental results.

In many animal experiments there is one statistical 'saving grace' that can be used to reduce the impact of high variability and small sample sizes, and that is the experimental design. Researchers usually have almost complete control over the experimental design used. For example, animals can be ordered so that they arrive from the supplier at set dates, unlike clinical trials where patients need to be enrolled. Researchers can also plan how the study is conducted. If the study is completed over two days, or two pieces of test equipment are used or two surgeons perform the surgery, then these can be taken into account when planning the study. Hypotheses that are to be tested are planned well in advance and so designs can be tailored to suit the questions being answered. Many characteristics of the animals are also recorded before the start of a study for welfare reasons, for example age and body weight. So there is extra information about the animals themselves that can be used in the analysis of the study data.

In conclusion, if the researcher is to avoid the statistical pitfalls of high variability and small sample sizes, then it can be argued that the use of good experimental design (and the appropriate statistical analysis of the data generated when using such designs) is more crucial in animal research than in many other scientific disciplines.

1.3 Pitfalls encountered when applying statistics in practice

There are many pitfalls that may trap the unwary researcher when carrying out animal research. The following examples are taken from a number of published sources, namely Festing *et al.* (2002, pp. 11–16), McCance (1995), Gaines Das *et al.* (2009) and Kilkenny *et al.* (2009), along with the authors' own experiences.

1.3.1 Pitfalls with experimental design

Using appropriate designs at specific points in the experimental process

Many researchers fail to employ the right design at the right time. This can lead to using more animals than is necessary and can undermine the reliability of the experimental conclusions. For example, when setting up a new animal model, or revising an existing one, there are certain types of design that can be used to investigate the many hypothesised factors that could influence the experimental results. These designs, the so-called large factorial designs, provide a quick, easy and systematic way of developing knowledge of the animal model. If the researcher fails to use these designs, then it may take longer to fully understand the animal model. Factorial designs are discussed later in this book (see Section 3.5).

Failure to account for nuisance effects in the design

Most researchers can probably list nuisance effects that could be accounted for in the study design. For example,

animals may be housed in different cages or rooms, be selected from two or more litters or be operated on by one of two surgeons. The list can go on. It is important to check if these nuisance effects have an effect on the measured response. If not then they can be ignored and future designs simplified, otherwise strategies should be developed that take them into account.

If a design is not planned in advance, then comparisons between the treatments may become influenced (or biased) by other unwanted nuisance effects that were not taken into account. It may be the case that a nuisance effect cannot be separated from the treatment effect in the statistical analysis and so the treatment effect cannot be reliably assessed. We say that the two effects are *completely confounded* with each other. In the worst case scenario the observed treatment effect may be wholly due to the nuisance effect.

Consider, for example, an experiment where the control animals were tested on one piece of equipment and the treated animals are tested on a second. Any treatment differences observed could be due to, or influenced by, differences between the two pieces of equipment. Unfortunately if such a design has been used then there is no statistical way of testing for this bias.

As a rule of thumb if the results from an experiment appear unusual, then there may be an underlying nuisance effect that is influencing the results.

Experiments done on an *ad hoc* basis

Some researchers do not take a systematic approach when planning a series of studies. Rather than plan them in advance, studies are carried out in a piecemeal fashion. For example, in a series of drug trials, higher doses of the compound are investigated by conducting extra studies, rather than including all doses in the design at the beginning of the experiment. In this situation, the dose-response relationships are assessed across studies, and hence any study-to-study differences will influence the assessment of the dose-response relationship.

Control groups not used correctly

The purpose of a control group is to allow treatment effects to be assessed in the absence of any other experimental effects. To achieve this, the control group must be exposed to exactly the same conditions as the treatment groups (to allow the treatment comparisons to be unbiased). For example, in rodent studies it is often the case that the animals are housed in racks of cages. Each rack is allocated to a single treatment to avoid cross-contamination. However, if the racks containing the control animals were placed nearest to the door of the animal room, then these animals may be more disturbed than the treated animals. This could bias the treatment comparisons.

Inefficient choice of treatment groups

If there are two or more factors of interest in a study, then it is recommended that all combinations of the factor levels are included in the design. For example, consider an experiment where there are two factors: Drug (levels: vehicle and compound) and Strain (levels: transgenic and wildtype). It is important that where possible all combinations of the two factors are included in the design, i.e. vehicle + transgenic, vehicle + wildtype, compound + transgenic and compound + wildtype. This is an example of a small full-factorial design, as discussed in Section 3.5.3. If a combination of the factor levels is not included in the final design, then drawing inferences from the analysis can become more difficult. The sensitivity of the statistical analysis to identify significant treatment effects can also be compromised.

Too few animals per group

If the sample size is too small, then the experiment will lack sufficient statistical power to detect a real treatment effect (see Section 3.7.2). Running a study with too few animals is a waste of animals as well as the researcher's time and resources (Button et al., 2013). A power analysis, as described in Sections 3.7.2 and 6.8, should be completed before running a study to confirm the sample size is large enough to achieve meaningful results. There is at least anecdotal evidence that suggests researchers generally underestimate the sample size required when conducting animal experiments. It is preferable to conduct one or two large

(and reliable) studies instead of a series of smaller inconclusive ones.

Too many animals per group

It should be remembered that, when running a statistical analysis, it is possible that a biologically irrelevant effect could be declared statistically significant if the sample size is too large. The researcher should begin the planning process by identifying the level of biological relevance. For example, perhaps a drug that causes a 20% change from control is of interest and merits further investigation. If an estimate of variability is available, then an appropriate sample size can be selected so that the statistical analysis should generate a statistically significant result only when a biologically relevant effect has been observed. Failure to take biological relevance into account when designing a study can lead to oversensitive tests. Such tests will declare statistical significance when the biological effect is not large enough to be of practical interest. In practice it is perhaps more likely that the sample size in animal experiments will be too small than too large.

Failure to recognise the true structure of the design

In some experiments complex experimental designs are used and it can be difficult for the researcher to recognise the structure. The replication of the factors in the study may not have been chosen using a suitable technique and hence the statistical analysis may be less powerful than it could otherwise have been. For example, an experiment was planned to assess two types of flooring in guinea pig cages. There were 30 guinea pigs available for inclusion in the study. Animals were group housed and their preference to the floor types assessed individually by measuring the time spent in either half of the cage. By considering the experimental design it was found that the sensitivity of the statistical tests could be improved, without increasing the total numbers of animals used, if the guinea pigs were housed in pairs rather than four per cage, as originally planned.

Trying to do too much with limited resources

Occasionally the researcher will try to achieve too much in a single study. This can cause problems if there are a fixed number of animals available to use. For example, a study was planned to assess the effect of a treatment on plaque deposition in the brains of a strain of transgenic mice. It was hoped that the treated group could be compared to the control group at five distinct time points (2, 3, 4, 6 and 12 months of age). However, only 40 mice from the transgenic strain were available for inclusion in the study. If the ten groups (five time points by two treatments) were included in the study, then there would only be four mice per group per time point. This would not have been enough to detect biologically relevant effects, assuming testing differences between treatment and control was the purpose of the study. Choosing three time points, say 2, 6 and 12 months, would allow either six or seven mice per group and still allow possible differences with age to be detected.

Ignoring the possibility of within-animal testing

In certain situations it is possible to administer more than one treatment to each animal. This can be achieved using a crossover design (i.e. testing a sequence of treatments over time on each animal; see Section 3.4.9) or a dose-escalation design (see Section 3.8.2). With such designs it is important to allow sufficient time gaps between test periods to allow the treatment effects to wash out of the animals' biological systems. In theory each animal should return to approximately its baseline level before receiving the next treatment.

Alternatively if treatments can be applied locally, for example when assessing the effect of cream treatments on a skin condition, then more than one cream can be tested at the same time in each animal. In both cases comparisons between treatments can be made within-animal. This removes any animal-to-animal variability from the assessment of the treatment effects and generally provides more sensitive tests. Ignoring the possibility of testing multiple compounds in the same animal could seriously compromise the experimental results and increase overall animal use.

Quality of responses

The type of response measured in the experiment should be considered at the planning stage. As a general rule numerically continuous responses contain the most information, see Section 3.2.1, as they can be observed at many values. The researcher can therefore differentiate subtle effects when using this type of response. A response that is discrete, ordinal or binary (see Section 3.2.1.1) will be measured on a scale that has fewer distinct values. It is therefore more difficult to observe experimentally induced small changes and hence these responses contain less information. Such experiments will require more animals to achieve the same level of statistical sensitivity (Festing *et al.*, 2002). Also the statistical tests available to analyse discrete, ordinal or binary responses can be less powerful than those available for continuous ones (see Sections 5.5.1 and 5.5.2).

For example, consider a study to assess the effect of transporting rats from a supplier to the test establishment on the formation of lesions in the liver. Let us assume the researcher wants to assess the severity of the lesioning. The initial plan was to count the number of animals showing lesions (a yes/no binary response). However, counting the total number of lesions per animal would contain more information (a count response is on a numerical scale). Such responses can be analysed using more powerful statistical analysis techniques, such as ANOVA (see Section 5.4.3), and hence fewer animals would be required. Better still, if an imaging technique such as magnetic resonance imaging (MRI) were used to measure the total lesion volume per animal (a continuous numerical response) then even fewer animals would be required.

Designs chosen through habit

The experimental design being used should always be questioned and may change as new information becomes available or practical techniques are refined. A review should be conducted after the initial study data have been analysed and any nuisance effects (either proven or suspected) should be accounted for in follow-up studies. A design should not be selected simply because it has been used extensively in the literature.

Unusual designs

It has been suggested that journal referees are unwilling to publish results from unusually designed studies. If the author has included a specific description of the design in the manuscript, and given reasons why it was selected, then we argue that referees should feel more confident in the results obtained. Perhaps in future as researchers become familiar with the benefits of using complex designs, then there will be fewer unusual cases.

Internal validity

Internal validity is defined as the extent to which the design and conduct of the experiment eliminates the possibility of bias (van der Worp *et al.*, 2010). If the experiment is internally valid then any observed treatment effects (when compared to a suitable control) should be purely due to the treatment itself and not other unforeseen effects. To avoid bias, studies should be randomised (to avoid selection bias) and blinded (to avoid performance and detection bias). The latter should ensure that the researcher's beliefs do not, however subtly, influence the outcome of the experiment. There is evidence that failure to blind an experiment correctly can result in an apparent increase in treatment efficacy; see Rooke *et al.* (2011) for example.

External validity

Assuming an experiment has been blinded and the randomisation performed correctly (hence the experiment has good internal validity), then there is still a risk that the external validity of the experiment will be questionable. Van der Worp *et al.* (2010) define external validity as: 'the extent to which the results of an animal experiment provide a correct basis for generalisation to the human condition'. In many areas of animal research there are, perhaps valid, concerns about

the reliability of animal models to predict responses in human patients. For example, the use of a model for inducing a disease that is not sufficiently similar to the human disease could result in development of test compounds that work in animals but not humans. While such practical considerations are beyond the scope of this text, a suitable experimental design can help avoid such problems. If both males and females were included in the experimental design and statistical analysis, for example, then this would avoid the problem described in van der Worp *et al.* (2010) where only male or female animals were used in an animal experiment whereas the disease itself occurred in both male and female human patients.

1.3.2 Pitfalls with randomisation

Randomising when designing is actually better

Sometimes it is easier to rely on the randomisation to remove the influence of a nuisance effect, rather than include a factor in the experimental design that will account for it. If a factor is included in the experimental design and subsequent statistical analysis, then the size of the effect can be assessed at the analysis stage and its influence on the experimental results removed.

Consider an experiment where rats are shown a series of visual stimuli over a set period of time, some of which provide a food reward. The stimuli could be shown to the rats in a random order. However, if the order was planned and controlled then the researcher could account for time and learning effects in the statistical analysis.

Failing to randomise

The process of assigning animals to treatment groups should be done at random, preferably using a randomisation technique such as picking balls from a bag. Selecting animals at random from the cage is not truly a random process and could introduce unwanted systematic effects that may influence the outcome of the experiment. For example, consider what happens when animals arrive from the supplier and are assigned to cages. If the inquisitive animals are picked out first, and these animals are assigned to the control group cages, then you may end up with all the active animals as controls. If one of the responses measured is loco-motor activity, then you may already have a group effect present at baseline (caused by the non-random alloca-tion), which will bias any treatment comparisons.

Incorrect randomisation

As we shall see in Chapter 4, the choice of randomisa-tion has implications on the type of analysis that can be performed. For example, the analysis of a full-factorial design (Sections 6.3.3.1 and 6.3.3.2) is different from that of a complete block design (Section 6.3.3.3) even though structurally they may be the same. The analysis of fac-torial designs includes additional factor interactions in the analysis whereas the analysis of block designs should not include treatment by block interactions. The difference in these two analysis approaches, as we shall see in Section 4.2.2, is based on the different randomisa-tions applied. Failure to employ the correct randomisa-tion may lead to an unreliable statistical analysis.

Blinding studies

One should be careful when randomising studies to ensure that all the scientists involved in the experiment are blinded to the treatment allocation (see Section 4.1.2). If the assessments are qualitative in nature, and the treatment the animal receives is known, then it is difficult for a scientist to remain impartial. There is now evidence that a failure to blind an experiment properly may induce an increased observed treatment effect (Macleod *et al.*, 2009). Observers assessing the treat-ment effect should be blinded to the treatment alloca-tion, as should those administering the treatments to the animals and anyone performing routine husbandry duties.

1.3.3 Pitfalls with statistical analysis

The *t*-test

The *t*-test is a simple and popular statistical test. This test involves comparing the difference between two treatment means with the variability of the responses from these two groups only. In the authors' experience, animal experiments are usually complicated affairs and hence the *t*-test is rarely the most appropriate test to use; see also Nieuwenhuis *et al.* (2011). The statis-tical analysis should reflect the experimental design employed and make full use of its properties. This is not to say the conclusions drawn from the results of *t*-tests are incorrect, just that more powerful tests could perhaps have been used, thus allowing sample sizes to be reduced. We contend that journal referees should always question the use of *t*-tests in submitted articles.

Using all information collected

The principal purpose of the statistical analysis of many animal experiments is to test the hypothesis that one group is in some sense different from another. However, there may be more information that can be recovered from the data collected. For example, use of graphi-cal tools to investigate interrelationships between the responses in a study can help the researcher under-stand more about the underlying processes in the ani-mal model. These insights, gained by an appropriate statistical analysis, may enable the scientist to reduce animal usage in future studies.

Data trawling

Sometimes it is tempting for a researcher to conduct a data-trawling exercise to try to find a statistical result that agrees with a preconceived idea of what the result should be. This strategy can lead to errone-ous false positive conclusions. Such approaches are perhaps more likely to occur when the researcher has freedom to choose (and change) the analysis meth-ods, for example in academic research or early drug discovery studies, as opposed to regulatory testing such as safety assessment and toxicology studies, where analysis strategies are predefined in advance in the protocol.

A commonly encountered example of this pitfall occurs when performing multiple comparison proce-dures. The researcher is confronted (usually by the com-puter package) with a long list of available tests and little information about their individual properties and when or where to use them. It may be tempting to try out many tests and choose the one that provides the 'best' result. We would not recommend this approach. However, it is important to have some degree of flexibility in the analysis performed. In animal experiments, with small sample sizes, there is always the risk that the predefined analysis is not suitable. We recommend that the researcher should define in advance (before running the experiment) exactly how the data will be analysed. Once the data have been collected and a different analysis strategy is required, then this should be reported (alongside the original analysis plan) together with a justification of why the strategy has changed. Such an approach will lead to transparency in the analysis and give the audience an idea of how much the results are data driven.

Using graphical tools improperly

There are many texts on the use and misuse of graphical tools; see for example Tufte (1983). It is a subject in its own right. Graphs should be as simple as possible and yet convey the message in a clear and concise way. In Section 5.3 of this book we will describe some graphical tools that, in the authors' experience, are of the most use to the researcher. We shall also discuss the limitations of some of the graphs that are commonly used.

Identification of outliers

The issue of outliers is a controversial one that we shall consider in Section 5.4.1.5. Some scientists always prefer to leave unusual observations in the dataset, others feel it is sensible to exclude them. We reserve comments about outliers to later in the book; however, we note here that usually the purpose of running a study is to estimate and compare certain group means. If an outlier artificially raises (or lowers) one of these means, then perhaps it should be removed. Furthermore if an observation artificially raises the variability that we test these means against, then again perhaps we are justified in removing it.

If an outlier can be explained biologically, then there is a greater justification for removing it. For example, in a study investigating the effect of two types of surgical technique on post-operative recovery, one of the individual operations was artificially lengthened. The increased time taken to complete the operation may have influenced the animal's post-operation recovery. Failure to remove this animal's results from the statistical analysis could have affected the conclusions.

Pseudo-replication

This problem occurs when a nested design has been employed in the study but then has been ignored in the statistical analysis (see Section 3.7.3.6). If the scientist fails to identify the pseudo-replication then, as discussed in Lazic (2010), this can result in a false estimate of the precision of the experimental results. This can undermine the conclusions of the statistical analysis.

Consider a 'simple' experiment where each animal receives one of the treatments and a single response is measured. The treatments are assigned to individual animals, so the treatment effects should be assessed against the (animal-to-animal) variability of the response, using a suitable statistical test. To calculate this animal-to-animal variability, as a rule of thumb, we require one observation per animal in the statistical analysis. If each animal has been sampled several times, then these samples should be summarised to give a single result per animal.

Lazic (2010) describes a study to assess the effect of a treatment on cells in the brain. Treatment or control was administered to a number of rats. The rat brains were sliced into sections and a number of cells from each section were assessed. A valid analysis is to summarise the results from all the cells from all sections within an animal (for example taking an average) and then carrying out a t-test using these summary observations. An incorrect analysis would involve completing a t-test on the individual cell observations recorded in the study. This is sometimes called false replication as the animal-to-animal variability has been mixed-up with the (usually smaller) within-animal measurement-to-measurement variability. One of the assumptions of this analysis is that individual observations are independent (see Section 5.4.1.4). This is clearly not the case if multiple responses are taken from the same animal.

The same is true of biological assays. Consider an experiment where the samples taken from one animal are assayed in triplicate on a 96-well plate. It is generally accepted that the three results (per animal) should be averaged before any formal statistical analysis is carried out. Only one response per sample is then used in the statistical analysis.

Analysis of repeatedly measured responses

A common mistake made by researchers is the failure to identify a repeated-measures structure in the data. For example, multiple measurements may be taken from the same animal but at specific time points or from specific brain regions. There could also be an experimental design structure imposed on the within-animal sampling. For example, when imaging the brain using an MRI scanner, images are taken from front to back of the brain. This constitutes non-random within-animal sampling.

The levels of the factor that define the repeated measurements cannot be randomised, for example, day 1 must come before day 2. So randomisation cannot be used as an argument to justify the assumption that the observations are not related to, or independent of, each other. The assumption of independence is discussed in Section 5.4.1.4. In such cases a repeated-measures analysis approach should be used to analyse the data, rather than taking each time point or brain region separately. One benefit of this approach is that if some of the data are missing completely at random, then in certain analyses we can use the rest of the observations taken on the animal to account for the missing data. This is particularly important if the purpose of the experiment is to investigate the effect of a treatment over time.

Misinterpretation of the p-value

Often a non-significant p-value is taken as an indication of no biological effect. However, it should be noted that although the result from the study was not statistically significant, there could still be a real biologically relevant effect. It could be the case that the statistical test was not sensitive enough to detect the real effect. This could

occur, for example, if the sample size was too small. Consider the analogy of a court case. Failure to prove guilt does not guarantee innocence (see Section 2.3.1).

Power analysis as an analytical tool

One of the questions raised by many researchers when faced with a non-significant statistical result is whether or not the statistical test result is reliable. In other words, although we have failed to observe a statistically significant effect, does this imply that there is really no biological effect or is it just that we were not able to detect the effect? It has been argued that one way to investigate this is to consider the statistical power of the test (the power to detect a true effect; see Sections 2.3.5.2 and 3.7.3). The argument goes that if the test lacks statistical power, then the failure to identify a statistically significant effect does not necessarily imply there is not a real underlying effect. Unfortunately this argument is incorrect (Hoenig and Heisey, 2001). Power analysis should only be used to predict the properties of future studies and not used to assess the result of the current experiment. We shall elaborate on this issue further in Section 3.7.2.

Analysing groups with no variability

Occasionally in animal experiments it may be the case that all the results obtained from animals within a group are the same. This can occur, for example, in a behavioural study where due to ethical constraints there is an upper limit on the length of time an animal can be tested. If the time-to-event is the response measured, then it is possible that all the animals in a group achieve this boundary. Hence the group mean has no variability. In such cases care has to be taken when carrying out an analysis to deal with this properly.

Groups excluded from the analysis

In many experiments a positive control is included in the experimental design alongside a control group and several treated groups (see Section 3.2.2). When data from such experiments are analysed it is common practice to exclude the positive control from the dataset prior to the analysis. However, as discussed in Section 5.4.3.2, the most reliable statistical analysis involves using all the animals. In particular, the variability estimate obtained when considering the results from all the animals in the experiment will be more accurate and reproducible (as more information is used to generate it). If the positive control is included in the analysis, and a multiple comparison procedure is applied to the statistical tests (see Section 5.4.8), then the researcher may decide to exclude any positive control comparisons from this procedure, even if the group is included in the dataset that is used to estimate the variance.

Sometimes the variability of the positive control group is different from those of the other groups. In this case (and we argue only in this case) the researcher should remove the positive control group prior to performing the statistical analysis, as otherwise the homogeneity of variance assumption will not hold (see Section 5.4.1.3).

It may also be the case that a more complicated experimental design, such as a row-column, crossover or incomplete block design, has been employed (see Sections 3.4.7, 3.4.9 and 3.4.5, respectively). In such cases the design has been specifically constructed to account for additional factors and removing one of the treatment groups from the dataset will adversely affect the properties of the design and hence the efficiency of the statistical analysis.

1.3.4 Pitfalls when reporting animal experiments

There has been a great deal of attention recently concerning the quality of the reporting of animal experiments; see Rooke *et al.* (2011) and Vesterinen *et al.* (2010) for example. Some of the concerns raised involve the non-reporting of information that readers may find useful. This includes information that would allow them to form their own opinions about the validity of the experimental methodology, the reliability of the results generated and the conclusions drawn. More generally, there has also been concern expressed regarding the overall publication bias in the literature. Such issues can, in the long term, cause animals to be tested unnecessarily. This can occur if false positive results are published and other researchers attempt to replicate them in further animal experiments. Failure to replicate a false

positive published result first time may result in additional experiments being carried out to try to refine the model and hence achieve the expected statistically significant result.

Publication bias

There is now anecdotal evidence for publication bias in the literature of animal experiments. The issue has been considered by several authors: for example, Sena *et al.* (2010) for *in vivo* stroke model studies. Publication bias can occur for diverse reasons. For example, much of the published research reports positive results, with journals less likely to accept papers that describe negative findings. Sena *et al.* (2010) report that in the 512 studies investigated, only 2% reported no significant results. This implies that, across all the literature, a skewed overall picture will develop. False positive results are more likely to get published than false negatives, and hence there will be a general overestimation of effects in the literature when it is taken as a whole. This overestimation will then be repeated in narrative and systematic reviews and hence the problem will be compounded. It can also be argued that false positive results are rarely retracted whereas false negative results are rarely identified (and hence the literature imbalance corrected). All this is in contrast to clinical trials data, which are routinely reported regardless of the outcome.

Bennett *et al.* (2009) comment that neuroimaging studies that employ multiple comparison procedures (as part of the statistical analysis) are less likely to get published than studies analysed using less strict tests. Analyses that do not adjust for multiplicity may, all other things being equal, contain more significant results, perhaps false positives, than studies that use more rigorous techniques. Hence differences between the strictness of the statistical tests employed could lead to publication bias as false positive results are more likely to be published when certain tests are used.

Publication bias can also be linked to the statistical power of the experiment. Sena *et al.* (2010) argue that, in many animal experiments, the sample size is small (for ethical reasons) but this can lead to inconclusive experiments that will not get published, even if biologically meaningful effects are observed. Small sample sizes can also lead to unusual and unreliable results (false positives) that will be published even if the study itself is underpowered.

Non-reporting of variance

To help the reader form an opinion on the reliability of the experimental results, a measure of the variability of the data should be given. This can usually be achieved by including error bars on plots, for example the standard error (see Section 5.2.2.3) or the confidence interval (see Section 5.2.2.4). It can also involve quoting either the standard error or the standard deviation (see Section 5.2.2.2) within the text. Quoting such values will allow readers to assess how comparable their own experimental processes are (in terms of reliability) and also assess the statistical power of the experiment described in the article.

Non-reporting of the sample size

The more animals that are used in an experiment, the more reliable the results generated will be. Failure to report the number of animals used will make it difficult for the reader to judge how reliable the experimental results are. If only three animals are used per group then the effect observed, however large, could be just a chance result in three animals and not a result that will be reproducible.

The researcher should also report how many animals were excluded from the experiment (and why). If the sample sizes are uneven across the experimental groups, then this should be reported alongside the initial group sizes. The will allow a reader to judge the robustness of the experimental procedures.

Non-reporting of the sample size calculation

Many researchers use the literature as a guideline for selecting a suitable sample size. This implies that sample sizes can become established with little direct evidence to support their use. If authors include information about their decision-making process (however rigorous) then that will help future researchers decide how much weight should be placed on the sample size used in the examples reported in the literature. If a power analysis was performed to select the sample size then this should be reported so as to encourage others to use these techniques.

Non-reporting of the randomisation applied

The validity of the results, both in terms of the statistical analysis and biases present in the observed results, is influenced by the randomisation performed. It is therefore important that the researcher describes exactly how and when the randomisation was performed. This will not only give readers more confidence in the reported results, but also aid them when using the animal model in their own work.

Non-reporting of the blinding

As with the randomisation, it is important that the researcher explain the techniques that were employed to blind the experiment. This will provide an indication of the likelihood that results were influenced by systematic bias. Such descriptions will also help the reader judge how well the experiment was conducted (the internal validity) and also the quality of the results generated. If blinding is routinely described in the published literature, then perhaps more researchers will apply more rigorous blinding in their experiments and hence improve the reliability of their results.

Non-reporting of the assumptions of the statistical analysis

There are always assumptions that have to be made when performing a statistical analysis. While in many cases it will be evident that these assumptions have been met, sometimes it is not so obvious. The researcher should not only discuss which assumptions were made, when performing the statistical analysis, but also explain how they were assessed and what the result of that assessment was.

1.4 So where does statistics fit in?

For many researchers the primary purpose of statistics is to assess whether two or more experimental groups are significantly different from each other. This involves the calculation of p-values and the inclusion of stars on a means with standard errors plot (see Section 2.3). There is, however, a lot more, in addition to the p-value, that the subject of statistics can offer.

To begin with, statistics can help the researcher understand the factors that influence the animal model and identify underlying relationships between these influential factors. Once important factors have been identified, then that knowledge will be beneficial when planning follow-up experiments.

There are many experimental designs that can be used during the experimental process to aid in the understanding of how the experimental factors influence each other. Making the most of these experimental designs (in the statistical analysis) can allow the researcher to uncover hidden relationships that may otherwise be missed. Such knowledge will improve and enhance the designs used in future studies.

The researcher should not ignore the graphical tools available. The use of simple plots, such as scatterplots and box-plots, can reveal information otherwise missed. For example, categorised scatterplots provide a visual assessment of the relationship between baseline and posttreatment responses and this can help the researcher decide whether or not to include baseline information in the statistical analysis (see Section 5.4.6).

There has been much discussion, and rightly so, about the correct sample size to use in a given study. This is a question that can be answered by statistical analysis. However, we can go further than this and look at other types of replication within the study. For example:

- How many samples should be taken per animal? Should these samples be assessed in duplicate or triplicate wells within the 96-well plate?
- How many histological slices of the brain should be assessed?

Statistics can help identify an appropriate replication of the levels of these factors, as well as the number of animals to use.

Thinking in a statistical way can also be beneficial when running a study. Standardising how an experiment is conducted should reduce variability in the responses. It may sound like common sense but standardising the time between the stages in the experiment, for example the time between dosing and sample collection, may help reduce the underlying variability of the data.

Finally statistics plays an important role when communicating experimental results to the wider scientific community. The researcher should report not only the statistical methods used, and the assumptions made, but also the experimental design employed. Information such as sample size, randomisation and techniques employed to reduce variability will not only allow readers to put the results into context but also may allow them to set up the animal model within their own laboratories in an efficient way.

1.5 The ARRIVE guidelines

To improve the quality of reporting of animal experiments, a set of guidelines (the ARRIVE guidelines – Animal Research: Reporting *In Vivo* Experiments) has been developed to provide a framework to help researchers report their results. The guidelines describe 20 subjects that should be included in scientific publications. Journals now routinely ask for this information, perhaps in electronic supplementary material.

Some of the subjects covered in the ARRIVE guidelines are not of direct relevance to this text, although all are useful and have at least an indirect bearing on the subject matter presented in this book. In this section we shall concentrate on a selection of the guidelines; for more details see Kilkenny *et al.* (2010).

Table 1.1 gives a selection of the items described within the ARRIVE guidelines along with links to relevant sections within this text.

Table 1.1. Selected items from the ARRIVE guidelines

ARRIVE guideline	Links with this text
Item 6 – Study design For each experiment, give brief details of the study design, including: a. The number of experimental and control groups. b. Any steps taken to minimise the effects of subjective bias when allocating animals to treatment (e.g. randomisation procedure) and when assessing results (e.g. if done, describe who was blinded and when). c. The experimental unit (e.g. a single animal, group, or cage of animals).	a. The researcher should consider the number of groups that can be accommodated, given the total animals available, and the type of control groups required (Section 3.2.2). b. A valid randomisation should be carried out (Chapter 4) and also the experimental design used should minimise bias, for example block designs (Section 3.4). c. A discussion of the experimental unit is given in Section 3.2.3.
Item 10 – Sample size a. Specify the total number of animals used in each experiment and the number of animals in each experimental group.	a. The total number of animals used, and the within-group replication, are needed as they give an indication of the sensitivity of the statistical tests (Section 5.4.3.1 – degrees of freedom). The within-group replication also influences the standard error of the mean, commonly quoted in papers (Section 5.2.2.2).
b. Explain how the number of animals was decided. Provide details of any sample size calculation used.	b. The choice of sample size should be based on sound scientific reasoning, as described in Section 3.7.2. Use of nested designs may help increase understanding of the sources of variability and therefore not only identify the number of animals required but also the level of within-animal replication (Section 3.7.3). Use of factorial designs may help increase the window of opportunity to observe drug effects and this allows sample sizes to be reduced (Section 3.5.4).
c. Indicate the number of independent replications of each experiment, if relevant.	c. When making multiple statistical tests there is always a risk of finding false positive results. One way to guard against this is to conduct multiple independent experiments (Section 5.4.8). If a positive result was observed in only one of several experiments, then the reader should be made aware of this as it could indicate a false positive result.
Item 11 – Allocating animals to experimental groups a. Give full details of how animals were allocated to experimental groups, including randomisation or matching if done.	a. Some form of randomisation should be used to assign animals to groups (Chapter 4), but this can only be carried out after an experimental design has been selected, for example a block design (Section 3.4). It should also be stated if a stratified randomisation (Section 4.2.1) has been used.
b. Describe the order in which the animals in the different experimental groups were treated and assessed.	b. It is important for the reader to know the order of testing. Testing in a non-random order can lead to unintentional systematic bias (Section 4.1.1).

Table 1.1. (*cont.*)

ARRIVE guideline	Links with this text
Item 13 – Statistical methods	
a. Provide details of the statistical methods used for each analysis.	a. A description of the statistical analysis used is essential as this allows the reader to assess the sensitivity and appropriateness of the analysis performed (Section 1.3.4).
b. Specify the unit of analysis for each dataset (e.g. single animal, group of animals, single neuron).	b. A discussion of the observation and experimental units is given in Section 3.2.3. Both should be identified by the scientist prior to running the experiment.
c. Describe any methods used to assess whether the data met the assumptions of the statistical approach.	c. Any statistical analysis will involve certain assumptions. A description of any analysis should include information about how the assumptions of the analysis were assessed (Section 1.3.4) and whether the assumptions were met.
Item 15 – Numbers analysed	
a. Report the number of animals in each group included in each analysis. Report absolute numbers (e.g. 10/20, not 50%).	a. When reporting the results of an animal experiment, it is recommended to include the number of animals used in each group. This gives the reader an indication of the sensitivity of the results. In Section 1.3.1 we discuss how too many animals can result in oversensitive tests and statistically significant results that are not biologically relevant.
	It is also recommended that researchers report absolute figures rather than percentages. The latter can be misleading. For example, consider one response changing from 1/1000 to 2/1000 and a second response changing from 3/10 to 6/10. The biological meaning of these results may be completely different even though the percentage changes are the same.
b. If any animals or data were not included in the analysis, explain why.	b. If any animals were excluded, an explanation should be given as to which method (either statistical or otherwise) was used to define exclusion criteria. For example, the researcher may use externally Studentised residuals (Section 5.4.1.5).
	Information should also be given about how many animals were excluded from the analysis as this will give the reader information about the reliability of the methods employed and the variability of the response (Section 1.3.4).
Item 16 – Outcomes and estimation	
a. Report the results for each analysis carried out, with a measure of precision (e.g. standard error or confidence interval).	a. Some measure of the variability of the reported results should be given, for example standard errors or 95% confidence intervals (Sections 5.2.2.3 and 5.2.2.4, respectively). Statisticians prefer the more flexible confidence intervals, although scientists tend to use standard errors, especially on plots of the data.

Statistical concepts

Before we describe the experimental designs and statistical analyses that may be of use to the researcher, a few fundamental concepts are introduced. While many researchers are familiar with these concepts, they are the foundation for the arguments that follow and hence are considered first.

2.1 Decision-making: the signal-to-noise ratio

Arguably the primary role of the statistical analysis of an animal experiment is to allow the scientist to draw reliable conclusions from the results obtained. Statistics provides the decision-maker with a framework for achieving this. Importantly it also quantifies the confidence that should be placed in that decision.

Example 2.1: Plasma glucose level

Consider the following two experiments, designed to assess the effect of two treatments A and B, on reducing plasma glucose levels in diabetic mice. Treatment A was tested in experiment 1, treatment B in experiment 2. Both studies also included a control group to allow a test of the treatment effect. The plasma glucose level of the two control groups was around 280 mg/dL. Animals dosed with treatment A had an average plasma glucose level of 227 mg/dL whereas those dosed with treatment B had an average of 185 mg/dL. Without any further information it appears that treatment B was more effective at decreasing plasma glucose level. A scatterplot of the four averages is presented in Figure 2.1.

But was this conclusion valid? It is always difficult to compare results across experiments, even if the control groups appear to be similar. Other effects, unique to each experiment, may be influencing the results. We shall comment further on this later, where it will be shown that other experimental designs may be more appropriate.

Assume that different researchers carried out the two experiments; a plot of the individual results is presented in Figure 2.2.

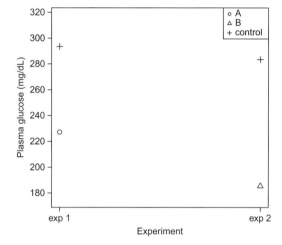

Figure 2.1. Plot of the four plasma glucose level treatment means for Example 2.1.

We can see now that although there was a bigger effect in the experiment involving treatment B (the average for treatment B was 41 mg/dL lower than treatment A), the results were actually more variable in the second experiment. Perhaps the first researcher was more experienced and hence generated less variable results, or perhaps the second batch of animals originated from more litters than the first batch. Due to this variability we would be more confident in a conclusion that treatment A is significantly better than the control, as opposed to the conclusion that treatment B was better than the control. This is the case even though the effect was biologically smaller for treatment A.

Example 2.1 is artificial, but it does highlight an important point when making a decision using a statistical analysis. We must take into account not only the size of the biological effect (the signal) but also the variability (the noise) of the effect. To do this we calculate

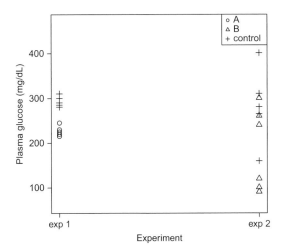

Figure 2.2. Plot of the individual plasma glucose levels for Example 2.1.

the size of the effect relative to the background variability. This is known as the *signal-to-noise ratio*.

The signal-to-noise ratio forms the basis of many of the formal statistical tests. The size of the ratio gives an indication of the level of confidence we have in the conclusions drawn. The larger (numerically) the ratio, the more certain we can be that our conclusions are correct. We will return to this ratio as we progress through the book.

There are two ways the researcher can increase the signal-to-noise ratio, and hence increase confidence in the experimental conclusions:

- Increasing the signal: The greater the size of the effect, the greater the signal-to-noise ratio.
- Decreasing the noise: The smaller the variability, the greater the signal-to-noise ratio. Hence the key to making confident decisions begins with understanding (and then controlling) the sources of variability in the study.

There are various techniques that can be used to reduce the variability in the experimental results, some of which are related to the experimental design. For example, it is well known that inbred strains are generally less variable than their outbred equivalents. The researcher can also use experimental design (and corresponding statistical analysis) to account for nuisance sources of variability introduced by practical constraints. For example, if the testing procedure was conducted over two days, then a suitable experimental design can account for any day-to-day differences that would otherwise have increased the variability of the data generated.

As a practical example of these ideas, consider giving a lecture to an audience of students. The signal in this case is the knowledge that you are verbally passing on to the students. Now assume there is an alarm (the noise) ringing in the background, which is drowning out your voice. It does not matter how loud you talk, if the alarm is louder than your voice then you will not be heard. Similarly, it does not matter how loud the alarm is, as long as you can talk louder than the alarm you will be heard. There are two ways you can improve the chance of getting your message across. You can either talk louder (increase the signal) or reduce the volume of the alarm (reduce the noise), for example by shutting the windows. Of course in real experiments there will probably be a number of alarms. The skill is to identify which alarm is the loudest and try to turn off that alarm first. The largest source of variability in a study may not necessarily be the animal-to-animal variability!

As we go through this book we shall see how the use of experimental design and statistics can help the scientist increase the signal as well as decrease the noise. If this can be achieved then animal numbers may be reduced while maintaining the same level of confidence in the experimental results.

In conclusion then, it is worth remembering that it is important to focus attention not only on the size of the response but on the size of the response compared to the underlying variability. The two do not always give the same impression! The selection of experimental design, in particular the choice of sample size, is critical in aligning these two measures of effect. A successfully designed experiment will only achieve statistical significance when biological relevance is reached, and vice versa.

2.2 Probability distributions

When conducting a statistical analysis we usually need to estimate how variable our observations are – the noise in the signal-to-noise ratio. As any researcher knows, animals within the same group will behave differently. This leads to the noise (or variability) in the

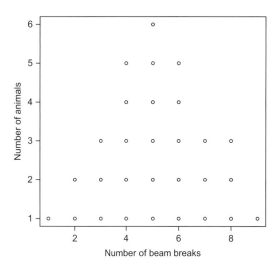

Figure 2.3. Scatterplot highlighting the distribution of the observed beam breaks.

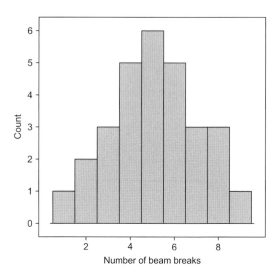

Figure 2.4. Frequency histogram highlighting the distribution of the beam breaking response.

experiment. As we shall see in Section 2.3, when conducting an analysis we need to consider not only the overall size of this noise, but also the pattern (or distribution) of the responses.

Example 2.2: Locomotor activity assessment

Consider the following experiment conducted to assess the locomotor activity of mice in an open field. The animals were placed in a testing arena fitted with infrared movement detector beams. The number of times each animal broke a detector beam was recorded. Figure 2.3 is a graphical illustration of the results from the experiment. The range of responses was between one and nine beam breaks (represented along the X-axis), with one animal breaking the beam once, another breaking the beam nine times, and six animals breaking the beam five times. Each point in Figure 2.3 corresponds to an individual animal (29 mice were assessed in total).

From this plot we can start to see how the responses are distributed around the central value (five beam breaks). Some animals were more active than others, hence a range of responses was observed. We can also see a pattern in the distribution of these responses. More observations were measured in the middle values (roughly between four and six), with fewer observations recorded as the response moved away from this range.

2.2.1 The frequency distribution

Figure 2.3 is a simple way of visualising the observed responses. Another way of visualising the distribution

of the responses is to produce a frequency histogram. In the frequency histogram the responses are separated into a number of bins, where each bin is represented as a bar in the histogram. The area of each bar reflects the number of responses within that bin. An example of a frequency histogram is given in Figure 2.4, where each bar corresponds to a distinct number of beam breaks. Note in this case that all the bars have an equal width (of dimension one) and hence the height of the bars reflects the number of animals within each bin. In general the response measured may be more continuous, i.e. not only consist of integers, and hence the bins would represent ranges of responses.

2.2.2 The density distribution

In Figure 2.4 the Y-axis on the frequency histogram plot reflects the number of animals within each bar, and hence this axis is labelled as 'Count'. However, let us now rescale the Y-axis in a way that the total area of all the bars within the plot equals one. The area of an individual bar now reflects the proportion of the 29 animals that achieved that number of beam breaks. We call this a density histogram (as opposed to a frequency histogram). Figure 2.5 is such a density histogram.

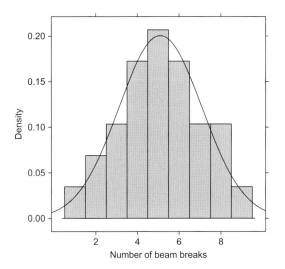

Figure 2.5. Density histogram highlighting the distribution of the beam breaking response.

2.2.3 The probability distribution

The height of the bars on the density histogram can be approximated by fitting a curve over the top of them. An example of such a curve is given in Figure 2.5. As the area of the bars added together equals one, so the area under the curve (AUC) equals one too. The curve is defined as the *distributional curve of the response* as it describes the distribution of the response.

It is usually the case that the curve fitted over the bars is a member of a specific family of curves. Curves in the same family are all slightly different from each other but share certain characteristics, for example they are bell-shaped, symmetric around a central maximum and so on. The family of curves therefore reflects the underlying theoretical distribution of the response. The specific member of the family, overlaid on the histogram plot, defines the estimated underlying distribution of the response. If the curve represents the estimated distribution then the bars of the histogram illustrate the distribution of the observations actually recorded. Note the curve smooths out the jaggedness present across the bars on the histogram, and so represents the expected frequencies of the response rather than the observed frequencies. Of course to be valid the fitted curve should reflect the observed distribution of the responses!

If we can make assumptions about the shape of the distribution, by choosing the family of the distribution curves, then we can predict the probability (or chance) of observing a response within a given range. We simply work out the percentage of the area under the curve that lies within this range. Consider the above density curve in isolation (without the histogram bars). The AUC of this curve, for a given range of X-axis values, represents the probability of observing a response within that range. For example the AUC for the whole curve (between X-axis values $-\infty$ and $+\infty$) equals 1 (or 100%). By calculating the AUC we can work out the probability of the response lying within a range directly from the AUC. Hence the curve defines the *probability distribution* of the response. The probability distribution is used in many statistical tests to generate, for example, *p*-values and confidence intervals (see Section 5.2.2.4).

Before we describe some of the approaches that can be used when analysing data generated from animal experiments, we shall consider some of the more commonly encountered probability distributions and their links to the statistical analyses described in this text.

2.2.4 The normal distribution

Perhaps the most important distribution, and certainly one that most readers will have encountered, is the Gaussian or normal distribution.

Many biological responses follow this distribution. If a response that is normally distributed is measured repeatedly, you would expect most of the responses to lie close to the centre of the distribution, with fewer and fewer observations observed as you move away from the centre. In theory you should see an equal number of responses above the centre as you see below it, hence the distribution will be symmetric around the centre.

Example 2.3: A normally distributed response

Consider an investigation conducted by an animal supplier to estimate rat body weight at a given age. The supplier weighed 100 animals from its stock. A distribution of the body weights was illustrated using a histogram (see Figure 2.6).

The height of the bars corresponds to the number of rats observed in the weight range defined along the X-axis. We can fit a smooth distribution curve on the plot to summarise this underlying pattern. Figure 2.6 shows a bell-shaped curve (the Gaussian or normal

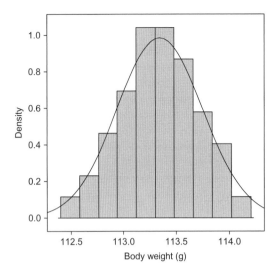

Figure 2.6. Histogram highlighting the distribution of rat body weights, with a normal distribution curve overlaid.

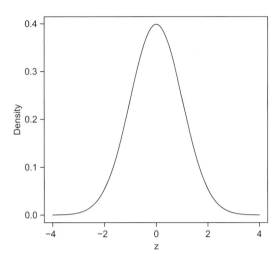

Figure 2.7. The standard-normal distribution.

curve) overlaid on the histogram. In this case the curve describes the height of the bars well. If the response is normally distributed, then the histogram bars will closely follow this smooth curve.

In certain statistical tests it is useful to change the scale of the horizontal axis. In the case of the normal distribution this transformation results in a distribution known as the standard-normal distribution (Figure 2.7). The process of changing the scale is known as standardising the response variable.

The transformation that standardises a response variable y is given by:

$$z = \frac{y - \mu}{\sigma} \tag{2.1}$$

where z is the standardised response, μ is the mean of the distribution (Section 5.2.1.1) and σ is the standard deviation (Section 5.2.2.2).

We shall make use of the standard-normal distribution in many of the tests described in Chapter 5.

2.2.5 The chi-squared distribution

Another useful probability distribution that we require in many statistical analyses is the chi-squared distribution. This distribution is useful because it is the basis for some of the more complicated statistical tests.

So far we have considered only one variable (the response variable) that is normally distributed. Assume it has been standardised using the equation above. If we now have several (k) standardised normally distributed variables $z_1, z_2, z_3, ..., z_k$, then the variable

$$x = z_1^2 + z_2^2 + z_3^2 + ... + z_k^2 \tag{2.2}$$

follows the chi-squared distribution with k degrees of freedom (see Section 5.4.3.1 for more details on degrees of freedom). Figure 2.8 shows the distributional curve for the chi-squared distribution with five degrees of freedom.

2.2.6 The *t*-distribution

Closely linked to the standardised normal and chi-squared distributions is the *t*-distribution. This distribution, as the name suggests, is used in the well-known *t*-test (see Section 5.4.2).

If z is a standardised normally distributed variable and x is a chi-squared distributed variable with k degrees of freedom, then the variable

$$t_k = \frac{z}{\sqrt{x/k}} \tag{2.3}$$

is *t*-distributed with k degrees of freedom.

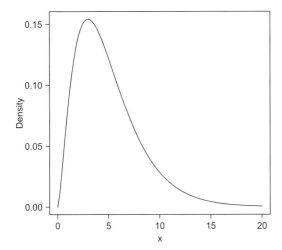

Figure 2.8. The chi-squared distribution with five degrees of freedom.

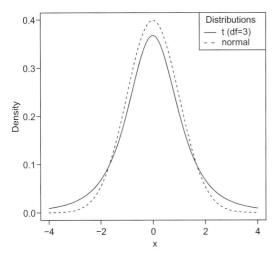

Figure 2.9. The t-distribution with three degrees of freedom alongside the normal distribution.

The t-distribution is similar to the normal distribution (in shape) but is slightly flatter and has larger tails to reflect greater uncertainty in the distribution of the response. An example of the distribution curve of a t-distribution with three degrees of freedom, along with the standard-normal distribution, is given in Figure 2.9.

The following result is required by many of the statistical tests described in this book. Assume $y_1, y_2, ..., y_n$ is a random sample taken from a normal distribution with mean μ and variance σ^2 (see Section 5.2.2.1). If the sample mean is denoted by $\bar{y}$ and the sample variance by s^2 then

$$t = \frac{(\bar{y} - \mu)}{\sqrt{s^2 / n}} \tag{2.4}$$

is t-distributed with $n - 1$ degrees of freedom.

2.2.7 The F-distribution

The final distribution we consider is the F-distribution. This distribution is required for many of the statistical tests described below, for example the tests produced within the analysis of variance approaches (see Section 5.4.3).

If x_1 and x_2 are two chi-squared distributed variables with k_1 and k_2 degrees of freedom, respectively, then the variable

$$F_{k_1, k_2} = \frac{x_1 / k_1}{x_2 / k_2} \tag{2.5}$$

follows the F-distribution with k_1 numerator degrees of freedom and k_2 denominator degrees of freedom.

The distribution curve of the F-distributions with 5 and 20 degrees of freedom is presented in Figure 2.10.

2.3 The hypothesis testing procedure

One of the primary roles of statistics in animal experimentation is to aid the researcher in the decision-making process. To appreciate some of the implications of using formal statistical tests, we need to understand the hypothesis testing procedure. This begins at the initial planning stage of the experiment with the formation of two hypotheses, the *null* and *alternative* hypotheses.

2.3.1 The null and alternative hypotheses

The null hypothesis, usually denoted by H_0, is the hypothesis that the experimental effect of interest has

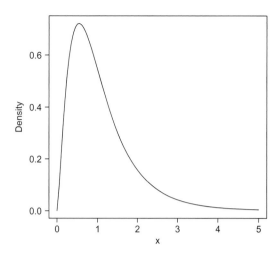

Figure 2.10. The *F*-distribution with five and 20 degrees of freedom.

no influence on the response being measured. For example, consider a scientist who wishes to investigate the effect of a novel treatment. Assume this can be achieved by comparing the mean of the responses in the treatment group to the corresponding mean in the control group. To begin with the null hypothesis is established (either consciously or not) as:

H_0: The treatment mean is equal to the control mean.

The alternative hypothesis, denoted by H_1, is that the response is influenced by the novel treatment. The alternative hypothesis H_1 can be one of two types. The most commonly tested is also the most general. This hypothesis states that there is an effect (of treatment), but that the direction of that effect can be either positive or negative. For example:

H_1: The treatment mean is not equal to the control mean.

This leads to a two-sided statistical test as the effect we are assessing can be in either direction.

If the scientist knows for certain the direction of the effect of interest, then the alternative hypothesis can be chosen to reflect this. For example, if the novel treatment is expected to increase the response, then the alternative hypothesis would be:

H_1: The treatment mean is greater than the control mean.

This leads to a one-sided statistical test.

In the formal statistical testing procedure we begin by assuming H_0 is true and attempt to disprove it (and hence by implication accept that H_1 is true). We do this by collecting sufficient evidence to reject the null hypothesis. The reader should be aware that the whole process is weighted in favour of the null hypothesis being accepted. The scientist has to prove that the null hypothesis is not correct.

There are three consequences of the decision-making process that should be apparent to the reader:

• The statistical decision-making process always favours accepting the null hypothesis as being true. To claim the alternative hypothesis is true, a certain body of evidence must be acquired.

• Just because we cannot disprove the null hypothesis, this does not necessarily imply it is true. It may just be that the experiment was not powerful enough to disprove the null hypothesis. This can happen, for example, if the sample size in the study was not large enough.

• The alternative hypothesis is the *hypothesis the researcher wishes to prove*. So if the purpose of the experiment is to prove that two drugs (A and B) are equivalent, then the null hypothesis should be:

H_0: Drug A has a different effect compared to drug B, i.e.

drug A mean ≠ drug B mean.

The alternative hypothesis would be of the form:

H_1: Drug A has the same effect as drug B, i.e.

drug A mean = drug B mean.

To assess this type of null hypothesis we require an equivalence test. This is a different procedure to the standard analysis approach used by most animal researchers.

From now on we shall focus on the more commonly applied hypothesis testing procedure, where the researcher is trying to prove an effect has occurred and hence the null hypothesis assumes that there is no effect.

2.3.2 The *p*-value

Once the researcher has decided on suitable hypotheses, the experiment is planned so that the null hypothesis can be assessed. The experiment is then conducted according to the plan and the data collected. Under certain assumptions about the properties of the data generated, a suitable statistical test is employed to attempt to disprove the null hypothesis. This decision usually involves assessing the *p*-values that are calculated as part of the statistical analysis.

The *p*-value is the probability that the experimental result will be at least as extreme as the one observed when running the experiment *if the null hypothesis were true*. It is the chance of being incorrect if you decide the null hypothesis is false.

So, for example, the *p*-value answers the question: 'What is the chance of achieving the result I have observed, or one even more pronounced, if there really is no difference between the treatments?' The *p*-value itself, as observed by Festing *et al.* (2002, pp. 15–16), is often misinterpreted:

A p-value is not the probability that the null hypothesis is true.

The *p*-value is a rather abstract quantity. One of the purposes of this book is to provide scientists with statistical tools, other than the *p*-value, to give them a greater insight into the decision-making process.

2.3.3 The significance level

It is common practice to reject the null hypothesis if the *p*-value is less than a certain value, usually 5% or 0.05. If the chance of obtaining a result at least as extreme as that observed in the experiment (when the null hypothesis is true) is found to be less than 5%, then this is sufficiently small for the researcher to reject the null hypothesis. In other words, the observed effect is so large that it is unlikely that the null hypothesis is correct. This 5% value is called the *significance level* and is generally denoted by α.

When conducting an experiment we can never entirely remove the risk of rejecting the null hypothesis when it is true. There is always a chance we will observe a large biological effect in our study (by chance) when

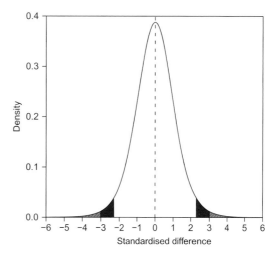

Figure 2.11. Calculations involved in performing a hypothesis test. The grey shaded areas (light and dark grey in each tail of the distribution) correspond to the area under the curve that defines the (null hypothesis) rejection region for the two-sided test. The two light grey shaded areas correspond to the area under the curve that defines the *p*-value for the two-sided test when the observed standardised difference was three.

in reality there is no genuine effect. A 5% risk is generally accepted as being a suitably low risk.

To highlight the link between the significance level and the *p*-value, consider an experiment that consisted of a treatment group and a control group, with $n = 9$ animals per group. Assume that the response was normally distributed (see Section 2.2.4).

The following stages (which correspond to the approach used to perform an unpaired *t*-test; see Section 5.4.2.1) are illustrated in Figure 2.11.

- We begin the hypothesis testing process by assuming the null hypothesis (that there is no difference between the treatment and control group means) is true. Let us also assume that the response is normally distributed. We can then determine the distribution of the difference between the means under the null hypothesis. If the transformation (Eq. (2.4)) described in Section 2.2.6 is applied to the observed difference (where $\mu = 0$ under the null hypothesis) so that

$$\text{standardised difference} = \frac{\text{difference}}{\sqrt{s^2 / n}}, \qquad (2.6)$$

where s^2 is a measure of the sample variance, then the standardised difference will be t-distributed with a bell-shaped distribution centred on zero, as shown in Figure 2.11.

- Assume we are performing a two-sided statistical test. The statistical test can now be carried out in two related ways:
- We can first calculate the region of the t-distribution where the null hypothesis will be rejected if the difference between the means (once standardised) lies within it. This area is known as the *rejection region* and is the four grey shaded areas in Figure 2.11. When added together, these correspond to the area under the curve equal to the significance level α (usually 5% of the area under the curve, with 2.5% in each tail). The X-axis values that define the boundaries of the rejection region of the t-distribution, in this example -2.3 for the lower rejection region and $+2.3$ for the upper rejection region, are known as the *critical values*.
- Now if we observe a (standardised) difference that is greater or less than the appropriate critical value (i.e. the standardised difference is in the rejection region) then we conclude the null hypothesis is probably not true. The chance of observing such a large or small difference (assuming the true difference between the means is zero) is small; hence we conclude that in reality it is highly unlikely that the true difference is zero. Hence we reject the null hypothesis.

As an alternative statistical analysis strategy, we can take the following approach (which is commonly applied in statistical software packages):

- For a positive difference we calculate the chance of observing such a result (or one larger) assuming that the null hypothesis is true. This can be achieved by considering the area under the curve of the appropriate t-distribution, where the observed (standardised) difference defines the lower X-axis boundary for the area. Assume a (standardised) difference of 3 was observed between the treatment and control means. The chance of observing an effect as large as this (assuming the true difference is zero) is denoted by the light grey area on the right-hand side of the curve in Figure 2.11, which starts at a (standardised) difference of 3.
- Now as we are performing a two-sided test we want to know the chance of finding a result as extreme as this,

so we also require the chance of observing a (standardised) difference less than -3. As the t-distribution is symmetric around zero the corresponding area under the curve has the same numerical value (it is the equivalent area in the opposite tail). This is illustrated by the light grey area on the left-hand side of the curve in Figure 2.11, where the shaded area ends at the standardised difference of -3.

- The two light grey areas added together correspond to the p-value for the two-sided test. As described above, it is the probability of observing a result, or one more extreme, as the one found by running the experiment if the null hypothesis were true.
- If the researcher is testing at the α significance level, then as long as the p-value is less than α the null hypothesis is rejected.

It can also be seen from Figure 2.11 that when the observed (standardised) difference equals the critical value, the p-value will equal the significance level α.

2.3.4 Significant stars

Once the analysis has been performed and the p-values generated it is common practice to quote stars rather than p-values when reporting results. These stars are also included on graphs to indicate where the significant effects are. Standard practice appears to be:

* $p < 0.05$ (5%), ** $p < 0.01$ (1%) and *** $p < 0.001$ (0.1%).

We do not recommend this practice. Statistical tests should not be seen as providing a yes/no decision. The p-value is a continuous numerical value that provides the scientist with an indication of the level of confidence that can be placed in the conclusion. A p-value of 0.060 is similar to 0.049 and although the former is 'not significant', it should be interpreted as giving a similar conclusion to the latter. As Rosnow and Rosenthal (1989) wryly commented:

...surely, God loves the .06 nearly as much as the .05.

2.3.5 Type I and Type II errors

There are two types of error that can be committed when following the decision-making process described above. These are commonly known as Type I and Type II errors.

Type I error

A Type I error occurs if the researcher rejects the null hypothesis when in fact it is true (a false positive conclusion).

If the significance level is set at 5%, then the null hypothesis should be rejected 5% of the time (when the null hypothesis is true). This is the probability of committing a Type I error.

Type II error

A Type II error occurs if the researcher does not reject the null hypothesis when it is false (a false negative conclusion). When considering the probability of committing a Type II error (sometimes denoted by β) it is more convenient to look at the power of the statistical test. The power of a statistical test is given by:

$$\text{Power} = 1 - \beta$$
$$= 1 - Pr(\text{committing a Type II error}). \quad (2.7)$$

The power of the statistical test is the probability of rejecting the null hypothesis when it is false. See Section 3.7.2 for a discussion of some of the implications of statistical power.

Calculating statistical power

To help understand the concept of statistical power we return to the example discussed in Section 2.3.3.

- As in Figure 2.11, we begin the hypothesis testing process by assuming the null hypothesis (that there is no difference between the treatment and control means) is true. Let us also assume that the response is normally distributed. We can then determine the distribution of the difference between the means under the null hypothesis. Assuming the transformation described in Section 2.3.3 (Eq. (2.6)) has been applied, then the standardised difference will be t-distributed with a bell-shaped distribution centred on zero. This is shown as the left-hand curve in Figure 2.12.
- We can now calculate the rejection region (the grey shaded areas in Figure 2.12). Once added together these correspond to the proportion of the area under the curve that equals the significance level α (usually set at 5%). If we obtain a (standardised) difference

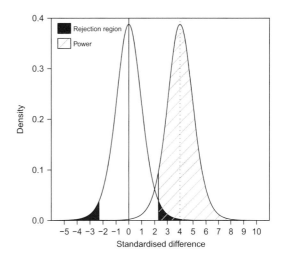

Figure 2.12. The power of a test. The grey shaded areas correspond to the rejection region under the null hypothesis and the hatched area corresponds to the statistical power if the true effect size is four (dotted vertical line).

that is so small or large that it lies within one of these two regions, then we assume the null hypothesis is not true (hence we reject the null hypothesis and accept the alternative).

- Assume the standardised difference between the treatment and control means was +4 (hence the null hypothesis is not true). This is represented by the dotted vertical line in Figure 2.12. Given the normality assumption we can now generate the actual distribution of the (standardised) difference. It is not centred on zero but is centred on +4 (represented by the bell-shaped curve on the right-hand side of Figure 2.12).
- Remember we reject the null hypothesis if we obtain a (standardised) difference that lies in the rejection region. If the null hypothesis is true this equals 5%, but given that the actual distribution is centred on +4 we can now calculate the actual chance of obtaining a standardised difference in the rejection region. This is the hatched area in Figure 2.12 and corresponds to the statistical power.

By considering Figure 2.12 it can be seen that as the risk of a making a Type I error reduces (and the rejection region is made smaller), so the statistical power reduces (and the risk of making a Type II error increases). This follows because to decrease the risk of a Type I error, the scientist will require more convincing evidence of an effect before rejecting the null hypothesis. Unfortunately this also means that genuine effects may be missed (by setting more stringent acceptance criteria). For example, if the significance level is set at 1%, i.e. the risk of finding a false positive result is fixed at 1%, then a comparison with a corresponding p-value of 0.02 is not declared significant. However, the treatment may have had a real effect but it has not been declared significant because of the strict significance level adopted. Type II errors are also more likely to occur when not enough animals are used in the study. As we discussed in Section 2.3.3, it is usually the case that we set the significance level at 5%.

Now as the curves included in Figure 2.12 are t-distributions, their shape is influenced by the sample size. The larger the sample size the tighter the distribution will be about the mean. We can therefore adjust the sample size in the study to make sure the power of the statistical test is suitably high (or the risk of a Type II error suitably low). To increase the statistical power (and reduce the Type II error to an acceptable level) more animals will be required (see Section 3.7.2).

2.4 Exploratory vs. confirmatory experiments

Most experiments can be categorised as either exploratory or confirmatory, and the researcher should be aware of the difference between them when conducting animal experiments. Both involve the hypothesis testing process described above, but in slightly different ways.

Experiments may be conducted to generate hypotheses (the exploratory experiments) or to test hypotheses (the confirmatory experiments); see Snedecor and Cochran (1989, p. 64) and Festing and Altman (2002). While both types of experiment may use the same experimental designs, they lead to subtly different statistical analysis approaches. When reporting the results of an experiment the researcher should make it clear to the reader which type of experiment (and statistical analysis) was performed.

When conducting an exploratory experiment, the researcher will want to assess many effects, explore

datasets in different ways and even perform data-trawling exercises. We should recognise when performing this type of statistical analysis that there will probably be false positive results generated. We recommend that the researcher does not adjust for multiplicity (see Section 5.4.8) and simply accept that there is a strong chance that some of the results generated will be false positives. These analyses provide an insight into the animal model, and allow the researcher to develop ideas. These ideas should be confirmed in an independent confirmatory experiment.

A confirmatory study is conducted to test specific hypotheses that were developed *a priori*. When performing a confirmatory study the researcher should, in theory, have a good idea which effects will influence the outcome of the experiment (i.e. the important blocking effects, see Section 3.4.1) and hence be able to construct a suitable experimental design. As the effects that need to be included in the statistical analysis are known, the strategy to conduct the statistical analysis will also have been planned in advance and, given an estimate of the variability of the response from exploratory experiments, an appropriate sample size selected. The statistical analysis should then only test those hypotheses planned in advance (the so-called planned comparisons, see Section 5.4.8.3). If more statistical tests are performed, then the researcher should either make adjustments to the results generated to reduce the increased risk of finding false positive results, see Section 5.4.8.1, or accept that these analyses are exploratory.

Example 2.4: MRI assessment of a transgenic phenotype

An experiment was conducted to compare the volumetric changes observed in the brain regions of wildtype and TasTPM transgenic mice (Maheswaran *et al.*, 2009). The size of several brain regions was measured at four time points using MRI. The difference between the volume of the brain regions in the wildtype and transgenic mice was assessed.

The researcher hypothesised that if the phenotype did affect the brain, then the volume change observed in certain brain regions over time would vary between strains. Hence it was planned to make comparisons only between the transgenic and wildtype animals in these brain regions. These comparisons therefore form a confirmatory analysis of *a priori* hypotheses.

However, by using the MRI imaging technique, the researcher was able to measure the volume of many brain regions. While not part of the hypotheses that were planned in advance, the researcher may want to investigate the difference between the strains in these other brain regions. The data was collected, so it seems sensible for the researcher to see if there were any phenotype effects in this part of the dataset. This second analysis could be considered as an exploratory analysis. As we shall see in Section 5.4.8.2, this can lead to two subtly different analysis approaches within the parametric analysis framework.

If there are significant results in the exploratory analysis, then the researcher should perhaps try to verify them in future experiments by including these brain regions in the planning stages of a future confirmatory experiment.

2.5 The estimation process

Many statisticians do not agree we should use the hypothesis testing framework described above when making inferences about experimental results. An alternative approach, and one that is certainly appealing, is the estimation approach.

Rather than try to test to see if the difference between two means is significant, we simply aim to estimate the size of the means (or the difference between them) and produce a range of values that will probably contain the true value (to a certain level of probability). This approach works particularly well when conducting pilot studies where the purpose of the study is not to test significant effects but merely to identify (and quantify) effects of interest.

The estimation process can be used in many scenarios though. For example, rather than produce a p-value to test the significance of the difference between the treatment and control group means, we estimate the size of the difference and a range of plausible values that the true difference should lie within. This, it can be argued, ties in better with the experimental process where experiments are conducted to discover the magnitude of an effect, rather than simply testing to see if there is a significant difference between the groups. The range that the difference lies within has a real biological meaning whereas a p-value does not.

In this text we shall highlight examples where we can use the statistical analysis to define the range of plausible values (the so-called confidence intervals) as well as generate p-values for hypothesis tests.

Experimental design

3.1 Why design experiments?

It has long been recognised that the use of experimental design is crucial in animal research. By using more efficient experimental designs we can maximise the amount of information gained, while reducing the number of animals required. Even seemingly straightforward experiments employ designs that have features that may, in certain cases, help reduce the number of animals. It is also true that if the scientist spends time considering the experimental design, then practical problems can be solved systematically. Experimental design provides a logical framework that will allow the scientist to develop and understand the animal model in a more refined way.

Experimental design is also a useful tool for researchers who do not feel confident running statistical analyses. As observed by Montgomery (1997, p. 18), if you plan the design carefully and correctly, using a little common sense, then the analysis will almost certainly be relatively straightforward. The validity of the results of many statistical tests relies on the underlying experimental design and randomisation.

We shall begin by considering in more detail some of the real benefits to be gained when using experimental designs, from both practical and statistical perspectives. We will then define the fundamental concepts that define an experimental design and finally describe some commonly applied families of designs.

3.1.1 Practical reasons

Experimental designs can help the scientist manage experiments more effectively. For example, the block designs described below give the scientist some degree of flexibility when running experiments. Experiments can be safely conducted over multiple days, using several pieces of equipment or by several technicians without affecting the scientific integrity of the study.

Experimental designs allow the scientist to investigate not only effects that may or may not affect the outcome of an experiment but also how these effects influence or interact with each other. While some of these effects may not be of direct interest, awareness of their influence can help improve the researcher's understanding of the animal model. The better the understanding of the animal model, the easier it is to tailor future experiments to answer specific questions. This will allow the researcher to achieve more reliable results from future studies and hence reduce the numbers of animals required (Festing and Altman, 2002).

Example 3.1: Age-dependent effect of nicotine on locomotor activity

A study was carried out to assess the age-dependent effects of nicotine on locomotor activity in rats (Belluzzi *et al.*, 2004). Early adolescent, late adolescent and adult rats were allocated to one of four nicotine treatment groups (n = 8 to 12 per group) and assessed for 20 minutes in a conditioned place preference trial. The tests were performed in four identical place-conditioning chambers. While any chamber effects may not be of particular interest, a difference in animal behaviour between the four chambers may indicate the animal model is being affected by external stimuli. This additional information may increase the researchers' understanding of the processes that influence the animals' response to nicotine. It could also aid in the design of future studies when deciding how to manage the behavioural tests across multiple place-conditioning chambers.

3.1.2 Statistical reasons: variability, the signal and bias

Consider the signal-to-noise ratio discussed in the previous chapter. If we can increase the signal-to-noise ratio, then by implication we can reduce the number of animals used while still achieving the same degree of statistical precision. Experimental designs can be used to increase this ratio by reducing the variability of the responses and/or increasing the signal. By including factors in the design that account for the nuisance sources of variability, we can reduce the noise in the signal-to-noise ratio. It is sometimes overlooked, but experimental design can also be used to select conditions that increase the size of the signal, again increasing the signal-to-noise ratio. This process will also give us a better understanding of the animal model.

Reducing the variability

If we discover that a nuisance effect is increasing the variability of the results, then perhaps we can reduce the influence of this effect by including a factor in the experimental design to account for it. For example, suppose it is discovered that there is a difference between the experimental results gathered on successive days. In many behavioural experiments, the results on a Monday (following two days of relative quiet in the animal house) will be different to other test days where the animals have been disturbed by general husbandry procedures. If we do not take this into account, when designing and analysing the study, then the day-to-day effects will increase the variability of the responses and hence decrease the signal-to-noise ratio. However, we can use an experimental design (and appropriate statistical analysis) to account for this source of variability. Such designs are called block designs and are discussed in more detail in Section 3.4.

By using more complicated designs, the so-called nested designs (see Section 3.7), the scientist can identify the amount of variability associated with different stages in the experimental process. Once the most variable stages have been identified, then the scientist can concentrate on improving the reliability of these processes. The use of nested designs to identify the sources of variability is commonly used in manufacturing processes, but there is no reason why such designs cannot be routinely applied in the field of animal research.

Increasing the signal

Experimental designs can also be used to increase the signal, or window of opportunity. If we can increase this window then this allows the scientist to reduce the number of animals used without risking loss of statistical significance. These designs, defined as factorial designs, can be used to assess which levels of the controllable factors, such as Gender, Age and Dose, should be selected to maximise the window of opportunity. For example, a study was conducted to assess an inflammatory response in dba vs. balb c strains of mice. This experiment allowed the scientist to select the strain that was most sensitive so that future experiments would have the largest window of opportunity when testing novel compounds.

When setting up a new animal model, while it may seem a waste of resources to run such pilot studies at the start of the experimental process, the long-term benefits can easily outweigh the initial costs. These designs are discussed in Section 3.5.4.

Reducing bias

Finally a good experimental design should reduce (as much as possible) the risk of biasing the comparisons of interest. If, for example, the scientist wishes to see if a novel drug has had an effect compared to the control, then the treatment group mean could be compared to the control group mean. But is this comparison a true reflection of the effect of the drug? Could the comparison be influenced by some other nuisance effect? In the worst case scenario the nuisance effect may be inseparable from, or completely confounded with, the effect of interest. If this is the case then there is no way of knowing what the treatment effect is because any comparisons will be biased by the nuisance effect. In such cases the experiment is probably ruined and will need repeating (assuming the problem has been identified).

The problem with experimental bias, unlike investigating the size of the signal or the variability of the response, is that it is difficult to identify. It is a hidden danger. If an experiment is conducted and the results are unusual or unexpected, then it may be the case that an unknown nuisance effect is influencing the results.

Example 3.2: A drug study where treatment effects are confounded with age effects

Consider an experiment where the oldest animals are allocated to the control group and the youngest animals are allocated to the treatment group using a non-random approach. As a result any observed treatment effects could be due to the difference in animal ages rather than any effect of the drug. The treatment effect is said to be *confounded* with the effect of age and hence we cannot tell whether the effect observed is due to treatment or age. Of course with the use of a little common sense it is unlikely that such a design would be used in practice. But how do we guarantee subtler biasing does not occur? For example, assume animals were randomised to treatments. It may be the case that most (but not all) of the control animals are the older animals. If we are not careful the age effects could bias the treatment effects. Perhaps the simplest way to avoid such issues is to use an appropriate experimental design, with a suitable randomisation.

3.2 What does an experimental design involve?

Before we begin to discuss the different types of design available to the scientist, a few fundamental concepts are introduced. These provide a framework for identifying and constructing the experimental designs that can be used in practice. Prior to finalising the study design, the scientist should consider the following.

3.2.1 Variables to be recorded

When planning an experiment one of the first things the researcher should do is consider the responses that will be measured. This can have an impact on the experimental design. Consideration should be given to how the responses will be reported and also the statistical analysis that will be performed once the data are generated.

As well as the responses of interest, the researcher should consider other variables that may need recording, such as body weight, cage position in the rack, health status, operators, handlers and so on. Such variables may prove useful when analysing the data and

drawing conclusions from the experiment. It is best to spend time before the start of the experiment considering these variables and putting plans in place on how to capture them.

3.2.1.1 Types of response

The choice of response to be measured may be an obvious one. Clearly it has as many practical implications as statistical ones. Responses measured must capture the biological effects in a meaningful way while imposing the minimal necessary level of harm to the animals. We have been involved in many discussions about suitable end points to measure. The choice of response is perhaps a subject in its own right, varying from animal model to animal model and is beyond the scope of this book. There are, however, a few statistical issues that the researcher should consider when deciding on which response to measure.

Given the small sample size used in most animal experiments, the researcher should aim to gather as much information as possible from the experimental animals. The type of response measured can influence this. Responses should also be selected that maximise the signal-to-noise ratio, as described in Section 2.1.

Responses can be categorised into a number of different types. These include the following.

Continuous responses are measured on a continuous numerical scale. Examples include body weight, time-to-event, level of cholesterol in the blood and so on. By continuous we imply that they can be measured at any numerical value. So for any two individual levels of a continuous response, it is always possible to record a value in between them. For example, if one animal weighs 9 g and another weighs 9.5 g, then it is possible to find a third animal that weighs 9.25 g. These responses contain the most information and hence require the smallest sample size to achieve a sufficiently sensitive statistical analysis.

Discrete responses are numerical but can only be measured at certain fixed values. The response is directional, so an increasing response indicates an increasing (or decreasing) effect. For example, if the response measured is a count of the number of

Table 3.1. Examples of different types of response

Continuous	Discrete	Ordinal	Nominal	Binary
Body weight	Litter size	Disease state (mild/	Genotype	Strauss tail
Organ weight	Number of correct	moderate/	Stress type	(yes/no)
Time-to-event	responses	severe)	Dog excitability	Paw withdrawn from
Blood or brain	Clinical score	Dog	state (fine/	hotplate (yes/no)
concentration	Number of rearings	excitability score	nervous/ excited/	Disease state (yes/
Body temperature	Arthritis score (scale	Sample appearance	uncontrollable)	no)
Latency in the water maze	0,1,2,3,4)			(present/absent)

events, then each observation can only be an integer (you cannot have 2.5 counts!). From a pragmatic point of view, it may be possible to treat a count response as a continuous response. As a rule of thumb, if the counts have a range of around 15 or more distinct values, then they can be treated as a continuous response (Festing *et al.*, 2002, p. 72). There should also be a wide range of counts present in each group. It would be difficult to justify the assumption that the data was continuous if all the counts in one group had the same value! As described in Section 5.4.1.3, if your response is a count response then you may also want to consider a square root transformation prior to analysis.

Ordinal responses are measured on an increasing or decreasing non-numerical scale that can only be measured at set values. For example, non-numeric disease severity scores (mild/moderate/severe) or animal behavioural scores (calm/normal/excited). Although these responses can only be measured at specific values they are at least directional. Moving from one category of response to another does have a biological meaning. It should be remembered that unlike discrete responses, the biological implication of moving from one level of the response to the next highest or lowest is not the same across all response levels. So, in the above example, the biological implication of moving from the mild to the moderate condition is not necessarily the same as moving from the moderate to the severe condition.

Nominal responses are non-numerical responses and are similar to ordinal responses. However, unlike ordinal responses they do not have an ordering to the measurement levels. For example, consider an

experiment to assess stress following injection. The response recorded may consist of the animals' reaction to the injection procedure. In such cases it may be difficult to order the reactions in terms of severity as many different type of reaction share a similar stress level. Hence the levels of the response do not follow a natural order. Such responses contain less information than the previous three discussed and the statistical analysis of such responses will therefore require more animals.

Binary responses are measured on a scale of only two levels. Examples include yes/no or present/absent responses. The analysis of such responses involves specific methodologies that tend to be less sensitive than other methods. Many more animals will be required to achieve statistical significance than would be needed if the response had been measured on a continuous scale.

Example 3.3: Arthritis score

In a study assessing the effect of novel compounds on the severity of arthritis in mice, the severity was measured over time on a scale of 0 to 4 for each paw. So the total for each mouse was a score between 0 and 16. Even though the response was in reality a discrete response, it was treated as continuous for the purposes of the statistical analysis.

Generally it is the case that continuous responses, while being information rich, take longer and more resource to measure. However, it is worth bearing in mind that if you choose a response that is not continuous then you will probably need more animals per group, everything else being equal, to account for the reduced information that the response contains.

Table 3.1 contains examples of responses found in animal experiments.

Example 3.4: Assessing kidney lesions induced by p-aminophenol

A study was conducted with rats to assess the effect of a single intravenous injection of p-aminophenol hydrochloride on the development of kidney lesions in rats (Green *et al.*, 1969). Following injection of 20, 40 or 60 mg of p-aminophenol hydrochloride, pairs of rats were humanely killed at 24, 48 and 96 hours and at 1 and 2 weeks post-injection and sections of the kidney taken and fixed.

While the original investigation did not include a statistical analysis of the results, let us assume the researchers planned to perform a statistical analysis. The researchers would have to decide upon the most appropriate response to measure. The total lesion area of a kidney section (a continuous response) would provide the most information, but would also be the most time consuming to measure. An alternative response that would be quicker to measure would be to count the number of lesions on a cross-sectional area of the kidney (perhaps still a continuous response). Simpler still, the researcher could classify the kidney lesions in an animal as mild, moderate or severe (an ordinal response) or perhaps simply record whether there were lesions present or absent (a binary response). Although the latter responses would be quick to assess, more animals would be required to achieve the same level of statistical sensitivity than would be the case for the continuous measures.

3.2.1.2 Reporting responses

When reporting the results of an animal experiment care must be taken to give as much information as possible to readers so that they can judge the biological relevance. If possible the original data should be presented. If you cannot present the actual data, then a suitable summary measure should be provided. These summary measures should be meaningful and reliable.

For example, for continuous data an estimate of the reliability of the results should be presented, in the form of either a standard deviation (SD) or standard error (SEM) (see Section 5.2.2), along with a suitable summary measure such as the sample mean. For other types of response the mean and SD may not be reliable, see Section 5.2.4, and the median may be more informative. For any response it is also helpful to give the reader an idea of the sample size used and the number of animals present in the final analysed dataset.

It is recommended (ARRIVE guidelines item 15) that data are not presented as percentages but as actual numbers. This is because it is easy for percentages to give a misleading picture or tell a specific story.

Example 3.5: Novel object recognition paradigm

A series of experiments were conducted to investigate the ability of typical and atypical antipsychotics to attenuate the effect of subchronic PCP-induced cognitive deficits in the novel object recognition task (Grayson *et al.*, 2007). On the day of testing the rats were shown two identical objects (the familiar objects) for three minutes. Rats were then returned to their home cage for a minute while one of the familiar objects was replaced with a novel object. Rats were then returned to the test box for a further three minutes. If the rats remembered the familiar object then they should, in theory, have spent more time investigating the novel object.

One of the responses analysed was the discrimination index (DI):

$$DI = (novel - familiar) / (novel + familiar) \times 100\%, \qquad (3.1)$$

where *novel time* is the time the animal spent investigating the novel object and *familiar time* was the time spent investigating the familiar object.

Consider an active rat that spent two minutes investigating the novel object and one minute investigating the familiar object. The DI index for this animal is 33%. Unfortunately the same DI index would also be recorded for an animal that was lethargic and spent only two seconds investigating the novel object and one second investigating the familiar object before falling asleep. The different behaviour of these animals is not reflected in the DI index and so care must be taken when making conclusions based on this response. The point is that a small biological change can show up as large percentage change if the numbers that are used to calculate the percentage are small. This is true regardless of the biological relevance of the responses.

3.2.1.3 Baseline responses

A decision must be taken prior to starting a study whether or not to take any baseline measurements. Baseline measurements can be beneficial in the statistical analysis. They can sometimes be used to reduce the between-animal variability. If baselines can be measured well in advance of the main part of the study, then they can also be used when assigning animals to treatment groups using a stratified randomisation procedure (Section 4.2.1).

Baselines can also highlight issues regarding the conclusions drawn from the statistical analysis. In Example 1.1, discussed above in Chapter 1, there were concerns with the validity of the experimental results that would not have been identified if the baseline blood cholesterol level measurements had not been recorded.

3.2.1.4 Recording conditions during the experiment

There are many pieces of information that the animal researcher should record and report alongside the responses of interest. Some of these will be considered beforehand, others during the experiment itself. The important principle is to try to collect as much information as possible, given the ethical and practical constraints, to help reduce animal use.

In most studies many external influences will affect the animals' responses. Some of these will be controlled, such as the treatment each animal receives. Some will have been predicted in advance and hence designed into the study, such as knowing there will be two observers recording animal behaviour. Others, however, will not be expected. It is important, when conducting the experiment, to record as many of these external influences as possible. They can be investigated later on in an investigatory analysis of the data and help in the design of future studies.

Keeping a record of exactly what happened in a study can also be used as a justification for excluding outliers. We note at this stage that it is always difficult to exclude unusual observations purely on statistical grounds. However, if there is a biological explanation, then the researcher will have a stronger case for excluding an observation that is a genuine outlier. See Section 5.4.1.5 for a more detailed discussion of strategies for removing outliers.

3.2.2 Set of treatments

Once the researcher has selected the variables to measure, the next design property to consider is the set of treatments. If too many groups are included in the design, while keeping the total number of animals fixed, then the sample size could be reduced to dangerously low levels.

The researcher also has to decide which control groups to include in the experimental design. It is worth spending time considering this issue as the conclusions that can be drawn from the experiment will depend on the choice of comparator control. Effectively control groups allow us to investigate the effect of a treatment by removing any known and/or unknown experimental effects when assessing the treatment effects. It is therefore important that the control group is treated in exactly the same way as the treatment groups, otherwise biases may be introduced.

It is common practice to quantify the size of the treatment effect by comparing the posttreatment response with the baseline response. These comparisons may appear appealing as they are within-animal comparisons; however, they might not reveal the true treatment effect. For example, they are not necessarily free of any time-related experimental effects and if the response drifts over time then they will be biased. It may also be the case that the change from baseline response is still influenced by differences between the groups at baseline (Karp *et al.*, 2012); see also Section 5.4.6.9.

Possible controls you may consider including in your experiment are set out below.

Negative control

The aim of the negative control is to ensure that an unknown variable is not influencing the experimental outcome. The use of such a control can help the researcher avoid false positives. However, there is an argument that it is not always suitable to use negative controls on ethical grounds, although this is perhaps more of a concern in clinical trials than animal experiments.

Vehicle control

Vehicle controls can be used if the compound is given in solution. They allow the researcher to assess treatment effects above and beyond any vehicle-related effects.

Positive control

Perhaps ethically more acceptable than the negative control, the purpose of the positive control is to show that the novel treatment is as good as or better than the positive control. By considering the results from the positive control we can also demonstrate that the experiment was successful as it was capable of detecting a known effect. If there is a known difference between the positive and negative controls, then we should be able to detect it. The positive control can also be used to

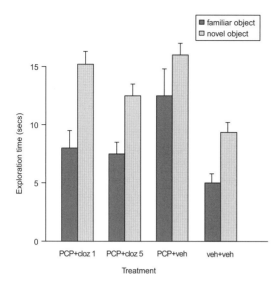

Figure 3.1. Plot of means with within-group standard errors for total time spent investigating the novel and familiar objects for Example 3.5.

confirm that the effects that you want to model (or have manipulated as part of the animal model) are present in the experiment.

Consider a situation where:

(i) The comparison between the novel compound and the vehicle control is non-significant.

(ii) The comparison between the positive control and vehicle is significant.

From (ii) we conclude that the experiment would be capable of detecting a treatment effect if there was one. However, from (i) the lack of significance implies that the compound did not have an effect. Unfortunately the researcher does not always have a 'gold standard' positive control available.

Sham control

Sham controls are useful if you want to mimic the experimental procedures, such as surgery, without involving test substances. They also allow the researcher to separate treatment effects from the effects of the surgery.

Comparative control

These are similar to a positive control. The aim of the study is to show a new therapy is as good as, or

equivalent to, an existing one. Care should be taken when running an analysis that involves comparing back to a comparative control. Remember that the null hypothesis (in most analyses) is to assume that there is no treatment effect. We then run an experiment to see if we can disprove this hypothesis. In comparative studies it may be preferable to use a null hypothesis that there is an effect with the test compound, and then to try and disprove this by running the study.

Naïve control

Animals in the naïve control group do not receive any treatments nor have any procedures carried out on them. The naïve control group provides information on the underlying animal response within the experimental protocol.

Example 3.5 (continued): Novel object recognition paradigm

In the study described above, animals received either the vehicle or PCP for seven days followed by a seven-day drug-free period. On the day of testing animals were administered either haloperidol, clozapine, risperidone or the vehicle 30 minutes prior to testing in the novel object recognition paradigm. From a simulated dataset, the average time rats spent investigating the novel and familiar objects, when administered clozapine at 1 and 5 mg/kg, is presented in Figure 3.1.

From the plot it can clearly be seen that in the clozapine-treated groups (PCP + cloz 1 and PCP + cloz 5) the time spent investigating the novel object was greater than the time spent investigating the familiar object. Unfortunately there was also some evidence of an effect in the PCP (PCP + veh) and vehicle (veh + veh) groups. So the effects observed in the clozapine-treated groups could simply be an artefact of running the experiment, rather than any specific effect of clozapine. Any assessment of the treatment effect, i.e. the difference in novel and familiar times in the treatment groups, should take into account the difference observed in the vehicle group. It is interesting to note that the recognition response discussed above, where

$$DI = (novel - familiar) / (novel + familiar) \times 100\%, \qquad (3.2)$$

revealed no statistically significant effect of clozapine in this experiment.

3.2.3 The experimental unit and the observational unit

When planning an experimental design it is important to identify the experimental unit and the observational unit. These ideas are the key to many statistical analyses.

An experimental unit for a treatment factor is *the smallest unit which a level of the treatment can be applied to*. For most animal studies the animals will be the experimental units, as each animal is individually treated.

Another example of an experimental unit that can be employed in animal experiments is the cage the animals are housed in. Cages would be the experimental units if a treatment was administered to a whole cage of animals, perhaps orally in the food. In aquatic studies the test compounds are usually administered to the tanks the fish are housed in. Hence it is the tanks that are the experimental units and not the individual fish within the tank.

An observational unit is *the smallest unit on which a response will be measured* (Bailey, 2008, p. 8). Again this is usually the animals, as we can measure the animals' responses individually. There are, however, examples where the animals may not be the observational units. If several histological slices of a target organ are taken, then the slices are the observational units even if the animals are the experimental units. In experiments where animals are repeatedly measured, the observational units correspond to the individual measurements but the experimental units may still be the animals, depending on the experimental design (see Table 3.2).

It is important to consider these two concepts when planning an experiment as the treatment effects are usually assessed against the experimental unit variability and not the observational unit variability. So it is the replication of the experimental units that is of primary importance. While not as influential, it is still the case that measuring the experimental units (animals) repeatedly will be beneficial. In Section 3.7.3 we consider higher-order nested designs. In these designs the experimental unit and the observational unit are usually different.

Example 3.6: Toxicology experiments

Bailey (2008, p. 128) describes two toxicology experiments where the observational units are different but the experimental units are the same. The experiments are conducted to assess how rats absorb the toxin bromobenzene over time. In each study, the rats are exposed to one of three doses of bromobenzene, the vehicle or a negative control and the level of toxin present in each rat measured.

In the first experiment nine rats per group were individually administered either a dose of bromobenzene or one of the controls. The rats were then humanely killed at three time points, three rats per group per time point. Using this approach the level of bromobenzene in the liver of the rats can then be assessed over time.

In the second experiment, rather than employing the invasive liver extraction approach, a non-invasive technique was used where the bromobenzene was measured in the rats' urine. In this experiment each rat was measured at all the time points, hence fewer animals were required.

In both experiments the rats were dosed individually, hence in both scenarios the experimental units were the rats. However, the observational units were different in each case. In the first experiment the observational units were the rats, as each animal provides one measurement. In the second experiment the observational units were the rats at each time point. Each animal therefore provides three observational units. The number of animals required for the second study (to achieve the same level of statistical sensitivity) will depend on the relationship between the within-animal variability and the between-animal variability. However, the second study will probably require fewer animals in total than the first.

3.2.4 Effects and factors

The results obtained from an experiment are influenced by a number of effects. These can be effects of interest such as treatment effects, which the researcher controls and manipulates, or nuisance effects, such as the effect of the room the animals are housed in. We begin the planning stage of any experiment by considering these effects in order to investigate and/or control for them. Once effects are identified we need to quantify them scientifically. We do this by constructing experimental factors that correspond to these effects. The levels of each factor represent specific examples of the underlying effect. The factors are then used to generate the experimental design that is employed to assess the effects.

For example, if an experiment consists of two drug groups with ten animals per group, then we say the study has two factors, Treatment (at two levels: drug and control) and Animal (at 20 levels: corresponding to the 20 animals). The researcher aims to assess the effect of the treatment and hence constructs the Treatment factor to quantify the effect and test it scientifically.

We distinguish between the experimental factors and the effects we are attempting to quantify by using a capital letter for the factor name. So the Treatment factor

Table 3.2. Seven different ways to measure an animal repeatedly

Scenario	Description	Examples	Relationships between factors	Experimental unit	Type of design	Section
1	Animals measured repeatedly: levels of the factor that defines the repeated measurements are shared across animals	Animals measured at specific time points or at specific brain regions	The factor that defines the repeated measurements is crossed with the Animal factor and any treatment factors	Animal	Repeated measures design	3.8.1
2	Animals measured repeatedly: levels of the factor that defines the repeated measurements are not shared across animals	Multiple trials per animal, blood samples assayed in triplicate, multiple cells tested from each animal	The factor that defines the repeated measurements is nested within the Animal factor – levels of the nested factor for the first animal are not related to the levels for the second and so on	Animal	Nested design	3.7.3
3	Treatments assessed at random positions within the animal.	Local anaesthetic skin creams tested on different positions on each animal	All within-animal factors crossed	Position within-animal	Block design	3.4
4	Two treatments: within-animal treatment levels are assessed at random positions within the animal and between-animal treatment levels are administered one per animal	Three types of implant placed within each animal. Movement of the implants assessed under various systemic treatments	All within-animal factors crossed, Animal nested within the between-animal treatment factor	Animal (for between-animal treatments) and position within-animal (for within-animal treatments)	Split-plot design	3.9
5	Animals receive multiple treatments over time in a different order for each animal	Husbandry studies testing several housing conditions within-animal	Animal factor crossed with the factor that corresponds to the test periods and the Treatment factor	Combination of the animal and test period	Crossover design	3.4.9
6	Animals receive multiple treatments over time in a non-random order	Escalating doses (to avoid toxicological effects) administered within-animal over time	Animal factor crossed with the factor that corresponds to the test period/Treatment factor	Combination of the animal and test period	Dose-escalation design	3.8.2
7	Multiple different responses measured for each animal	Many parameters measured on each animal (body weight, organ weight, …)	–	–	Any type of design	–

is created to assess the effect of the treatments. Factor levels are also usually presented lower case.

In this book we will consider the experimental factors in more detail (Sections 3.5 and 3.8.1). However, at this stage we should remember that the experimental factors are a tool for investigating the underlying effects that influence the results of an experiment. If an experiment is designed well, then the scientist will have confidence that the levels of the experimental factors describe (in some sense) the effects that are influencing the responses. In such experiments the statistical analysis should be able to separate out the important effects. This is not always the case in poorly designed experiments.

3.2.4.1 Defining factor level labels

As a rule, throughout this book we assume that the factor level labels must be uniquely specified and have a practical meaning within the experiment. So for example, if an experiment consists of eight animals in total, and each animal receives both treatment and control, then the levels of the Animal factor are labelled 1 to 8 in the treatment group and 1 to 8 in the control group. If the eight animals assigned to the control group are different from the eight assigned to the treatment group, then the Animal factor has 16 levels, and the labels are 1 to 8 in the treatment group and 9 to 16 in the control group.

This may seem rather counter-intuitive but it does help when setting up the analysis within a statistical package. Assume that the animals are labelled 1 to 8 in both groups, even though the eight animals in the control group are different from the eight in the treatment group. As we shall see later, to carry out the appropriate analysis you would need to tell the statistical package that there are 16 animals in the study, not just the same 8 animals assessed twice. While this is not a problem with many types of design, it can become a problem in some of the more complicated designs.

This method of defining factor levels will also help the researcher decide which type of design is being employed. For example, by considering the factor levels within the design it may be identified as nested (Section 3.7) or repeated measures (Section 3.8.1).

3.2.4.2 Defining the factors in an experimental design

An experimental design is defined by the experimental factors it contains, the nature of these factors and the relationships between them.

- Factors can be categorised as *random* or *fixed*. Whether factors are defined as random or fixed will influence the statistical analysis and the conclusions drawn.
- Factors can be either *categorical* or *continuous*. Most factors considered in this text are categorical factors, although some can be considered as either.
- The relationship between any pair of factors within the design can be described as either *crossed*, *partially crossed* or *nested*.

Understanding these three simple concepts will allow the scientist to make the best use of experimental design and also provide strategies for the statistical analysis. Before going on to describe the types of experimental designs available, we consider these concepts in more detail.

3.2.5 Fixed and random factors

Experimental factors can be categorised as either fixed factors or random factors. Deciding on whether a factor is random or fixed will depend on the nature of the underlying effect and the conclusion that the scientist wishes to draw from the study. It may also depend on the experimental design and the randomisation used.

Both types of factor can lead to changes in the response measured. A biologist would say both can cause variability in the data. With fixed factors there are fixed differences between the levels of the factor (that we may want to test to see if they are significant) whereas with random factors the differences are random.

For example, assume a colony of marmosets is housed in more than one room in the animal facility. The researcher believes that the responses of the marmosets may be influenced by the room in which they are housed. If marmosets from only two rooms are required for a study, then an investigation could be conducted to see if there is an overall difference between the two rooms. In this case Room should be categorised as a fixed factor at two levels as there may be a fixed change in the experimental results obtained from marmosets housed in one room compared to the other. As only two rooms are assessed, we cannot generalise any conclusions to all rooms in the facility. If, however, the study animals are housed in many rooms (rooms that are randomly selected from all available in the facility) then we may consider Room to be a random factor. We can then see how the marmosets' responses vary from room to room (in a random fashion). This conclusion can be generalised to all rooms in the facility as it represents the random room-to-room variability.

In this text we shall reserve the term variability to describe the random variability of the response that is introduced by the random factors and not the fixed differences caused by the fixed factors.

3.2.5.1 Fixed factors

Fixed factors are usually factors that quantify the effects that the researcher is investigating. For example, the Treatment factor is always a fixed factor. With fixed factors we assume that the levels that are present in the experimental design consist of all the possible levels of the factor. For example, if both sexes are used in a study, then Gender will be defined as a fixed factor. It has two levels, male and female, both of which are present in the design.

When using a fixed factor we assume there may be 'fixed' differences between the factor levels. The purpose of the experiment, if the factor is of interest to the researcher, is to estimate these differences and perhaps perform a suitable statistical test to assess their magnitude.

Consider an experiment to test the difference between a novel drug and a control. The fixed factor Treatment has two levels (drug and control). We assume that these are the only two levels possible (and they are, given that the purpose of the experiment is to test whether the effect of this dose of treatment is different from that of the control). We can also say that the two levels of the Treatment factor adequately describe the treatment effect in this experiment. The researcher believes there will be a fixed difference between the

animals receiving the drug and those receiving the control. This difference can be assessed by comparing the treatment and control group means, using a suitable statistical test.

Other examples of fixed factors include Strain of animal (wildtype vs. transgenic), Age of animal (2 months vs. 4 months vs. 6 months), Time, Diet, Supplier and so on. In fact most factors the animal researcher will need to consider can be defined as fixed.

3.2.5.2 Random factors

The most commonly encountered random factor in an animal experiment is the Animal factor. With random factors we assume that each level of the factor present in the experiment was selected (or sampled) at random from a population of levels. So when carrying out a statistical analysis we assume (to some extent) that we have taken a random sample of animals from the wider population of animals. We also assume that the effect at each level of the random factor is the same, apart from some random variability. So we assume that two animals, everything else being equal, should give the same results apart from the animal-to-animal variability.

As we have randomly sampled from a wider population, then we are justified in projecting the conclusions of the experiment onto the wider population that the experimental animals were sampled from. In other words, if we see a treatment effect in the animals in our experiment (with the results obtained from a small fraction of the total population of that species or strain) then we can assume the effect is present in the wider population of animals too. Care must be taken when projecting outside this population though. If the experiment was conducted with male animals, and hence the experimental animals were randomly selected from the population of male animals, then it would be dangerous to predict how females will react based on these results.

The goal of many statistical analyses is to compare the difference between the levels of the fixed factors (the signal) to one or more of the random factors (the noise). Sometimes, however, we may simply want to investigate the magnitude of the variability associated with a random factor. When investigating random factors we are therefore interested in the amount of variability accounted for by the levels of the random factors.

Most animal experiments involve at least one random factor, namely the Animal factor, but there may be others. Examples of random factors the authors have observed in animal experiments include: Section (histological sections or slices taken at random from a brain), Sample (multiple measurements taken at random on an animal) and Assay (each sample from an animal being assayed in triplicate wells on a 96-well assay plate). The other random factor that the animal researcher may encounter is Cage. If animals were group housed and dosed in their food, then cages are the experimental units and treatments should be assessed against the cage-to-cage variability, i.e. Cage needs to be defined as a random factor.

Example 3.7: Mouse selection

Consider the Animal factor, with levels corresponding to the individual mice. We assume in the analysis that we have randomly selected the mice from the population of mice, and that each animal will give the same result, apart from the usual animal-to-animal variability. If there is any reason why one group of mice should give higher results than another, for example we have two observers assessing the animals in the study, then it may be appropriate to try to account for this in the analysis. This can be achieved by including an additional factor (Observer in this case) in the experimental design to account for this effect.

3.2.5.3 Random or fixed?

Certain factors may be considered as random or fixed, depending on the questions the researcher wishes to answer.

For example, consider the test arena in a behavioural test.

- We may say that we have taken a sample of arenas at random from a population of arenas. We assume each arena has the same effect on the results, apart from some random arena-to-arena variability. If we can estimate this variability, then we can predict what would happen if we use different arenas in the next experiment. We have estimated (in general) how variable arenas are.
- Alternatively we might assume the Arena factor is a fixed factor. Perhaps there were only three arenas used within the experiment. Trying to assess the arena-to-

arena variability using such a small number of arenas would result in an unreliable estimate of the overall arena-to-arena variability. In this case we calculate the fixed differences between the three arenas in the experiment and fit Arena as a fixed factor in the analysis.

Defining Arena as a fixed factor in this example allows the researcher to investigate differences between the arenas in the experiment. Defining Arena as a random factor allows the researcher to draw conclusions about the variability of test arenas in general. Conclusions from this latter analysis will therefore be valid if we want to include other arenas, not present in the current study, in future experiments.

As well as Arena other factors that could be defined as random or fixed include Cage, Room, Operator, Surgeon, Test box and so on. In this book we shall assume, unless otherwise stated, that these factors are defined as fixed. More advanced statistical analyses are possible which assume that these factors are random. However, such tests are not necessarily more sensitive and are beyond the scope of this book. For a description of such approaches see Montgomery (1997, pp. 470–91). Most analysis packages, by default, assume all factors are fixed, although the more powerful packages do have the option to declare factors as random.

Interestingly it is worth remembering that all studies contain both random and fixed factors. The grand mean or intercept (the overall average of the responses recorded in an experiment) is usually considered to be a fixed factor. Experiments also require at least one random factor (where the levels of the factor correspond to the observational units) to allow us to carry out statistical tests. Designs that contain both fixed and random factors are defined as *mixed designs*. It can be argued that all experimental designs are mixed designs.

Example 3.8: Wheel-running experiment

The following experiment is based loosely on two experiments described in Festing *et al.* (2002, p. 46 and p. 51). An experiment was conducted to test the hypothesis that the density of neurones in the hippocampus of the mouse brain is affected by exercise. To test this hypothesis, 15 male mice and 15 female mice were assigned to one of three groups, each group was then allowed varying degrees of exercise. Each group has access to a running wheel for a different amount of time:

- No running (non-rotating wheel placed in the cage for 30 minutes per 24 hours);
- Moderate running (access to a running wheel for 30 minutes per 24 hours);
- Marathon running (access to a running wheel for 3 hours per 24 hours).

Histological sections were prepared from the hippocampus of each mouse and the number of neurones in four microscope slides from each animal counted. The mice were the experimental units and the microscope slides were the observational units.

In this experiment the fixed factors were Treatment at three levels and Gender at two levels. We assumed there was a fixed difference between the three treatments, and that these three levels were all the levels required when deciding if there was an effect of exercise on neurone density. Similarly Gender was a fixed factor as we assessed the hypothesis that the neurone density varied depending on the gender of the animal.

The other two factors in the design, Animal and Microscope slide, were both random factors. Fifteen animals per sex were randomly selected from the population of mice, and the four microscopic slides were randomly selected from each mouse.

Alternatively if we had assumed the four microscope slides taken from each mouse had been one from the front, two from the middle and one from the back of the hippocampus (rather than four selected at random), then we could have defined Section as a fixed factor at four levels: front, middle-front, middle-back and back. We could then have investigated the effect of exercise on neurone density across the hippocampus. This highlights the different hypotheses that can be assessed depending on the design used and the factor designation.

3.2.6 Categorical factors and continuous factors

Most experimental factors described in this text are categorical. They consist of a number of distinct levels (or categories). The scientist is then interested in either the fixed differences between the levels of the factor (for fixed factors) or how much they randomly vary (for random factors). Examples of categorical factors include Gender, Treatment, Genotype and Animal.

For some factors though, the levels are numeric. For example, if the doses of a compound included in an experiment are 0, 3, 5 and 10 mg/kg. We could assume that the corresponding Dose factor was at four levels (a categorical factor) and we could then test to see if there is a significant difference between the 3, 5 and 10 mg/kg treatments compared to the 0 mg/kg control. Alternatively we could assume the Dose factor was continuous, i.e. it can take any numerical value. We can

then estimate the dose-response relationship across the range we have observed (0 to 10 mg/kg). This way we could predict what the effect of, say, a dose of 7 mg/kg would be. To do this we need to assume some underlying relationship between the response and the dose of the compound, for example a linear relationship. We can then use the data generated to estimate the exact relationship. We shall expand on this in Sections 3.5.5 and 3.6 where continuous factors are used for factorial designs and dose-response designs, respectively.

Another example of a factor that can either be categorical or continuous is the baseline body weight of the animal. It can be assumed to be a categorical factor (levels: low, medium and high) and used as a blocking factor in the design and analysis (see Sections 3.4 and 6.3.3.3, respectively). We could though assume baseline body weight was continuous (and hence assume it is a response variable rather than a factor) with levels that are the actual baseline body weights. We could then fit baseline body weight as a covariate (see Section 5.4.6) to help reduce the animal-to-animal variability.

3.2.7 Crossed factors and nested factors

The relationship between any pair of factors within an experimental design can be described as either *crossed*, *partially crossed* or *nested*. Partial crossing is a special case of crossing, so in general we say that factors are either crossed or nested with each other. As there are only two fundamental types of relationship it should be easy to work out which ones are present in your design. By understanding these different relationships, and how the factors within a given design are related, we can make better use of our experimental designs.

As a rule of thumb (and this really is only a rule of thumb) random factors tend to be nested within either fixed or other random factors, whereas fixed factors tend to be crossed with each other.

3.2.7.1 Nested factors

Nested relationships are present in even the simplest designs. Consider the design described above, where there are eight animals in the treatment group and

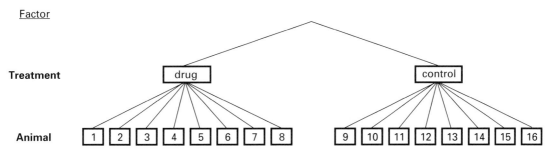

Factor

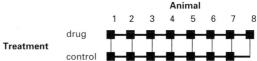

Figure 3.2. A nested design involving two treatments (levels: drug and control) with eight animals per group.

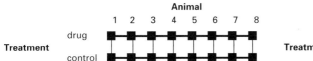

Figure 3.3. A design involving two crossed factors: Treatment (levels: drug and control) and Animal (levels: 1 to 8).

Figure 3.4. A design involving two crossed factors: Treatment (levels: drug and control) and Animal (levels: 1 to 8) with one missing combination.

eight animals in the control group. The design con-sists of two factors, Animal and Treatment. If the eight animals in the treatment group are different from the eight animals in the control group, then we say Animal is nested within Treatment. It should be noted that in many cases Animal is nested within the Treatment factor(s).

Nested relationships can be easily described using a diagram. A simple example is presented in Figure 3.2, corresponding to the experiment involving two treat-ments and eight animals per treatment.

Note that in Figure 3.2 we have labelled the animals 1 to 16; 1 to 8 in the drug treatment group and 9 to 16 in the control group. If we had labelled the animals 1 to 8 in both groups, then this would imply (using the rule described in Section 3.2.4.1) that there were only eight animals in total in the study, with each animal receiving both drug treatment and the control at some point dur-ing the experiment.

3.2.7.2 Crossed factors

Along with the nested relationships between factors, as described in the previous section, the second way that factors can be related to each other when they are crossed.

In the example described in the previous section, let us now assume that the study consisted of eight animals rather than sixteen. Each animal received both treatment and control and hence provided two experimental units, one per treatment. As each animal was associated with both treatments, and each treat-ment was associated with all animals, the Treatment factor was crossed with the Animal factor. Assuming only one observation was taken on each animal/treatment combination, i.e. the observational units were the combinations of the Animal and Treatment factors, then the crossed relationship between these factors can be represented using a grid diagram, as given in Figure 3.3. Each black square corresponds to a combination of the levels of the two factors present in the design.

As well as all combinations of the levels of the two factors being present in the design, if the number of observational units at each of the combinations of the two factors is equal then the two factors can be said to be *fully crossed*. So in the above example, Animal and Treatment were fully crossed as there was one obser-vational unit at each combination of the Animal and Treatment factors.

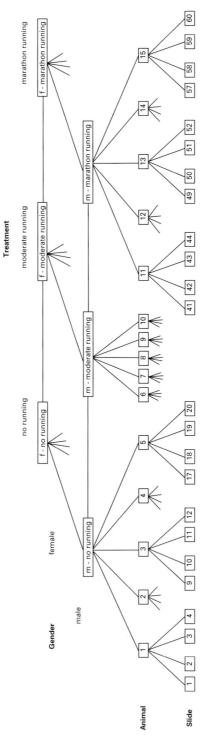

Figure 3.5. A design involving two crossed factors: Gender (levels: male and female) and Treatment (levels: no, moderate and marathon running) with two factors nested within combinations of these factors: Animal (levels: 1 to 15) and Slide within Animal (levels: 1 to 60).

3.2.7.3 Partially crossed factors

In practice the conditions required for two factors to be fully crossed may appear to be rather strict. In many experiments it will be the case that while there is some degree of crossing between two factors, the number of observational units is not the same at every combination of the levels of the two factors. It may also be the case that not all combinations of the factor levels are present in the design. This could be due to practical constraints on the design or simply missing data.

In the above example, assume animal 8 is taken out of the experiment after the drug is administered but before the control is given. The drug level of the Treatment factor occurs with eight levels of the Animal factor, but the control level of the Treatment factor only occurs at seven levels of the Animal factor. A diagram of the design is given in Figure 3.4.

The replication is unequal across the design and hence we say that the Animal and Treatment factors are partially crossed.

It is perhaps more likely that pairs of factors will be partially crossed, rather than fully crossed or nested. For example, if a study is conducted over two days, and all treatments are administered unequally on both days, then the Day factor is partially crossed with the Treatment factor. If two strains or both sexes are used in the study, but there is some missing data, then it is usually the case that these factors will be partially crossed with Treatment.

3.2.7.4 Designs containing nested and crossed factors

For simplicity, when introducing the different types of experimental design, it is standard practice to focus on the properties that differentiate each type of design. This usually involves considering only the crossed or nested factors within a design. We shall take this approach in the following sections when we introduce each type of design in more detail. However, it should be noted that in practical situations the researcher will employ designs that contain a combination of both crossed and nested factors. Hopefully once the reader is familiar with the types of designs described below, then the

generalisation to more practical yet complex designs will be straightforward.

Example 3.8 (continued): Wheel-running experiment

The relationships between the factors present in this design are a combination of crossing and nesting. The factors present in the study are Treatment (no running/moderate running/marathon running), Gender (male/female), Animal (30 mice were used) and Microscope slide (four slides assessed per mouse).

The first two factors, Treatment and Gender, are crossed. All treatments were tested in both males and females. As each animal is assigned to only one treatment (and obviously can only be of one sex) then the Animal factor is nested within the combination of the Treatment and Gender factors.

Each microscope slide is for only one animal; hence Microscope slide is nested within Animal. Other nesting relationships also hold but follow automatically and hence need not be stated specifically. For example, as Microscope slide is nested within Animal, and Animal is nested within Treatment, then Microscope slide is also nested within Treatment.

Drawing such a design is complicated; however, an illustration of the design is presented in Figure 3.5. Due to limitations of space the diagram shows the full nesting structure for six male animals: 1, 3 and 5 (in the no running group) and 11, 13 and 15 (in the marathon running group) but not for the five male animals 6–10 (in the moderate running group) or any of the nesting structure in the female groups. Note the crossed grid structure at the top of the diagram and the nesting structure underneath this grid.

3.2.8 Repeatedly measuring the animal

It is common practice in animal experiments for each animal to be measured multiple times. There are many ways that we can repeatedly measure an animal, depending on the treatment allocation to the animals, the nature of the repeated measurements and the randomisation(s) performed. We differentiate between seven practical scenarios in this text:

1. Measurements taken over time, but at the same identifiable time points for all animals. For example, day 1 post-dose, day 2 post-dose and so on. Similarly measurements may be taken on multiple identifiable positions within an animal (such as brain regions, left/right-hand side). We define these as examples of repeated measures designs (see Section 3.8.1).

2. Multiple measurements taken from an animal but unlike the previous example the repeated levels are not the same across the animals. For example,

blood samples taken from an animal are split into triplicate vials and each vial is assayed separately. There are three measurements per animal but there is no relationship between the measurements across animals. The first assayed vial from one animal is not related to the first assayed vial from any other animal. These are examples of higher-order nested designs (see Section 3.7.3).

3. Multiple treatments are administered to an animal at random positions, with one measurement taken per treatment per animal. For example, local anaesthetic skin creams tested on five 'random' positions on an animal. This is an example of a block design with Animal as a blocking factor (see Section 3.4).

4. The previous scenario can be generalised to include a second treatment administered systemically to the animals, with one level of the systemic treatment administered to each animal. As well as this between-animal treatment a second within-animal treatment is administered to sites randomly within the animal. This is an example of a split-plot design (see Section 3.9).

5. Each animal receives a sequence of treatments over time, one treatment per test period. One measurement is taken per animal per test period. The sequence of treatments is different for each animal. These designs are defined as crossover designs (see Section 3.4.9).

6. Each animal receives a sequence of treatments over time, one treatment per test period. One measurement is taken per animal per test period. The sequence of treatments is the same for each animal and is given in a non-random order (usually increasing doses of a compound over time). These designs are defined as dose-escalation designs (see Section 3.8.2).

7. Multiple end points are measured for each animal in the same experiment.

Designs based on Scenarios 1 to 6 above can be differentiated from each other by considering:

- the relationships between the experimental factors;
- the experimental and observational units;
- the randomisation.

Each scenario leads to a different type of experimental design and also a different recommendation for the

statistical analysis. A summary of the different ways we can measure an animal repeatedly is given in Table 3.2. The designs given in Table 3.2 are discussed in more detail in later sections of this chapter.

3.3 Summary of design types

Experimental designs can be separated into a number of distinct classes. In this text we differentiate between seven different types of design that are commonly encountered by the animal researcher: block, factorial, dose-response, nested, split-plot, dose-escalation and repeated measures. Each of these types of design can help us reduce animal use and refine our experiments in different ways. In the remaining sections of this chapter we will introduce each type of design, describe its properties in detail and explain how and where these designs should be applied. We aim to give many practical examples of their application to highlight their usefulness.

Experimental designs employed in practical situations are rarely from only one of the classes introduced above and can involve characteristics from two or more of these designs. We will show how to construct more complex designs that contain features from these simpler designs. We begin though by giving the reader an overall picture of the classes of experimental designs, and how the different classes are related to each other.

3.3.1 Block designs

Block designs form a useful class of designs that can be used in nearly every animal experiment. They allow the researcher to improve the precision of the experiment by reducing the influence of any nuisance effects that would otherwise increase the variability of the data. The textbook definition of a block design is one where the experiment is broken down into a set of mini-experiments or blocks. Each block contains a subset of the experimental units that are more alike, compared to the remaining experimental units. A factor can then be included in the analysis, with levels corresponding to the blocks, which effectively accounts for the differences between the experimental units from different blocks. These differences, if left unaccounted for, would potentially increase the underlying variability of the response.

Blocking factors may be generated due to the practicalities of the study, such as the need to use two pieces of equipment, or perhaps the need to run a study over three days. Other blocking factors may be included in the design at the researcher's discretion, such as blocking by body weight. Such decisions will depend on previous experience, literature evidence and knowledge of the kind of effects that may influence the outcome and potentially increase the variability. It is also possible to block by animal, where animals receive different sequences of treatments over time. These designs are defined as crossover designs.

Blocking factors are usually crossed with the Treatment factor(s). They can be defined as random factors, but for simplicity within this book they are always assumed to be fixed factors.

3.3.2 Factorial designs

Factorial designs are useful when the researcher has many different factors that may or may not influence the response. We define these as *factors of interest*. An investigation is therefore required to assess the effect of these factors of interest and how they relate to each other. We shall distinguish between two types of factorial design, namely the *large* and *small* factorial designs. In a factorial design, large or small, all factors of interest are crossed with each other, and all are considered fixed.

Large factorial designs are employed when the researcher wants to investigate the effect of many factors and how they interact with each other. The researcher may also want to identify those factors that can be ignored as having no significant effect on the response. These designs are particularly useful, for example, when setting up a new animal model. At this stage of the experimental process there may be many unanswered questions, such as which level of the factors give the most variable response. Large factorial designs necessarily involve many individual groups but, as we shall see, because we are only interested in the overall effects, the individual sample sizes can be small. In some fields of experimentation, perhaps with smaller underlying variability, a sample size of one or two per combination is routinely used. However, due to the large animal-to-animal variability, it is probably best not to use such small sample sizes in animal research.

Small factorial designs consist of usually no more than two or three factors. The purpose of studies that are based on these designs is to compare one group mean to another, using a suitable statistical test. Hence a sufficiently large sample size is required at each combination of the factors.

Both types of design are examples of factorial designs, but they are used to answer different questions. The small factorial designs are used regularly in practice. The large factorial designs are perhaps not utilised as much as they could be.

3.3.3 Dose-response designs

Dose-response designs, as the name suggests, are employed to allow the researcher to understand the effect of increasing the dose of a compound on the measured response. These effects can be modelled by a simple linear trend, but in practice are more likely to involve non-linear relationships. The choice of non-linear curve to fit to the data can be based on prior theoretical knowledge of the underlying biology or can be selected once the data has been generated. In this text we consider the logistic curve, as there is strong theoretical justification for using it. We describe the principles that should be followed to construct designs for estimating the dose-response relationship using this and other types of non-linear models.

3.3.4 Nested designs

Nested designs consist of a number of factors and, as the name implies, the relationship between at least one pair of factors is nested rather than crossed. In the extreme case we have the so-called *hierarchical nested designs*. With these designs all relationships between factors are nested and hence no crossed factors are allowed.

Factors that are nested within other factors are usually assumed to be random. When analysing data generated using nested designs we can investigate the amount of variability due to each of the random factors. This is important because the amount of variability associated with a random factor is linked to the replication of the levels of the factor that is needed to achieve scientifically valid results. In particular we can investigate the sample size (i.e. number of animals) required by considering the design as a nested design.

3.3.5 Split-plot designs

Split-plot designs are applied in many areas of research (they were originally developed for agricultural trials – hence the name) but their use is less common in animal research. These designs involve two treatment factors and are required when, for example, all the levels of one of the treatments are administered to each animal (the within-animal treatment factor) but only one level of the second treatment is administered to each animal (the between-animal treatment factor). These designs are seldom used, perhaps because it is unusual to administer multiple levels of a treatment simultaneously to an animal. If multiple treatment levels are administered to an animal, then it is usually carried out over time using either a crossover or dose-escalation design. Split-plot designs are discussed in Section 3.9.

3.3.6 Repeated measures and dose-escalation designs

In Section 3.8 we consider Scenarios 1 and 6 described in Table 3.2, the repeated measures design and the dose-escalation design. For both of these designs the levels of the factor that index the repeatedly measured responses (the so-called repeated factor) are:

- shared across all animals in the experiment;
- not randomised.

In repeated measures designs the experimental unit is measured at each level of the repeated factor. For example, each animal receives one of the treatments and then is measured at specific time points. Hence animals are the experimental units. The repeated factor is Time and all animals should be measured at each level of the Time factor, if possible. Also as day 1 must come before day 2, so the levels of the repeated Time factor cannot be randomly assigned within-animal.

In dose-escalation studies all doses of the compound are administered to each animal in an increasing dose order. The order is the same (and non-random) for each animal so that if toxicological effects are observed or safety concerns raised, at one of the doses, then the treatment regime can be adjusted or reduced for ethical reasons. As each dose of compound is assigned to one test period (and vice versa) the Dose factor cannot be estimated separately from the Test period factor (the repeated factor). The animals in each test period are the experimental units.

The difference between these two types of design is that it is the experimental unit (usually the animal) that is measured repeatedly in the repeated measures design whereas in the dose-escalation study the experimental units change across the levels of the repeated factor (each animal receives the same sequence of multiple treatments).

3.3.7 Designs applied in practice

The reader may already be thinking of the limitations of running an animal study based on only one of the above designs. In practice a combination of two or more will be required. In Example 3.8 there is a factorial part to the design (Treatment and Gender) and a nested part to the design (Animal and Microscope slide). In Example 3.35, a dietary study involving ducklings, the design involved block, factorial and nested components. Many of the designs considered in this text could involve measuring the animals over time and hence can be considered repeated measures designs too.

By making use of each part of the design, the scientist can answer different questions. If we consider the factorial part of the design we would be considering questions such as:

- Is there a treatment effect?
- Does the treatment effect vary between sexes?

The nested part of the design can be used to answer different questions:

- How many animals do we need in the study?
- Should we replicate more microscope slides?
- If we measure more slides can we reduce the number of animals needed without affecting the sensitivity of the experiment?

For a given experiment certain questions will naturally be of more interest than others. At this stage though it is worth noting we can investigate different aspects of the animal model using experimental designs, other than simply testing treatment effects. We shall return to consider examples of designs applied in practice at the end of this chapter.

3.4 Block designs

Possibly the most important class of designs available to the animal researcher is the block designs. A block design is an experimental design that contains at least one blocking factor. Including these factors in the design allows the researcher to account for corresponding nuisance sources of variability in the statistical analysis. This can then help reduce the sample size required. From a practical point of view, block designs provide the researcher with additional flexibility when planning animal experiments. Experiments can also be managed more effectively when a block design is utilised.

3.4.1 Practical reasons to block

When an experiment is carried out it is often the case that conditions cannot be kept constant for the whole experiment. For example, two pieces of equipment may be employed to test the animals' responses, several operators may be required to ensure the trial is completed in a reasonable time frame or perhaps the study needs to be conducted over two or more days.

Blocking, to put it simply, involves dividing the experiment into a series of mini-experiments. Each mini-experiment should ideally contain all the treatments, but have less replication of each of the treatments than the full design. From a practical point of view, by blocking the experiment into a set of mini-experiments, the scientist can more easily manage the study. The easiest way to include blocking factor(s) in the experimental design is make sure that all the treatments are administered to at least one experimental unit within each block and hence each block can be considered an experiment in its own right. Common sense suggests

that each of the treatments should be equally replicated within each of the blocks. In most cases such a rule will provide the researcher with an efficient, as well as a sensible, design.

A list of possible blocking factors that the authors have employed is presented in Table 3.3.

3.4.2 Statistical reasons to block

As discussed above there are many practical benefits to employing block designs; however, there are also important statistical advantages too.

3.4.2.1 Variance reduction

By using block designs, or to put it another way, to include blocking factors in the experimental design and statistical analysis, we aim to reduce the underlying variability in the data collected. This implies we can reduce animal numbers while maintaining the scientific integrity of the study.

When we include a blocking factor in an experimental design we try to make sure that all the experimental material (usually animals) and experimental conditions within each block are as similar as possible. We then include a factor in the statistical analysis whose levels correspond to the individual blocks. The difference between experimental units that receive the same treatment, but are assigned to different blocks (differences that would otherwise increase the underlying variability), can then be accounted for by including the blocking factor in the statistical analysis. For example, if we block by animal then the differences between the animals, which would usually be included in the underlying variability that we test treatments against, can be assigned in the statistical analysis to the Animal blocking factor. In other words treatments are tested against the within-animal variability rather than a combination of the within- and between-animal variability.

If there are differences between operators, pieces of equipment, days of the week and so on, then this will inflate the underlying variability of the response. Using a block design and including the blocking factor in the analysis will account for this, reduce the variability of the response, and hence help reduce the sample size.

Table 3.3. Examples of blocking factors

Blocking factor	Comments
Room	In long-term studies, the researcher may be forced to house animals in two or more rooms, for example rabbits in long-term studies to investigate the effect of novel compounds on the development of atherosclerosis.
Cage	Animals housed in cages that are placed near the door can be more disturbed than those housed away from the door. It may be possible to account for this by housing animals on different treatment regimes together within a cage. One should bear in mind though that there is a risk that cross-contamination may occur if animals with different treatments are housed in the same cage.
Arena	Due to practical constraints, such as in fear conditioning experiments, more than one test arena may be employed. This may influence the results, perhaps due to the arena position in the room.
Observer	Consider a study where the response measured is the length of time that an animal expresses a specific behaviour. Different observers may record different times even if they are observing the same animal. If more than one observer is employed in the study, then this observer effect would need to be accounted for.
Animal	If all or some treatments can be administered to each animal, then we can block by animal using, for example, a crossover design.
Batch	Do you have more than one batch of animals, where animals from different batches may have different ages or originate from different suppliers or mothers? Would the results be different between batches?
Litter	If you have recorded the litter numbers, this can be used in the design to remove any litter effects.
Age/body weight	If body weight is thought to be a source of variability, then define three blocks: small, medium and large animals and include the body weight blocking factor in the experimental design. This block information can then be used in the analysis to reduce the effect of body weight on the variability of the response.
Day of week	Studies that are conducted over a number of days may have day-to-day differences that can be accounted for by using a block design. In some behavioural trials the results taken on a Monday may be different from those recorded during the rest of the week. This can occur, for example, when running the five-choice reaction time test as the animals are left relatively undisturbed over the weekend (Hille et al., 2008).
Phase	Due to practical limitations the study may be carried out over a number of phases. A difference between the measurements taken in each of the phases could be due to any number of practical effects (Bison et al., 2009).
Time of day	Will the time of day influence the results? In which case you should block by time of day (AM/PM) or only carry out experiments in the morning. For example, if body weight is your measure of choice, then rat and mice body weights naturally decrease during the day.
Object	In experiments such as the novel object recognition paradigm, the choice of novel object (from a pair of objects) could influence the animals' reactions and hence may be suitable for inclusion as a blocking factor.
Object position	With cognition studies, such as the novel object recognition paradigm, should the test objects be placed on the left- or right-hand side of the arena?
Batch of test compound	Does all of the test substance originate from the same batch?
Order of operation	When assessing a novel surgical procedure, it was found that the order of the operations influenced the results. It was hypothesised that there may be a learning effect (for novice surgeons).
Plate	In gene expression studies, it may be possible to block by the assay plate. Also on 96-well assay plates there may be edge, row or column effects across the wells of the plates. These effects could be accounted for by using a block design across the wells.
Rack	Are there differences between the racks the animals are housed in? Animals housed in racks nearer to the door may be more disturbed than animals housed in racks further away from the door.
Position in rack	Animals housed in cages at the top of the racks may have different reactions to those housed towards the bottom (Gore and Stanley, 2005).

Example 3.9: Lymphocyte counts in mice

A study was carried out to assess the effect of three novel compounds on lymphocyte counts in mice (Mead *et al.*, 2003, p. 71). Given the variability of the lymphocyte counts it was decided to use five mice per group. A placebo control group was also included in the study, hence 20 mice were required. The researchers also felt that animals within the same litter might have similar underlying lymphocyte counts. Thus 20 mice were taken from 5 litters, 4 mice per litter. The four animals per litter were then randomly assigned to one of the four treatments. If the background lymphocyte counts were higher in the mice from one of the litters, thus increasing the between-animal variability, then this design would allow the researchers to account for the litter-to-litter variability in the statistical analysis.

3.4.2.2 Bias reduction

The second important benefit of blocking is that it reduces bias. When we compare treatments with the control, for example, we want to be sure that we are really assessing the treatment effect. We assume that the difference between the treatment group and the control group is not influenced (or biased) by one or more nuisance effects. Such treatment comparisons are said to be *unbiased*. A block design can help the researcher achieve this.

For example, consider a study conducted over two days to compare the effect of a treatment to a control. If we include Day as a blocking factor in the design, then common sense tells us we should equally replicate the treatments over the two days. Hence half the animals on day 1 would have received the drug and half the vehicle (similarly for the allocation on day 2 and so on). This would provide the best possible design. The Treatment factor is crossed with the Day blocking factor. When assessing the effect of the treatment, we can be confident that the size of the difference between treatment and control is not influenced by any day-to-day differences.

Now consider a different allocation of treatments to the animals. If we had unwisely given all the animals on day 1 the novel drug and all the animals on day 2 the control, then the treatment comparison would be biased by the day effect. When we make comparisons between treatment and control we are also comparing the difference between day 1 and day 2. This could bias the treatment comparison, especially if the day-to-day

difference is larger than the treatment effect we are interested in. Unfortunately there is no way of separating the treatment effect from the day effect in this case. We say the two factors are *completely confounded*.

Complete confounding, with all controls tested on the same day, is probably the worst case scenario. It may be the case that the majority of controls were tested on the same day. This could occur, for example, if the allocation of animals to days were left to the randomisation. In such cases we still run the risk of biasing our results, especially if we have not identified the nuisance effect.

Readers may consider the points raised in this discussion to be fairly obvious; the real difficulty is identifying the nuisance effects beforehand and including blocking factors in the experimental design and statistical analysis to deal with them. If there are two, three or more blocking factors required, then constructing the most efficient block design to include all these blocking factors becomes more of a challenge.

3.4.3 How to block

It is easy to include one or more blocking factors in an experimental design:

- Begin by identifying a source of variability within the study that you wish to take into account.
- This source of variability is then separated out into a number of distinct levels that quantify the nuisance effect. This breakdown is usually easy to define. For example, if the study was conducted over three days, and it was felt that there was going to be day-to-day variability, then it is sensible to define Day as a blocking factor with three levels, namely day 1, 2 and 3. If you wish to block by body weight, then there is more flexibility over the number of levels. You could choose two levels (low/high body weight) or perhaps three levels (low/intermediate/high body weight).
- These levels form a new factor to be included in the experimental design and statistical analysis.
- The experimental units (usually animals) are assigned to blocks so that each block of experimental units corresponds to one of the levels of the blocking factor.
- Finally treatments are allocated to the experimental units (animals) within each block.

Hopefully all treatments can be equally replicated within each block. However, this is not always the case. In some situations only a few experimental units are present in each block and so only a subset of the treatments can be allocated within any given block. If this is the case then the choice of design becomes important. There may be several competing designs that have the same number of blocks and the same experimental units within each block. However, some designs may be better or more efficient than others. Avoiding a formal mathematical definition, the efficiency of a design is a measure of the accuracy of the estimates of the treatment comparisons that can be generated using the design compared to other designs with the same number of blocks and the same experimental units within each block. Some designs will provide more reliable estimates than others, even though they are the same size. While the choice of block design should not influence the estimate of the difference between two treatments, the variability of these estimates will be lower, all other things being equal, if a more efficient design had been used.

There is a simple rule of thumb for assessing the efficiency of a block design without using any mathematical formulae. Assume a study is conducted to investigate the difference between two treatments, A and B. To assess the reliability of the treatment comparisons when using the block design, consider how many times treatment A occurs in the same block as treatment B. The more within-block occurrences, the more efficient the design will be for assessing the difference between A and B.

Example 3.9 (continued): Lymphocyte counts in mice

We return to the experiment conducted to measure lymphocyte counts, as discussed above and consider three scenarios.

Scenario A

The most efficient design will have an equal replication of treatments within each litter. This design provides the most accurate estimates of the pairwise treatment comparisons. These comparisons are all estimated equally efficiently because pairs of treatments occur equally often (once) within litter.

Scenario B

Consider what happens if the within-litter treatment replication is not equal. As the within-block pairwise treatment occurrences become more unequal (within the design), then the efficiency of certain treatment comparisons will decrease as the occurrences of these treatment pairs within block decrease.

Scenario C

Taken to the extreme we arrive at a design where almost all the control animals are from a single litter, similarly for the other treatments with the other litters. While not quite possible in this example (the sample size is five and the litter size is four), if the sample size was four then you could end up with a design where all the controls were from the same litter. In this case the treatment effect is confounded with the litter effect.

Scenarios A and C in Example 3.9 correspond to extreme designs, which stand at opposite ends of a sliding efficiency scale (with Scenario B somewhere in the middle). Usually we begin by planning a design at the most efficient end of the scale and then, due to missing data, we end up with a design that is less efficient with unequal pairwise treatment occurrences within block. Obviously the number of missing observations will depend on many factors including the animal model itself. However, if the researcher starts off with an efficient design it would be unlucky if the treatment comparisons in the statistical analysis were not unbiased and reliable.

Let us now consider another practical example, involving blocking by initial body weight of piglets.

Example 3.10: Anti-microbial medication assessment

Following the cessation of sow's milk, and the passive immunity it provides, weanling pigs are more vulnerable to disease. A study was carried out to assess whether spray-dried animal plasma (SDAP) in the diet could be used as an alternative to anti-microbial medication containing colistin sulphate for weanling pigs challenged with *Escherichia coli* K99 (Torrallardona *et al.*, 2003). The study design involved four treatment groups consisting of all combinations of SDAP (at two levels: 0% and 7%) and colistin sulphate (at two levels: 0 mg/kg and 300 mg/kg). As one of the responses measured was the gain in the body weight of the piglets over a set period of time, it was felt that the pre-treatment animal body weight could be an important source of variability in the study.

We consider three possible approaches the researcher could take to deal with the variability associated with pre-treatment body weight. The first two do not involve blocking and hence would probably result in less sensitive statistical tests. More animals would therefore be required to achieve statistical significance in these scenarios.

Scenario A

In this scenario, and not one to be recommended, the animals are assigned to treatment groups based on body weight. The largest animals receive the vehicle, the smallest animals receive the 7% + 300 mg/kg combination treatment and the remaining animals are assigned to the other two treatment groups. As the animals were dosed in mg/kg, this approach does at least require a small amount of the compound! Unfortunately if this study is carried out this way then the researcher has no way of knowing whether the treatment effect observed is due to the treatment itself or simply animal size. The effect of body weight and treatment are said to be confounded.

Scenario B

In scenario B animals are randomly assigned to the four treatment groups. While this approach is theoretically justified, there is the risk that we may end up with an uneven replication of treatments across the animal body weights. We could even be unlucky and end up with an allocation identical to that used in scenario A.

Scenario C

An alternative (and recommended) approach involves blocking by animal body weight.

To begin with we break down the body weights (in this case a continuous variable) into a number of levels. There is no rule as to how many levels the researcher should select in such cases. However, the ease of including the blocking factor in the design and analysis should be considered. In this case we have 48 pigs in total and so we could separate the animals into three blocks of 16 pigs each. The three levels of this blocking factor would then be light, medium and heavy animals. So all the light animals would be assigned to the first block, all the medium-sized pigs to the second block and the heaviest animals to the final block. Body weight is now considered a fixed factor in the design, at three levels. The 16 animals within each block are now assigned to four pens (four animals per pen) taking the litter into account. We then equally replicate the four treatments within each of these three blocks, randomly assigning the four treatments to four pens within each block. Treatments are administered in the diet and so the pens are the experimental units. Each occurrence of the vehicle occurs with one replicate of each of the other treatments. Hence we know that all treatment comparisons will be estimated with equal precision.

The Treatment factor is crossed with the Body weight blocking factor while the Pen factor is nested within Block and Treatment. We would recommend this approach.

3.4.4 Complete block designs

We now consider the different types of block design. In most cases the researcher will be able to use the *complete block* designs and these designs are described first. Complete block designs are the most efficient designs available and the easiest to apply in practice.

In a complete block design, all treatments are administered to at least one experimental unit within each block. Each block can be said to constitute a single trial or mini-experiment (Cochran and Cox, 1957, p. 106).

Example 3.10, described above, is an example of a complete block design. Each of the three blocks consists of four pens, with one pen per block receiving each of the four treatments.

3.4.4.1 Efficiency

Complete block designs provide the scientist with an efficient family of designs. As all treatments are present in all blocks, then all treatment comparisons can be made within block. This implies that all treatment comparisons will be reasonably sensitive, and certainly more accurate than if comparisons were made between blocks (assuming the block-to-block differences are large). If the replication of the treatments is the same within each block, then we also know (using the rule of thumb described above) that the variability of each of the treatment comparisons will be the same. This makes these designs a useful and reliable family of designs.

3.4.4.2 Randomisation

When employing a block design, the randomisation required to assign the treatments to the experimental material is a relatively straightforward procedure. Assuming each block consists of a number of animals, and animals are the experimental units, then *separately for each block*, the treatments are randomly assigned to the animals within that block.

We shall make further comments on the implication of this randomisation strategy in Section 4.2.2.

Example 3.11: Spinal cord injury

It has been suggested that, following an injury to the spine, if the axons can traverse the injury site then they may regrow in unscarred regions. A study was conducted to assess the benefit of using a polymer scaffold seeded with neural stem cells, see Teng *et al.* (2002), to aid recovery following a spinal cord injury. In the experiment 50 adult female Sprague Dawley rats underwent surgery to create a lesion in their spinal column. The rats were then implanted with either a scaffold implanted with neural stem cells or one of three controls: a polymer implant without neural stem cells, the stem cells only (with no implant) or lesion control (no implant or stem cells). The sample sizes across the four groups in the experiment were $n = 13, 11, 12$ and 12 (one died during surgery and another was excluded because it showed incomplete paralysis). For this discussion it is assumed that there were 12 animals in each group and hence 48 animals were required in total.

Table 3.4. Possible experimental design for the spinal cord injury experiment

Order	Surgery day 1	2	3
1	implant only	implant only	implant only
2	implant only	implant + neural stem cells	implant only
3	neural stem cells only	neural stem cells only	implant only
4	neural stem cells only	neural stem cells only	implant + neural stem cells
5	implant + neural stem cells	sham	neural stem cells only
6	implant + neural stem cells	sham	sham
7	neural stem cells only	implant only	implant + neural stem cells
8	implant + neural stem cells	implant only	neural stem cells only
9	sham	implant + neural stem cells	sham
10	sham	neural stem cells only	implant + neural stem cells
11	implant only	sham	sham
12	implant + neural stem cells	sham	neural stem cells only
13	implant only	implant only	implant + neural stem cells
14	sham	implant + neural stem cells	sham
15	sham	implant + neural stem cells	implant only
16	neural stem cells only	neural stem cells only	neural stem cells only

It was felt that there was some risk that any refinement in the surgical technique during the course of the study could influence the outcome. While not defined in the original article, let us assume that the surgeries were conducted over 3 days. It was therefore felt that the results from the animals operated during day 3 could be different to those from day 1. To account for this effect, the surgeries were performed using a complete block design. To begin with the 48 animals were assigned to the three surgery days, 16 per day. Within each day the 16 rats were randomly assigned to one of the four treatment groups, four animals per treatment per day.

A possible design is given in Table 3.4. Notice the order within each day is randomised to avoid surgical bias and so the order within day is not controlled in any way. This design allows the scientist to remove any day-to-day variability caused by improvements to the surgical technique.

All the researcher needs to do now is include the Day blocking factor in the statistical analysis (see Section 6.3.3.3).

3.4.4.3 Statistical analysis of block designs

The statistical analysis of data generated when using block designs is considered in Section 6.3.3.3. If the researcher has blocked the experiment, then an indicator variable should be included in the final dataset that contains the levels of the blocking factor. This factor can easily be included in all the parametric statistical

analysis described in Section 5.1.2. As discussed in Section 4.2.2.2, it is recommended that the researcher exclude any interactions between the treatments and the blocks from the statistical analysis. An example of the benefit of including a blocking factor in the statistical analysis, in terms of reducing the sample size required, is described in Section 3.7.2.

3.4.5 Incomplete block designs

Unfortunately it may be the case that the researcher does not have the luxury of being able to assign all the treatments within each of the blocks. For example, the researcher may wish to include Litter as a blocking factor in the experimental design. Unfortunately the litters were not the same size, hence it was not possible to replicate all treatments equally within each litter. Some litters had fewer animals than the number of treatments within the study, hence only a subset of the treatments could be allocated to the animals in these litters.

The choice of which treatments to include within each block, and which to leave out, will affect the accuracy of the pairwise comparisons. As commented above, the more often a pair of treatments occurs within a block the more accurate the comparison between them will be. In other words, one allocation of treatments to the blocks may allow sensitive comparisons of, say, treatment A back to the control but not treatment B back to the control. A different allocation of treatments to blocks may allow the researcher to test both treatments A and B back to the control with equal precision.

The general rule of thumb described above can be useful in this situation. When deciding on a design, count the number of times the comparisons of interest can be made within block. The higher the number the more precise the comparison will be.

Example 3.12: Assessing the effect of LPS challenge in rats

An experiment was conducted to assess the effect of lipopolysaccharide (LPS) challenge on the behavioural, physiological and neuroendocrine responses in the rat (Bison *et al.*, 2009). The experiment consisted of a saline control group and six doses of LPS: 1, 5, 15, 50, 125 and 250 μg/kg. Responses assessed included social interaction, home cage activity, saccharin preference test, body temperature, body weight, hormone and cytokine levels. The experiment was conducted over two cohorts of animals and it was hypothesised that there may be differences between the cohorts that would be an additional source of variability. It was therefore decided to employ a block design with Cohort as the blocking factor at two levels. Both cohorts included the saline control group but only a subset of the six LPS dose groups were included in each block, hence the design was an incomplete block design. As each block contained the saline group, the most reliable treatment comparisons were the comparisons of the LPS dose groups back to saline. By using this design the researchers were able to show that LPS significantly reduced body weight, social behaviour, preference for saccharin and home-cage activity while increasing ACTH and serum corticosterone levels, serum interleukins and tumour necrosis factor-alpha.

The researcher may be interested in making all pairwise comparisons between the treatments. If so then all comparisons should be made equally precisely (as is the case with the complete block designs). In such cases we require a special type of incomplete design, namely the *balanced incomplete block design*.

3.4.6 Balanced incomplete block design

3.4.6.1 Efficiency

A balanced incomplete block design (BIBD) is an incomplete block design that allows all pairwise treatment comparisons to be made with equal accuracy.

To achieve this, the design has to have the following properties:

- equal replication of treatments within the design;
- equal block sizes (not vital, but makes life easier!);
- every pair of treatments occurs together in the same number of blocks.

The third condition is an example of the rule of thumb described above.

As can be guessed from these strict conditions, BIBDs exist for only certain combinations of the number of treatments and size/number of blocks. A description of methods that can be used to construct these designs is given in Clarke and Kempson (1997, pp. 212–15) and an example of the use of a balanced incomplete block design is given by Manser *et al.* (1998) when testing the preference of laboratory rats for nest boxes.

3.4.6.2 Randomisation

As with the complete block designs, the randomisation of the experimental material to the blocks follows a similar process. *Separately for each block*, the set of treatments for that block (as defined by the incomplete block design) are randomly assigned to the animals within the block.

3.4.6.3 Statistical analysis

The statistical analysis of data generated when using an incomplete block design is considered in Section 6.3.3.3. Assuming the incomplete block design is balanced, or nearly balanced, then including a blocking factor in the statistical analysis should not cause any difficulties. The analysis follows the same procedure required as for the analysis of complete block designs.

Example 3.13: Lamb dietary study

An experiment was carried out to assess the effect that vitamin A and a protein dietary supplement have on the weight gain of lambs over a 2-month period (Anderson and McLean, 1974, p. 248). There were four treatments in the study:

  A Vitamin A low dose, protein low dose
  B Vitamin A high dose, protein low dose
  C Vitamin A low dose, protein high dose
  D Vitamin A high dose, protein high dose

It was felt that a replication of three lambs per treatment would be sufficient, so six pairs of sibling lambs were used in the study.

Table 3.5. Experimental design for Example 3.13

Lamb	Sibling lamb pair					
	1	2	3	4	5	6
First	A	A	A	B	B	C
Second	B	C	D	C	D	D

It was expected that the sibling lambs' responses would be similar to each other, so it was decided to use a block design for the study, with Lamb pair as the blocking factor. There were 12 lambs in total, divided into six blocks, where blocks correspond to the pairs of lambs. Each treatment was replicated three times, but only two treatments could be administered to lambs within each block. The final design chosen was a balanced incomplete block design and is given in Table 3.5.

Each treatment occurs with each other treatment once within a block (sibling lamb pair), hence all treatment comparisons can be made equally accurately. By using this design the researcher was able to conclude that the protein supplement did influence weight gain whereas vitamin A had no effect.

3.4.7 More than one block: the row-column block design

In practical situations there may be more than one possible blocking factor in an experiment. If there are two nuisance sources of variability, then we require a block design that allows us to account for both sources. Such a design is called a row-column block design. The rows of the design correspond to one blocking factor; the columns of the design correspond to the second blocking factor.

Row-column block designs occur in many experiments. For example, assume the researcher ordered animals with a wide range of body weights from a supplier. By blocking by body weight, as recommended above, any additional variability caused by requesting this wide range can be accounted for in the experimental design and statistical analysis. If the testing phase of the experiment is conducted over a single day, the researcher may believe that the time of testing may influence the results. Hence it may be decided to block by time of day as well as body weight. In this case there are two blocking factors that need to be included in the experimental design. Alternatively there may be two pieces of equipment used to conduct the testing, or

maybe the study was conducted over multiple days. All of these effects could be accounted for by including a second blocking factor in the experimental design.

Consider animal cages arranged in racks. If multiple treatments can be administered to the animals within each rack, then the rack of cages forms a row-column block design. If the response is influenced by cage position in the rack, then it may be worth blocking by cage position to account for these effects. Animals housed in cages near the door may be more disturbed than those housed towards the back of the room. Alternatively those housed near the computer terminal in the room may be more disturbed than those housed elsewhere. By blocking by the position in the rack, we would then be able to take this source of variability into account.

3.4.7.1 Efficiency

In situations where the experimental design includes multiple blocking factors, constructing the design becomes trickier. As a rule of thumb, if the researcher can make sure that every treatment is administered at every combination of levels of the blocking factors, then the design will be an efficient design.

3.4.7.2 Randomisation

To randomise a row-column block design
1. Randomly permute the rows of the design.
2. Randomly permute the columns of the design.
3. Randomly assign treatments to the animals within each row/column combination.

3.4.7.3 Statistical analysis

The statistical analysis of data generated when using row-column designs is the same as that for complete block designs, as described in Section 6.3.3.3. The scientist should include two indicator variables in the dataset containing the levels of the row and column blocking factors. As with the analysis of block designs involving single blocking factors, we recommend excluding any interactions involving the blocking factors in the statistical analysis (see Section 4.2.2).

Table 3.6. Possible experimental design for Example 3.11

Period	Order	Surgery day		
		1	2	3
1	1	implant + neural stem cells	sham	implant + neural stem cells
1	2	neural stem cells only	neural stem cells only	neural stem cells only
1	3	sham	implant + neural stem cells	sham
1	4	implant only	implant only	implant only
2	5	implant only	implant only	implant + neural stem cells
2	6	neural stem cells only	implant + neural stem cells	sham
2	7	sham	neural stem cells only	implant only
2	8	implant + neural stem cells	sham	neural stem cells only
3	9	neural stem cells only	sham	implant + neural stem cells
3	10	implant + neural stem cells	implant only	sham
3	11	implant only	implant + neural stem cells	neural stem cells only
3	12	sham	neural stem cells only	implant only
4	13	implant + neural stem cells	implant only	implant only
4	14	sham	implant + neural stem cells	sham
4	15	neural stem cells only	neural stem cells only	neural stem cells only
4	16	implant only	sham	implant + neural stem cells

Example 3.11 (continued): Spinal cord injury

In Example 3.11 described above, a study conducted to investigate the effect of scaffolds on spinal cord injury recovery, the researcher decided to block by day to remove any day-to-day variability. However, upon closer inspection of the randomised block design, it can be seen that the implant only treatment will be administered first on each of the three days. In fact the implant only treatment features a disproportionally high number of times in the early surgeries. Perhaps it would have been better to block in two directions when constructing the block design.

In the following design we have blocked in two directions, day (as before) but also order within day. The order of the operations was separated into four periods of time (two in the morning and two in the afternoon) and each surgical procedure was applied once within each period on each day. A possible design is given in Table 3.6.

The spread of surgeries within day is now much more evenly spaced. Both blocking factors (Day and Period) can now be included in the analysis to reduce the variability caused by time effects.

3.4.8 Row-column block designs based on Latin squares

Consider the situation described in the previous section where there are two nuisance sources of variability.

Ideally the researcher would like to account for these two sources of variability using a row-column block design. However, it may not be possible to replicate all treatments at each combination of the blocking factors. In the extreme case it may be possible to only administer one treatment at every combination of the levels of the two blocking factors. In such situations we can make use of Latin squares to construct efficient row-column block designs.

Formally a Latin square of order t is an arrangement of t symbols in a t by t square array in such a way that each symbol occurs once in each row and once in each column (Bailey, 2008, p. 106).

Examples of Latin squares are:

3 by 3 square	5 by 5 square
A B C	A B C D E
B C A	B C D E A
C A B	C D E A B
	D E A B C
	E A B C D

If the allocation of treatments across the rows and columns of the block design are made using a Latin square, then the rows and columns of the Latin square define the two blocking factors and the t elements of

Table 3.7. Possible experimental design for the learning ability experiment

Time	Body weight		
	Small	Medium-sized	Large
09.00–10.00	no running	moderate running	marathon running
11.00–12.00	marathon running	no running	moderate running
14.00–15.00	moderate running	marathon running	no running

the square define the treatments. With these designs the effect of the two nuisance sources of variability can be removed before the treatments are compared. This is because each treatment is administered to one animal in each row of the design and to one animal in each column.

Example 3.14: Housing conditions

Gore and Stanley (2005) discussed an example where Latin squares were employed to allocate five treatments to cages. The experiment was conducted to assess four doses of a compound (and control). Three racks of cages were required, where each rack contained 25 cages arranged in five rows and five columns. As part of the statistical analysis the researcher observed that the rack that the mice were housed in influenced their water intake and also that the body temperature of the mice depended on the row (within the rack) that the cages were placed in. This was not a problem in this experiment, as the treatments were assigned to cages using Latin squares. These effects could therefore be taken into account in the statistical analysis. However, if each treatment had been allocated to a single row of cages, then any environmental effects could have biased the treatment assessment.

In future trials they advocate using a row-column block design based on Latin squares to allocate treatments to cages. This, they argue, should remove any bias on the treatment comparisons caused by cage position. If the researcher uses more practically appealing designs such as:

- putting all replicates of a treatment in the same row of cages in each of the three racks;
- placing all replicates of a treatment in the same rack, perhaps in adjacent cages.

then there is a risk of making false positive conclusions due to this bias.

3.4.8.1 Efficiency

Latin squares can be used to construct efficient experimental designs when there are two blocking factors that need to be taken into account. These designs have been compared to other types of design such as complete

block designs (see Giesbrecht and Gumpertz, 2004, p. 125). It has been shown that they are more efficient than the alternatives and hence should be used, where possible, as fewer animals are required to achieve similar levels of statistical sensitivity.

3.4.8.2 Randomisation

Once a Latin square has been selected (at random from a suitable set of Latin squares), then

1. The rows of the square are randomised.
2. The columns of the square are randomised.
3. The treatments are randomly assigned to the treatment labels of the square.
4. The animals are randomly assigned to the row/column combinations of the square.

3.4.8.3 Statistical analysis

The statistical analysis of data generated from experimental designs based on Latin squares is the same as the row-column block design analysis, as described in Section 6.3.3.3. The scientist should include two indicator variables in the dataset, corresponding to the row and column blocking effects. Due to the lack of replication within the experimental design, it will probably not be possible to estimate any interactions between the blocking and treatment factors.

Example 3.8 (continued): Wheel-running experiment

We now consider a variation of Example 3.8, as discussed above and considered in further detail in Festing *et al.* (2002, p. 59). The experiment was conducted to investigate whether exercise influenced the learning ability of mice in a maze. Three treatments were tested: no running, moderate running and marathon running. In this example nine mice were available. Unfortunately there were two other nuisance sources of variability in the experiment that could affect the results. Firstly there may be an effect due to the time of day (caused by circadian rhythm) and secondly the body weight of the animals may influence the results. Two blocking factors were included in the experimental design, Body weight and Time of day. As there were nine animals in the study the blocking factors were defined using three levels each, with three animals per level of each blocking factor. So Body weight has three levels: small, medium sized and large, and Time of day has three levels: 09:00–10:00, 11:00–12:00 and 14:00–15:00.

We can now use a Latin square to define the allocation of animals to the experiment. An experimental design that may have been employed is given in Table 3.7.

One animal is assigned to each of the nine entries in the square. If we now include these two blocking factors in the statistical analysis we can take account of the variability caused by the body weight and time of day.

3.4.9 Crossover designs

The largest source of variability in any animal experiment is probably going to be the animal-to-animal differences. This animal-to-animal variability, as discussed above, is one of the biggest problems (from a statistical point of view) that animal researchers face. So why not block by animal at the design stage? If the researcher can block by animal, then we can account for the animal-to-animal variability in the analysis.

Blocking by animal necessarily involves administering multiple treatments to the animals. There are two ways that this can be achieved. If multiple treatments can be administered to an animal at the same time (for example, skin creams administered locally to regions of skin) then we can randomly assign treatments within the animal and use a standard block design as described above. This is Scenario 3 in Table 3.2. In this section we shall consider the more common situation where multiple treatments are administered over time to the animal. Such studies involve the use of a crossover design (Scenario 5 in Table 3.2). A study is defined as a crossover study if the subjects, in our case animals, are administered a sequence of treatments over several test periods, one treatment per test period.

When using these designs it is important to leave sufficient time between test periods, the so-called *washout periods*, to make sure that one treatment does not influence future responses (see Section 3.4.9.5 for more details). If animals are permanently changed by a treatment, then it is not possible to employ such designs. It may also not be possible to use these designs due to ethical constraints, especially if the individual procedures are distressing to the animal.

It is worth remembering that this is only a special type of block design and hence the ideas described in the previous section apply to crossover designs as well as to block designs.

The statistical analysis of crossover trials is described in Section 6.3.3.4 and is similar to the analysis of data generated from experiments that include blocking. The Animal and Time factors are included in the statistical analysis as blocking factors to account for these effects. Note that while the Animal factor is usually defined as a random factor in most analyses described in this text, in the analysis of crossover trials the Animal factor can be defined as fixed. This does not jeopardise the validity of the analysis as all treatments are tested against the within-animal variability.

Animals are measured on multiple occasions, either once per test period or multiple times within each test period, and so this family of designs is an example of an experiment involving repeatedly measured responses (Scenario 5 in Table 3.2). The experimental units are the animals within a test period as different treatments are administered to each animal, one per test period. The designs are similar to the dose-escalation designs (Scenario 6 in Table 3.2) except that with crossover designs the sequence of treatments administered is usually different for each animal and is, in some sense, randomised.

Crossover designs are also different to repeated measures designs (see Section 3.8.1) where in the latter each animal is administered a single treatment and then measured repeatedly, i.e. animals are the experimental units. However, repeated measures can be taken within each test period of a crossover design. These are usually known as repeated measures crossover designs (see Section 3.8.1.4).

3.4.9.1 Complete crossover designs

As we are blocking by animal (and test period), if each animal can receive each of the treatments at some

Table 3.8. Possible experimental design for Example 3.15[*]

| Test period | Rat | | | | | | | | | | | |
	1	2	3	4	5	6	7	8	9	10	11	12
1	veh	A	B	C	veh	A	B	C	veh	A	B	C
2	A	veh	C	B	C	B	A	veh	B	C	veh	A
3	B	C	veh	A	A	veh	C	B	C	B	A	veh
4	C	B	A	veh	B	C	veh	A	A	veh	C	B

[*]A = 5-HT4 partial agonist at 0.1 mg/kg, B = 5-HT4 partial agonist at 1 mg/kg, C = nicotine at 0.2 mg/kg.

point during the study then the crossover design will be a complete block design (blocking by animal). Hence every pairwise treatment comparison will be made with the same level of accuracy. Examples can be found in Hedenqvist *et al.* (2001), Bate and Boxall (2008) and Miyazaki *et al.* (2005).

Example 3.15: Five-choice serial reaction time task

5-HT4 agonists are currently being developed as candidate treatments for Alzheimer's disease. While the effect of this family of compounds on cognition has been demonstrated, no tests had been conducted specifically to assess their effects on attention. To investigate this, an experiment was conducted (using the five-choice serial reaction time task) to assess the effect of a 5-HT4 partial agonist on attentional deficit in rats (see Hille *et al.*, 2008).

Rats were trained over a number of sessions (around 30) to react to a visual stimulus. The rear wall of the test chamber contained five holes, which could be illuminated from behind. To receive a food reward, a rat had to learn to poke its nose into a (randomly) illuminated hole. Each animal was shown 100 visual stimuli in 100 trials and, amongst other responses, the total number of correct trials and average correct latency was recorded for each animal. Animals were tested on either a baseline protocol (days 1 to 4) or a variable stimulus (day 5).

It takes a lot of time and effort (on the part of the researcher) to train the rats to perform this task, hence they are considered a valuable resource. It follows that it would be preferable if the trained rats could be treated more than once. Luckily in this experiment the treatments had a short-term effect, and so animals could receive a sequence of treatments over time. In this example, two doses of the 5-HT4 partial agonist (treatments A and B), a nicotine positive control (treatment C) and the vehicle were administered to 12 rats over four weeks. A 2-day wash-out period was included between the test periods.

All treatments were administered to each rat, and so the design applied was a complete block design with regards to the animals. Similarly three rats in each test period received each treatment;

hence the design was also a complete block design with regards to the test periods.

The easiest way to construct the design was to make use of three four-by-four Latin squares. This guarantees the design was a complete block design in Animals and Test periods. A design that may have been used is given in Table 3.8. This design is based on a set of three squares given in Bate and Boxall (2008).

By using this design the researchers were able to show that the 5-HT4 partial agonist reduced incorrect and perseverative responses while the percentage of correct trials and latency during incorrect trials were increased.

3.4.9.2 Incomplete crossover designs

It may not be possible, either ethically or practically, to administer all treatments to all animals. In this case the researcher will need to consider using an incomplete crossover design. The exact choice of design may require the help of a statistician as there has been much research conducted on constructing incomplete crossover designs, for example Afsarinejad (1983) and Godolphin (2004). However, consider the common experimental situation where we want to compare all treatments with the control. Remembering that we are blocking by animal, and the more times a treatment pair occurs together in a block the more accurate the pairwise treatment comparison will be, then it is sensible to make sure each animal receives the control treatment at some point during the experiment.

Example 3.16: PCP challenge

Administration of phencyclidine (PCP) produces locomotor hyperactivity in the rat. It is thought that this provides a behavioural sensitisation model of aspects of schizophrenia. The model is sensitive to treatment with antipsychotics (Kalinichev *et al.*, 2009).

Table 3.9. Incomplete crossover design for Example 3.16[*]

Test period	Rats											
	1	2	3	4	5	6	7	8	9	10	11	12
1	veh	A	veh	B	veh	C	A	B	A	C	B	C
2	A	veh	B	veh	C	veh	B	A	C	A	C	B

[*]A = low dose, B = intermediate dose and C = high dose of antipsychotic.

Rats were administered PCP (5.0 mg/kg, intraperitoneally) twice daily, for seven days. This makes them permanently hypersensitive to further PCP challenges. On the day of testing the rats were given either the test compound or vehicle and baseline locomotor activity was recorded. This was followed by the PCP challenge. Post-challenge locomotor activity was then recorded for up to 60 minutes.

Kalinichev *et al.* (2009) describe three strategies for constructing a suitable experimental design for the study.

Strategy 1: One treatment per animal

This is a simple design where each animal receives one and only one of the treatments. While such designs have benefits in terms of animal welfare, it should be immediately apparent that there are some statistical limitations with using such a design. Treatments are tested against the between-animal variability. As this is usually larger than the within-animal variability, this design will require many animals to achieve the desired experimental sensitivity. For example, it was found that in a study consisting of four treatment groups, an estimated 20 animals per group, or 80 in total, were required. As the effect of the PCP challenge is permanent, and compounds wash-out quickly, this experiment is an ideal candidate for using a crossover design to assign the treatments to the animals.

Strategy 2: Complete crossover design

In the second strategy a complete four-period crossover design was proposed, with each animal receiving all four treatments during the study. This design produces a major saving in total animal usage, reducing the predicted number from 80 down to six. However, there are ethical issues with using such a design. Should each animal be challenged with PCP four times within a study?

Strategy 3: Incomplete crossover design

As a compromise a third strategy was proposed. This involves using an incomplete crossover design where each animal receives only two of the four treatments during the experiment. This family of designs is discussed in Afsarinejad (1983). As all treatments are not administered to all animals, then the treatments cannot be compared within-animal as often as in a complete crossover design. This will inevitably lead to an increase in animal numbers. In the

example described in Kalinichev *et al.* (2009) a total of 12 animals were required, still a substantial saving on the 80 needed for strategy 1. The final design is given in Table 3.9.

In this design all pairwise treatment comparisons were made with equal sensitivity. The researcher was able to show, using the design described in Strategy 3, that the antipsychotics haloperidol, risperidone and quetiapine all reduced hyperactivity in a dose-dependent manner.

3.4.9.3 The benefits of crossover designs

Crossover designs are some of the most useful designs available to the animal researcher. This is because:

1. Animals are used more than once in an experiment. So the experimental units in such studies, the unit of material that receives a treatment, are not the animals but the animals within a test period. Hence we have more experimental units per animal. This can allow us to reduce the total number of animals significantly. If a three-period crossover design is used, each animal receives three treatments during the study and the number of experimental units will be three times the number of animals.

2. All treatment comparisons can be made within-animal. This implies that differences between the animals will not influence, or bias, the treatment comparisons.

3. Treatments are tested against the within-animal variability. Such comparisons are usually more accurate as the within-animal variability is, generally, smaller than the between-animal variability. Hence it follows that when using crossover designs we require fewer animals to achieve the same statistical sensitivity.

3.4.9.4 The issues with crossover designs

Of course crossover designs are only applicable in certain experimental situations:

- If the treatments have a permanent effect on the animal, or take a long time to wash-out of the animal, then they might not be an appropriate choice of design.
- Studies based on crossover designs take longer to complete than other types of design. Obviously the more test periods the researcher wishes to include in the study design, and the longer the wash-out periods between the test periods, then the longer the study will be.
- A pitfall when using crossover designs that has received a lot of attention in the statistical literature is that of treatment carry-over effects (Jones and Kenward, 2003, p. 4). As this is an important issue in its own right we shall discuss it in more detail in the next section.
- Finally there are also ethical issues with using crossover designs. While we may reduce the overall number of animals required, each individual animal will inevitably receive multiple treatments or go through multiple procedures. The scientist must decide whether this is an ethically acceptable compromise. Such issues are of less importance in studies that do not involve animal discomfort, such as some husbandry studies.

Example 3.17: Nest box preference

Rumble *et al.* (2005) described a husbandry study to assess which type of nest box the common marmoset preferred. Four types of nest box were evaluated, the Cin-Bin and three nest boxes made from wood, plastic or metal. Marmoset behaviour was recorded using video cameras and the total time spent in each nest box over a 24-hour period was used as a measure of preference. It was felt that each marmoset could be assessed in all nest boxes, allowing the researcher to make within-animal comparisons between the boxes. Hence a four-period crossover design was employed. The design itself was a multi-factor crossover design (Bate and Boxall, 2008), which allowed the researchers to assess the effect of a second effect, in this case the video camera. While the cameras themselves were similar, it was felt that one particular camera could cause more disturbance than the others and hence this should be taken into account in the design. The conclusions from the study were that the marmosets prefer wood and plastic nest boxes to those made of metal. As expected, the video cameras used did not influence marmoset behaviour.

3.4.9.5 Treatment carry-over effects

If the effect of a treatment administered in a test period continues into the following test period, and hence influences the response of the animal to the treatment administered in that test period, then this is defined as a first-order treatment carry-over effect. We use the terminology 'first order' because the effect of a treatment continues into the following test period only. Of course higher orders of carry-over are possible but are beyond the scope of this book (Jones and Kenward, 2003, p. 8).

Although not discussed in this book, treatment carry-over effects can be dealt with at the analysis stage (Jones and Kenward, 2003, p. 212). However, we contend that it is more appropriate to try to remove these effects at the design stage. The researcher should try to include wash-out periods of suitable length to make sure that each treatment has been completely metabolised by the animal before the next treatment is administered. Of course this will make the experiment longer, but it is worthwhile to ensure that the experimental results are not influenced by treatment carry-over effects.

Another useful technique when trying to minimise the effects of carry-over is to use a *balanced crossover design* (Williams, 1949). A crossover design is said to be balanced for first-order treatment carry-over effects if no treatment is immediately preceded by itself, and each treatment is immediately preceded by every other treatment equally often (Bate and Jones, 2008; Stufken, 1996).

Example 3.18: Assessing drug transit in the gastrointestinal tract

The rate of gastrointestinal transit is known to be influenced by physiological conditions, diseases, drugs and food. While not a major safety concern, adverse drug side effects, such as diarrhoea, constipation and vomiting, could result in problems such as reduced patient compliance and quality of life. As part of the safety assessment of new drugs, the effect of the drug on the rate of gastrointestinal transit may need to be investigated. Paracetamol is poorly absorbed in the stomach but rapidly absorbed in the duodenum, so by measuring the rate of absorption of paracetamol we can model gastric emptying. The following example is based loosely on an experiment described in Sjödin *et al.* (2011).

An experiment was carried out in dogs to assess whether it would be possible to use pharmacokinetic modelling to quantify the rate of gastrointestinal transit in response to two compounds that are

Table 3.10. Possible experimental design for paracetamol absorption study

Test period	Dog					
	1	2	3	4	5	6
1	vehicle	erythromycin	atropine	vehicle	erythromycin	atropine
2	erythromycin	atropine	vehicle	atropine	vehicle	erythromycin
3	atropine	vehicle	erythromycin	erythromycin	atropine	vehicle

known to affect gastric emptying. Two compounds and a control were tested in the study:

1. vehicle (saline)
2. erythromycin (1 mg/kg)
3. atropine (0.06 mg/kg)

Dogs received a single dose of a test compound or vehicle as a 15-minute intravenous infusion. Thirty minutes after the start of the infusion, paracetamol (24 mg/kg) was administered into the stomach by a gavage using a rubber tube. The maximum paracetamol concentration (C_{max}) in the blood was taken as a summary measure of the absorption profile.

Six dogs were used in the study and each dog received all compounds over time, one per test period. The sequence of treatments may have been defined by a balanced three-period crossover design, such as the design given in Table 3.10.

Notice that vehicle precedes erythromycin and atropine twice within the design (dogs 1 and 3 for erythromycin; dogs 4 and 5 for atropine).

A wash-out period of at least three days between test periods was used; however (in our simulated example), let us assume there was some evidence that the effect of erythromycin was carried over into the following test period (see Figure 3.6). The results for vehicle and atropine were lowest when they were given in the test period after administration of erythromycin. This appears to have increased the variability of these treatment groups.

The effect could be a treatment carry-over effect, but it could also be a chance result. Care must be taken as there are not many replicates of the treatment carry-over effect. The best solution is to lengthen the wash-out period and see if this finding is reproducible in future studies.

3.5 Factorial design

In this text we make a distinction between two types of factorial design, namely *small* and *large*. While both types of design are members of the family of factorial designs, we make this distinction to highlight their different uses. Small factorial designs are applied routinely by many scientists, large factorial designs, however, have not been utilised as often and so their benefits might not be so well understood.

Researchers regularly employ small factorial designs when two or more categorical factors of interest are included in the experimental design, for example Strain and Treatment. By defining a factor as categorical we imply that it consists of a number of distinct levels. It is usually the case that an experiment is carried out to investigate differences between the levels of these categorical factors. When using small factorial designs a suitably large sample size is required at each combination of the factor levels to give a powerful enough experiment to detect biologically important differences between the various factor levels.

Large factorial designs are simply more complex and larger examples of small factorial designs. These designs consist of many more factors, and hence the number of combinations of the levels of the factors can be quite large. With large factorial designs we do not necessarily intend to test differences between each level of any given factor. Instead the researcher uses these designs to investigate the overall effect of, and any interrelationships between, many different factors. This can be achieved in a single pilot study. Factors that are found to be of no importance can be ignored when planning future studies. When using large factorial designs we do not need a large sample size at each combination of the levels of the factors, as the purpose of the experiment is not to compare individual levels of the factors but to assess their overall effect. The sample size in large factorial designs can be as little as two per group.

With both the small and large factorial designs, the factors of interest are crossed with each other. Many designs are said to have a factorial component, which implies that the factors in question are crossed with each other.

Before discussing the issues specific to small and large factorial designs, we shall consider some general

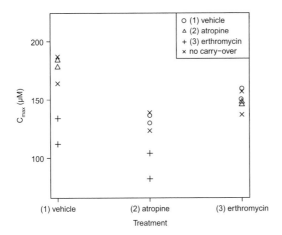

Figure 3.6. Scatterplot of the C_{max} response, categorised by the treatment administered in the previous test period.

issues. To begin with we consider how to conduct a valid randomisation of a factorial design. Next, as most factorial designs involve investigating the relationship between two or more categorical factors, we discuss this general issue. We then go on to consider small factorial designs. Using common sense we develop rules for constructing sensible designs. We then apply these rules to large factorial designs. Finally we consider the special case where the factors are not categorical but continuous.

3.5.1 Randomisation

The randomisation employed when using a factorial design is straightforward. Once all the combinations of the factor levels have been selected, and the replication at each level combination decided upon, then, where possible, the animals are randomly assigned to these levels. Only a single randomisation is required, unlike the randomisation of block designs where a separate randomisation is required for each block. As we shall see in Section 4.2.2.1, this has implications for the analysis of the data generated using factorial designs.

Note in certain situations it is not possible to assign animals randomly to the combinations of the levels of all the experimental factors. For example, if the factors

Strain or Gender are included in the factorial design, then animals cannot be randomly assigned to these factors. We believe the design can still be considered as a factorial design as Gender and Strain are usually crossed with the other factors of interest.

3.5.2 Categorical factors and interactions

Categorical factors consist of a number of distinct levels, for example Gender (males and females) or Strain (wildtype and transgenic). Factors on a continuous numerical scale can also be viewed as categorical. For example, Body weight is measured on a continuous numerical scale, but can also be assumed to be a categorical factor with, say, three levels (very heavy, heavy and light). These categorical factor levels also have a natural order, and this may need to be taken into account in the statistical analysis.

As a general rule when using a factorial design, we try to include as many combinations of the factor levels as possible. In fact the 'best' design will almost always include all combinations of the levels of the factors. So if a study design involves two factors, such as Gender and Strain, each at two levels, then there are four combinations of the factor levels of the two factors: male wildtype, male transgenic, female wildtype and female transgenic. The 'best' design will involve all four combinations of the levels of these factors.

In this section we shall assume that the researcher is able to include all combinations of the factor levels in the experiment. Such designs are called *full-factorial* designs. Designs where some of the combinations of the factor levels are intentionally excluded, the so-called *fractional factorial* designs, are briefly discussed at the end of the section.

All categorical factors of interest in a factorial design will be crossed with each other. For the purposes of the analysis we usually assume these factors are all fixed factors. The scientist is interested in investigating the fixed difference between the factor levels and the relationships, or interactions, between the factors.

Two factors are said to interact with each other if the effect of one factor depends on the level of the other factor. In other words an interaction is the failure of one factor to produce the same effect on the response at difference levels of a second factor. The benefit of using factorial designs, when investigating the effect of more than one factor, is that they allow the scientist to assess the size of the interactions between the factors.

Example 3.19: Assessing markers of atherosclerosis development

A study was conducted to assess whether the serum chemokines JE (the murine homologue of the human CCR-2 chemokine monocyte chemoattractant protein-1) and KC (the murine homologue of the human CXCR-2 chemokine Gro-α) could be used as markers for atherosclerosis development in mice (Parkin *et al.*, 2004). Two strains of mice, C3H apoE[-/-] and C57BL apoE[-/-], were used in the study. These mice were fed either a normal diet or a diet containing cholesterol (the Western diet). After 12 weeks the animals were humanely killed and their atherosclerotic lesion area determined by assessing Oil-Red O stained aortic sections.

The study design consisted of two categorical factors, Strain and Diet. The Strain factor consisted of two levels, C3H apoE[-/-] and C57BL apoE[-/-]. The diets used in the study were the normal rodent diet and the Western diet, and these define the two levels of the Diet factor. In total there were four combinations of the factor levels:
1. C3H apoE[-/-] + normal diet
2. C3H apoE[-/-] + Western diet
3. C57BL apoE[-/-] + normal diet
4. C57BL apoE[-/-] + Western diet

The effect of strain and diet can relate to (or interact with) each other in a number of ways. These are described hypothetically below.

No interaction

In this case the difference between the two diets is the same regardless of the mouse strain. A plot of the observed mean with standard errors when there is no interaction between strains and diets is presented in Figure 3.7.

If there is no interaction between strains and diets, the lines on this plot will be parallel. In this case there is an overall effect of diet. The lesions are larger in those animals fed the Western diet, regardless of strain. There is also an overall effect of strain. Lesions are generally larger in the C3H apoE[-/-] strain compared to the C57BL apoE[-/-] strain. However, the effect of diet is the same in both strains. The introduction of the Western diet causes a similar increase in lesions in both strains and hence there is no interaction between them. Alternatively it can be said that the difference between the diets is the same regardless which strain of mice they are fed to.

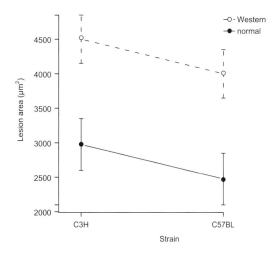

Figure 3.7. Plot of lesion area (μm²) means with standard errors for the case where there is no interaction between strains and diets.

If the scientist wishes to compare the overall effect of administering the Western diet vs. a normal diet, then it is appropriate to average the results from each diet across both strains (and hence make a single comparison between the diets) rather than making the comparison between the diets separately for each strain. This is effectively assessing the vertical difference between the two lines on the above plot. Why carry out the same test twice? This will effectively reduce the sample size by half for no obvious benefit!

Moderate interaction

A *moderate* interaction occurs when the overall effect of the first factor is the same regardless of the level of the second factor, but the size of that effect may vary with the level of the second factor. So, for example, introducing the Western diet may increase the lesion size in both strains of mice, but the size of this increase varies depending on the strain (see Figure 3.8).

In this example the effect of the Western diet is more pronounced in the C3H apoE[-/-] strain compared to the C57BL apoE[-/-] strain. While the lines on the interaction plot are not parallel, the slopes of the lines are both negative. If we wish to select a strain for use in future studies that maximises the effect of the Western diet,

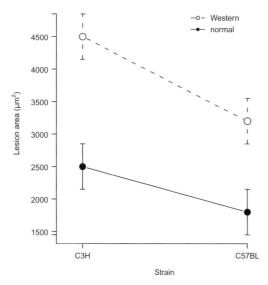

Figure 3.8. Plot of means with standard errors for the case where there is a moderate interaction between strains and diets.

then this plot indicates that selecting the C3H apoE$^{-/-}$ strain should be the most appropriate strategy.

Strong interaction

A third possibility is that the effect of the first factor is entirely dependent on the level of the second factor. Assume we discover that feeding the Western diet to the C3H apoE$^{-/-}$ mice has little effect on the size of the aortic lesions, whereas this diet has a much greater effect in the C57BL apoE$^{-/-}$ mice. This is an example of a *strong* interaction. Figures 3.9 and 3.10 are graphical representations of such interactions. In Figure 3.9 the slope of one line is positive whereas the other is negative indicating the effect of strain depends on which diet is fed to the animals. The Western diet, however, always results in bigger lesions than the normal diet.

The lines may also cross over, as in Figure 3.10. In this case the effect of diet is different, depending on the strain. Again the effect of strain depends on which diet the animals are fed on.

These findings may be of biological interest in their own right. If, however, the purpose of the experimental was to select a strain that maximises the difference between diets, then clearly C57BL apoE$^{-/-}$ would be the best strain to use in future studies.

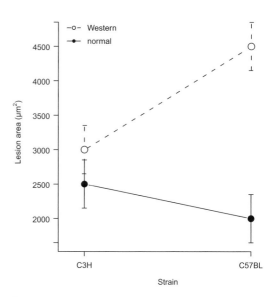

Figure 3.9. Plot of means with standard errors for the case where there is a strong interaction between strains and diets.

3.5.3 Small factorial designs

Factorial designs, in their simplest form, are often used in animal experiments. As mentioned above they are employed whenever the researcher has two or more factors in the study, each at a number of levels, which are to be investigated. In such designs these factors of interest will be crossed with each other. Examples of the use of such designs are given by Festing *et al.* (2001), Curtin *et al.* (2009) and Slotten *et al.* (2006).

It is usually the case that the purpose of these studies is to make pairwise comparisons between the combinations of the levels of the factors of interest. So the researcher will need to consider using a suitably large sample size for each combination. The analysis of data generated when using small factorial designs is discussed in Section 6.3.3.2. More generally, factorial experiments can be analysed using the parametric approaches described in Section 5.4.

Example 3.20: Assessing the effects of autoclaving diets on reproduction A

An experiment was conducted to see if autoclaving rodent diets had an impact on the reproductive success of mice; see Ford (1977) for more details. It was decided to test the effects of autoclaving on three different diets (each diet having a different physical structure)

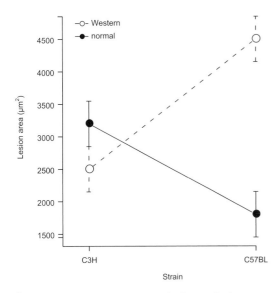

Figure 3.10. Plot of means with standard errors for the case where there is a strong interaction between strains and diets.

in two different strains. The factors in the experimental design were therefore:

- Treatment (levels: autoclaved or not);
- Diet (levels: pelleted and two expanded rodent diets);
- Strain (levels: LACA and DBA/1).

In total there were $2 \times 3 \times 2 = 12$ combinations of the levels of the above factors. All combinations were included in the experiment, with two breeding pairs per combination. However, assuming the researcher wanted to perform comparisons between the groups then (with a sample size $n = 2$) the power of the statistical tests may have been too low. Even if there were biologically relevant differences between the groups (i.e. the null hypothesis was false) then the statistical analysis may result in Type II errors (i.e. a failure to reject the null hypothesis when it was not true).

If the researcher wanted to make comparisons between the means of the 12 factor level combinations, then they may have found that to have sufficient statistical power (the probability of rejecting the null hypothesis when it is false; see Sections 2.3.5.2 and 3.7.2) then they would need around eight animals per group. In this case the total number of animals would be 96. In the actual experiment use was made of the properties of a full-factorial design, and this allowed the researchers to employ a sample size of two without undermining the scientific validity of the experiment. The results of the analysis revealed there was no effect of diet on reproduction but mice fed the pelleted diet did consume less food. The autoclaving increased the intervals between litters and there was also evidence of an interaction between autoclaving and diet, with a significant reduction in food consumption observed in the autoclaved/pelleted diet.

In studies such as the one described in Example 3.20 it is advisable to include all combinations of the levels of the factors in the design, i.e. to use a full-factorial design. It is true that due to practical reasons the researcher will occasionally exclude some of the combinations. This, however, may reduce the information gained from the experiment, as can be seen in the following example.

Example 3.21: Antipsychotic activity in the mouse

A study was conducted to investigate which of the mGlu2 and mGlu3 receptors mediate the effect of an mGluR2/3 agonist (LY379268) in two animal models of antipsychotic activity (phencyclidine and amphetamine-evoked hypersensitivity); see Woolley et al. (2008). The strains of mice tested, in separate experiments, included C57Bl/6J, mGluR2 knockout and mGluR3 knockout mice. We shall consider the experiments involving the C57Bl/6J mice in this section.

Mice were administered either the vehicle, phencyclidine (PCP) or amphetamine (AMP), where the latter two compounds effectively constituted two different animal models. Animals were placed in a test arena (for the habituation phase) and their locomotor activity measured. Following the habituation phase, either LY379268 (LY) at one of three doses (0.3, 1 or 3 mg/kg) or the vehicle was administered. The study consisted of ten treatments, five per animal model.

Phencyclidine model: vehicle/vehicle, vehicle/PCP, LY0.3/PCP, LY1/PCP, LY3/PCP

Amphetamine model: vehicle/vehicle, vehicle/AMP, LY0.3/AMP, LY1/AMP and LY3/AMP

The data from the two animal models were analysed separately. For each model the design was a factorial design involving two factors: PCP challenge (or AMP challenge) and Treatment. The two designs are illustrated in Figure 3.11.

Note some combinations of the factors are missing (for practical reasons), and this has weakened the design from a statistical viewpoint (see Section 5.4.3.5). In the analysis it is not possible to assess the interaction between the Treatment factor and the PCP (AMP) challenge factor.

The ten distinct treatments could also be considered as the combinations of three factors: the Hyperactivity factor (levels: compound challenge and vehicle challenge), the LY factor (levels: vehicle, 0.1, 0.3 and 3 mg/kg) and the Model factor (levels: phencyclidine and amphetamine).

There may be genuine reasons why six combinations were excluded from the experimental design. However, there are disadvantages when employing such a design. By using this incomplete design the researchers were not able to assess the interaction between the Model factor and the Treatment factor. Also it was not possible to make overall comparisons between the means of some of the two-way interactions (see Section 6.3.3.5). However, assuming the sample size at each of the factor level combinations is suitable, it was possible to make pairwise comparisons between

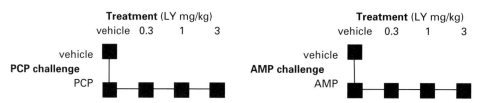

Figure 3.11. Two incomplete factorial designs used to assess antipsychotic activity in the mouse.

the group means of the ten combinations present. The research-ers were able to show that the mGlu2 but not the mGlu3 receptor mediates the actions of the mGluR2/3 agonist, LY379268 in this experiment.

Small factorial designs, such as those described above, are commonly used in practice. However, in the statistical literature the term factorial is usually reserved for designs that contain many factors. It is this type of factorial design that will be discussed in the next section. The reader should be aware that all the ideas presented in the next section also apply to the simpler case where the scientist wishes to investigate two or three factors in the conventional way.

3.5.4 Large factorial designs

While many experimental designs used in animal experiments have factorial components, large factorial designs are rarely used in practice. This is despite attracting some attention in the literature; see Shaw (2004) for example. By defining a design as large we imply that the researcher is planning to include many factors within the study.

The purpose of the study is not to test hypotheses regarding the differences between the factor levels, as with the small factorial experiments, but to investigate whether there is an overall effect of each factor. Many designs also allow the scientist to explore the interactions between the factors. The statistical analysis procedure is similar to that required for small factorial experiments (see Section 6.3.3.1). However, the purpose of this analysis, and the results that the scientist should concentrate on, are different. For example, the overall tests of effects should be investigated and

not the pairwise differences between the predicted means.

Consider factorial designs where all combinations of the levels of the factors are included, the so-called full-factorial designs. For example, if there are five factors, each at two levels, then there are 32 combinations of the levels of the five factors. It is easy to see that if a conventional number of animals were used at each combination of the five factor levels, then the experiment will involve a prohibitively large number of animals in total. If a sample size of ten per combination were used, then 320 animals would be required in total! However, the purpose of these experiments is to test hypotheses involving the overall effects of the factors, so only a small number of animals are required at each combination of the factor levels.

In other areas of research, where variability is not such an issue, then a replication as small as one or two can be used. It is the authors' experience that three animals per combination of the factor levels should be enough to identify outliers and also ensure that the design involves a suitably small number of animals in total.

3.5.4.1 Strategies when setting up a new animal model

When setting up a new animal model, the scientist should aim to maximise the window of opportunity to see a treatment effect (Shaw *et al.*, 2002). This will greatly reduce the total animal usage in the long run (see Section 3.7.2). But which level of each of the factors should be selected to maximise the window of opportunity? Does it make a difference which level is selected? For example, do you get a larger response in males than in females? If you do then it would be advisable to only use males in future studies. If it turns out that males and females both give a similar window of opportunity, then it may be possible to include both sexes in future studies.

In practice there may be many factors that influence the outcome of the experiment and hence the size of the window of opportunity. There are several strategies that can be used to investigate these factors, as described in Montgomery (1997, pp. 3–5).

Approach 1: The best guess approach

This is a commonly used approach where the scientist starts by selecting a reasonable set of levels for the experimental factors. This decision is usually based on previous knowledge gained by studying the animal model over a period of time. This unquestionably provides a good guide when setting up a new model. There are, however, two problems with this approach. If the scientist's first guess at the levels of the experimental factors give unsatisfactory results, then a second guess is required. Presumably the scientist originally believed this second guess would give worse results than the first (otherwise the second would have been tried first!). This can lead, in the end, to a waste of resources. The second problem occurs when the results from the first experiment are acceptable. The scientist might then be tempted to stop investigating the animal model further and hence miss the chance to identify a better combination of the levels of the factors that gives a larger window of opportunity.

Approach 2: One factor at a time approach

This involves running a series of experiments to assess the effect of the various factors. Each experiment investigates how one of the experimental factors influences the response. In each experiment all of the other factors are held constant by selecting only one of their levels to include in the study. The levels of the factor of interest are then varied to see how changing the levels of the factor influence the response. Unfortunately, as we shall see, this approach has serious drawbacks. Not only does it imply a non-systematic way of investigating a new animal model, but it can result in using far more animals and resources than are necessary. The

one factor at a time approach also provides the scientist with no information on how the factors influence or interact with each other.

Approach 3: Factorial approach

This approach, and it is the one recommended by most statisticians, involves using a large factorial design to investigate all of the experimental factors systematically in a single experiment. In such experiments we first decide on a number of levels for each of the factors we wish to investigate. We then investigate all of the factors together by running a study that contains most or all combinations of the factor levels. By definition these factors will be crossed with each other within the design.

Using a factorial design allows the scientist to carry out these preliminary investigations in a systematic way. Rather than assessing the effect of experimental factors in a piecemeal fashion, investigations can be conducted efficiently in one experiment. Those that are deemed important can be included in further studies. Those that are shown to be unimportant can be ignored, simplifying future designs and experiments. The benefit for the scientist is that by using more animals to start with, in a pilot study, the total number of animals used in future experiments can be reduced.

Example 3.22: MRI measurements of nasal cavities

A team decided to set up a new animal model for assessing the effect of compounds on nasal inflammation in guinea pigs. Animals were administered an inflammatory challenge (by inhalation) and the change in nasal cavity measured using the MRI scanning technique. When setting up the model they wanted to investigate possible factors that may influence the guinea pig responses. These factors included:

- Age of animals: Should we use older larger animals with larger nasal cavities?
- Gender: Can we use both sexes?
- Strain: Is there a particular strain that is more sensitive than others, leading to a larger window of opportunity?
- Dose (of challenge): Does a smaller dose produce a more consistent effect?
- Time (between challenge and dosing with anti-inflammatory compound): When is the optimum time to get the most consistent results?
- Time (post dosing for testing): When is the optimum time to get the most consistent results?

If we wish to answer each question in turn we would have to conduct many studies and hence use large numbers of animals. However, we could answer all these questions with just one study using a large factorial design.

To investigate the influence each factor has on the response, the researcher begins by selecting two levels for each of the six factors. There are therefore $2^6 = 64$ combinations of the levels of the six factors that can be included in the design. If we decide to run a full-factorial design with one animal per combination of the factor levels, then 64 guinea pigs would be required. This may be a prohibitively large number of animals. We will consider strategies (in the following sections) that may allow the researcher to reduce this number.

3.5.4.2 Graphical representation of large factorial designs

Perhaps the easiest way to explore the underlying structure of a factorial design is to produce a schematic diagram of the design. Factorial designs can be best represented using a grid-like diagram. These diagrams contain nodes corresponding to the combinations of the factor levels and edges that define the factor levels. The number of animals at each combination of the levels of the factors can also be included in the diagram by entering the sample size within each node.

Figure 3.12 shows two-factor, three-factor and four-factor full-factorial designs. The Gender, Housing type and Strain factors are all at two levels whereas the Diet factor is at three levels. Each example consists of 48 mice.

Figure 3.12(i) is a two-way factorial design with 24 knockout and 24 wildtype mice. For each strain 12 mice were group housed and 12 were isolated. In the design shown in Figure 3.12(ii) along with Strain and Housing we now have three diets in the study. The study consists of 48 animals as before, with 16 animals on each of the three diets, four per combination of Strain and Housing. Figure 3.12(iii) illustrates a development of the two previous designs. We now have included Gender in the experimental design. The four animals per combination of Strain, Housing and Diet consist of two males and two females. The total number of animals in this study is still 48 but we can now consider all four factors. More importantly we can also investigate how the factors influence or interact with each other.

Example (i) is a small factorial design. Depending on the underlying variability it should allow reliable comparisons between the group means to be made (as $n = 12$). Examples (ii) and (iii) are examples of large factorial designs as we should only investigate overall effects and interactions (as $n = 4$ and 2 per combination respectively). While not shown on these diagrams, the sample size for each combination could be entered in the grey boxes.

3.5.4.3 Hidden replication

It was noted above that in large factorial designs we could perhaps reduce the number of animals per combination to as little as two or three. While reducing the sample size to such small numbers per combination may seem dangerous, large factorial designs do benefit from the safety net of *hidden replication*.

Consider case (i) described in the previous section, the two-way factorial design with factors Housing and Strain, illustrated in Figure 3.12(i). Assume that there is no interaction between strains and housing conditions, i.e. the difference between the grouped and isolated housing means is the same for knockout and wildtype mice. Figure 3.13 shows the pattern in the results in such situations.

As the interaction was not significant, to test the overall effect of housing we can compare the overall group-housed mean to the overall isolated mean, averaging over the two strains. When comparing these housing means the effect of each strain will influence both housing means equally (see Figure 3.14). In other words the effect of strain cancels out when comparing housing level means.

This is an example of hidden replication. When assessing the overall effect of each factor, we have a larger sample size than simply the numbers within each combination of the factor levels. We achieve this by averaging over the other factor(s) in the experimental design. The more factors investigated within a factorial design, the more hidden replication will be contained within the design and hence the more powerful the design becomes.

The following example explores the effect of reducing the sample size at each combination of the factor levels.

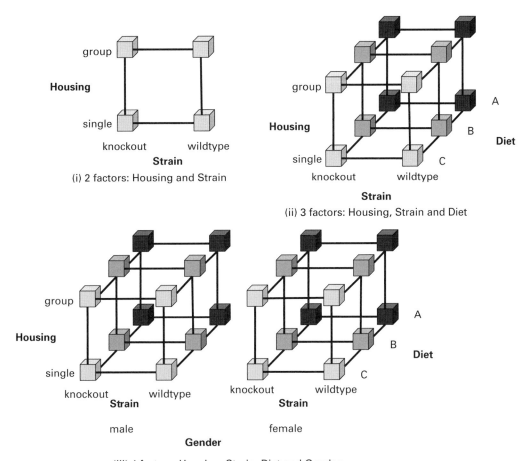

(i) 2 factors: Housing and Strain

(ii) 3 factors: Housing, Strain and Diet

(iii) 4 factors: Housing, Strain, Diet and Gender

Figure 3.12. Two-, three- and four-factor full-factorial designs involving 48 mice.

Example 3.23: An animal model for testing agents that may reduce cancer

Multiple lung tumours can be induced in certain strains of mice by exposing them to a carcinogen such as urethane. Animals that develop tumours can then be used as a model to test compounds that might prevent or reduce the incidence of cancer. In a study described by Shaw *et al.* (2002), a test compound or vehicle was administered to mice prior to exposing them to the carcinogen. After a period of time the animals were humanely killed and the number of lung tumours recorded.

There are many factors that can influence the outcome of such an experiment, so to develop the model the researcher decided to use a factorial design to investigate these factors. The factors included in the design were:

- Strain: Two strains of mice were thought to be susceptible (A/J and NIH).
- Gender: Is there a difference between the sexes? (Males and females were included in study.)
- Diet: Does the diet influence the results? (Two diets were used, the RM1 expanded diet and the RM3 pelleted diet.)
- Carcinogen: Two carcinogens were tested (urethane and 3-methylcholanthrene (3MC)).
- Treatment: Diallyl sulphide or vehicle were used to assess the effect of diallyl sulphide.

In total there were 32 different combinations of the above factors. The researcher included all combinations in the experiment, and hence a full-factorial design was employed. It was also decided that two animals would be allocated to each of the factor level

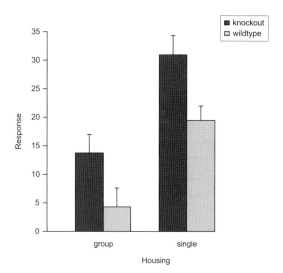

Figure 3.13. Plot of means with SEMs for the combinations of Housing and Strain when the two factors do not interact.

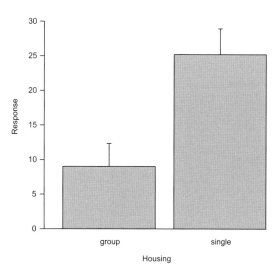

Figure 3.14. The pattern for Housing means averaged over Strain.

combinations; hence 64 mice in total were used in the experiment. The design is illustrated in Figure 3.15.

For the purposes of this discussion, simulated means with standard errors are shown in Figure 3.16. We can see from the plot that the difference between diallyl sulphide and the vehicle was more pronounced when the carcinogen urethane was administered to the mice. Also the A/J strain appears to be more susceptible than the NIH strain when administered urethane. Perhaps only this strain should be used in future (with urethane) as this will maximise the window of opportunity for observing treatment-related effects.

One problem with running a full-factorial design such as this is that a large number of mice are required. Although the researcher was able to investigate five factors (and eliminate Gender and Diet as being of less importance) it is still the case that 64 mice were used. As an exercise one of the two mice from each combination was randomly selected and excluded from the dataset. This results in a dataset containing data from 32 mice, one animal per combination of the levels of the five factors. The statistical analysis was then repeated.

Interestingly the analysis gave almost identical results to the analysis performed on the full dataset. For example, the observed means with standard errors plot is almost identical to the original (see Figure 3.17). This is mainly due to the hidden replication within the factorial design. In this example we would have arrived at the same conclusion if only 32 mice had been used: there was no need to use 64.

As mentioned above, in the authors' experience it is probably best not to go below a sample size of three animals per combination of the factor levels.

However, it is interesting to note that it is possible, depending on the underlying animal-to-animal variability and the hidden replication in the design, to use as few as one animal per combination without undermining the validity of the conclusions drawn from the analysis.

3.5.4.4 Fractional factorial designs to reduce animal use

The designs considered so far have been full-factorial designs. Every combination of the levels of the factors of interest are included in the design and hence the factors are fully crossed with each other (assuming an equal number of animals are assigned to each combination of the factor levels). As the number of factors increases, then so does the number of combinations of the levels of the factors. Given that the animal-to-animal variability is usually quite high then, as discussed above, it is unwise to use a sample size of less than three per combination. Unfortunately, even when using a sample size of three the total number of animals required (when using a large factorial design) may be prohibitively high.

If there is a limit on the number of animals available, then one way of testing many factors in a

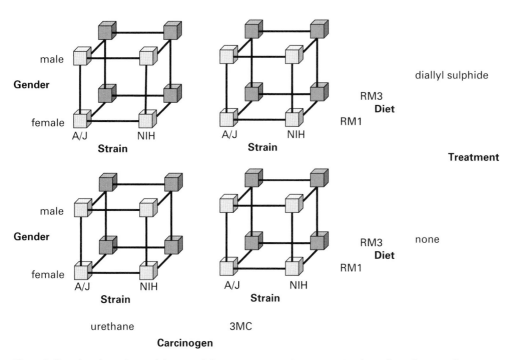

Figure 3.15. A four-factor factorial design with factors Treatment, Carcinogen, Gender and Diet for Example 3.23.

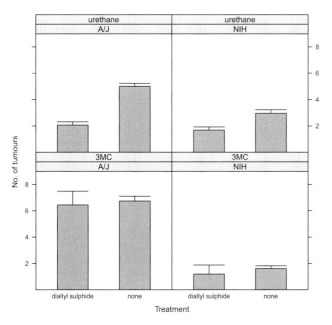

Figure 3.16. Plot of means with SEMs for the combinations of Strain, Carcinogen and Treatment for Example 3.23 – dataset with 64 mice.

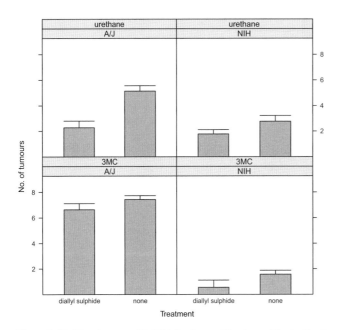

Figure 3.17. Plot of means with SEMs for the combinations of Strain, Carcinogen and Treatment for Example 3.23 – reduced dataset of 32 mice.

study is to use a fractional factorial design. In these designs only a subset of the levels of the factor combinations are included. It should be noted that once combinations are omitted from the design, then the researcher will lose the ability to test certain hypotheses. For example, it may not be possible to assess the highest-order interaction (the interaction involving all the factors).

One common design applied in this situation is the half-fraction factorial design. With this design only half of the combinations of the factor levels are included. There is plenty of mathematical theory about choosing the factor level combinations (Montgomery, 1997, Chapter 9). While it is outside the scope of this book, it is worth noting that the factor level combinations included in the design will have a large impact on the properties of the final design. One needs to be careful when constructing such designs and make sure they will allow you to answer all your questions.

A simple non-mathematical way of visually identifying which combinations of the factor levels to include

in a half-fractional factorial design is to use the graphical plots described in the previous section. As a rule of thumb it is best to try to spread the missing combinations across the design. Figure 3.18 illustrates two half-fraction factorial designs with three and four factors, respectively.

Example 3.24: Bioavailability testing

Kuentz *et al.* (2003), case study 3, described the use of a fractional factorial design when assessing the biopharmaceutical properties of a novel compound. Six factors, each at two levels, were screened: Mill, Dose, Excipient, Dosage form, Food and Class of animal. As Kuentz *et al.* (2003) commented, using the 'one factor at a time' approach to carry out the investigation would require at least 48 animals. Alternatively the large full-factorial design (for six factors at two levels) involved testing 64 combinations of the factors. Given a suitable sample size at each combination of the factors this would require too many animals, although all interactions between the factors could then be assessed. The approach recommended by Kuentz *et al.* (2003) was to use a special type of fractional factorial design called a Plackett–Burman design (Plackett and Burman, 1946). This design involved only 12 animals. It should be noted, however, that this design does not allow the researcher to assess any interactions between the factors. An example of a Plackett–Burman design is presented in Figure 3.19.

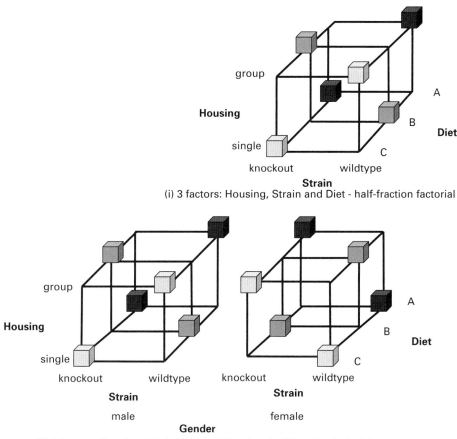

(i) 3 factors: Housing, Strain and Diet - half-fraction factorial

(ii) 4 factors: Housing, Strain, Diet and Gender - half-fraction factorial

Figure 3.18. Three- and four-factor half-fraction factorial designs with factors Housing, Strain, Diet (and Gender).

3.5.4.5 Two-stage procedure to reduce animal use

Another strategy to reduce the total number of animals required when using a factorial design is to employ a two-stage approach. To begin with the researcher runs a screening study to investigate all the factors considered important. The design applied at this stage should involve little replication at each combination of the factor levels as there are many factors (and hence many factor level combinations) in the design. Once the researcher has identified the most influential factors, then a second factorial experiment can be carried out investigating only those factors deemed important in the

first screening study. In this second study, larger sample sizes are used (as there are fewer combinations of the factor levels present in the design) and the aim now is to investigate the interactions between the factors.

Example 3.25: Hypothermia in mice

Hypothermia in mice was observed during a dosing study involving a novel compound. The compound was administered, in combination with an existing drug (drug X), to male mice of a particular transgenic strain. In the original dosing study a sample size of six mice per group was used.

Following this study it was deemed necessary to identify what caused this hypothermia. Was the side effect:

- A specific effect of the compound or did other compounds in the same chemical series have similar effects?

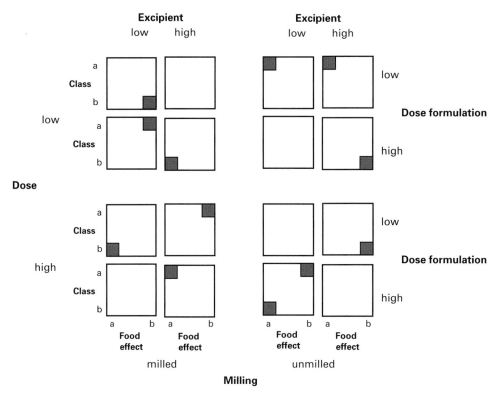

Figure 3.19. Example of a Plackett–Burman design with six factors and 12 animals for Example 3.24.

- Related to the activity of drug X and the central nervous system (CNS) exposure of the compound?
- Specific to the strain of mouse?
- Seen in both males and females?

A series of experiments was initiated to investigate these questions. Two possible strategies were considered.

Strategy A: One factor at a time

It was decided to compare three compounds (with the vehicle) that were in the same family as the initial compound. The study would involve eight groups in total, the three compounds (and the vehicle) with and without drug X.

Assuming the sample size was six mice per group, 48 mice would be required. This seemed reasonable as 48 mice could be tested in a single day. It was initially planned to carry out the experiment separately in male transgenics, male wildtypes, female transgenics and female wildtypes. If this approach was adopted, then 192 mice would be required to complete the four separate experiments.

Strategy B: Using a factorial design

All of the above questions can be answered using a four-factor factorial design, the four factors being:

- Treatment factor at four levels: three compounds (in the same family) and vehicle;
- Drug factor at two levels: with or without drug X;
- Strain factor at two levels: transgenic and wildtype;
- Gender at two levels: male and female.

There are 32 combinations of these factors levels and these combinations make up the full-factorial design. It was decided to assign either one or two mice to each combination of the factor levels so that three mice were assigned to each combination of compound, drug and strain. The three mice at each combination consisted of either two males and one female, or two females and one male. An experiment based on this design only required 48 mice in total and hence could be completed in one day. The final design is illustrated in Figure 3.20. Note there are an equal number of mice from each gender in each compound/drug/strain combination.

The benefits of Strategy B over A include:

- The experiment can be conducted in one day, hence day-to-day differences will not increase the variability or influence the conclusions. Strategy A would take four days.
- We can make within-day assessments of the interactions between gender and genotypes. We cannot do this for Strategy A as each sex/genotype combination would be tested on different days.

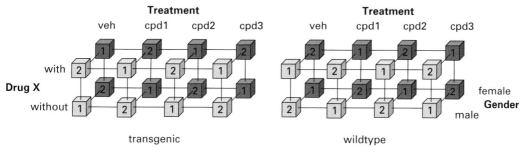

Figure 3.20. The four-factor factorial design with factors Strain, Compound, Gender and Drug for Example 3.25.

- The total number of animals used is 48 compared to 192 for strategy A.

The final experiment, using Strategy B, involved:

Day 1: Mice were implanted with a telemetry device to measure body temperature (subcutaneous injection).

Day 2: Mice were orally dosed with drug X or the control. Body temperature was recorded before and after dosing

Day 3: Mice were orally dosed with compound 1, 2, 3 or the vehicle. Body temperature was recorded immediately before dosing and every hour for three hours after dosing. The mice were then humanely killed and blood and brain samples taken for analysis of systemic and CNS exposure of the compounds.

The factorial design also allowed the researchers to investigate how these four factors interacted with each other. Figure 3.21 was part of the statistical analysis. It is an illustration of some of the results observed at 3 hours post dose. As there was no effect of strain, the means were calculated ignoring the strain of the mice.

From the results of the study, the side effect seemed larger in the females. The experiment also revealed that hypothermia was not restricted to the first compound (compound 1), although it was strongest in this compound. So it was hypothesised that it was either a property of this chemical series or due to inhibition of the target gene in general.

To test the second of these hypotheses, a study was planned to test compound 1 in a mouse where the target gene had been knocked out. If hypothermia was observed then it must be due to the compound's activity on a different substrate.

Data from the previous study was used to maximise the chance of demonstrating this effect. The researcher decided to use:

- female mice (which showed more of an effect than males);
- drug X (there was little effect without drug X);
- compound 1 or vehicle (compound 1 showed the largest effect in females);
- both knockout mice and the background strain.

It can be seen that we are using the results of the first experiment to reduce the number of factor level combinations required to be tested in the second experiment. We are concentrating the resources at the levels of the factors that should give the researcher the best possible chance of answering the second question.

Only six female knockout mice were still available from the colony, so the design employed for the second experiment involved 12 animals in total, six per strain, as illustrated in Figure 3.22. The experiment was carried out as described above. Figure 3.23 is one of the plots from the analysis of the data generated.

The temperature was reduced in those animals dosed with compound 1, but not those receiving the vehicle. The same effect was observed in knockout mice as in the wildtype mice. This suggests that the temperature reduction is due to some mechanism other than inhibition of the target gene.

The use of the two stage approach allowed the researcher to initially screen the factors to:

- investigate the interactions between the factors;
- identify which factors were important;
- identify which levels of the factors give the biggest reduction in temperature.

The second experiment was then designed to answer a specific question generated by the first experiment. The conclusion from these studies was that hypothermia was not due to inhibition of the target molecule but was CNS driven. There appeared to be a complex interaction between Compound, Treatment and Gender. All of this was achieved with 60 mice, not the 192 originally envisaged.

3.5.5 Factorial designs with continuous factors

In the factorial designs discussed so far, all of the individual factors within the design are assumed to be categorical. The levels of each of these factors consist of a set of distinct values. Sometimes, however, the researcher may want to include factors in a design with levels measured on a numerical scale. Such factors are called continuous factors. For example, consider a Litter size factor consisting of three levels: 5, 6 and 8 mice per litter. We could assume the factor has three categorical levels and hence the actual numerical levels (and their ordering) would be ignored when

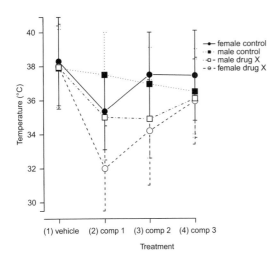

Figure 3.21. Plot of observed means with SEMs for the combinations of Gender, Treatment and Dose for Example 3.25.

constructing the design. We could, however, take the numerical levels into account.

Whilst the underlying structure of factorial designs with continuous factors is the same as those that consist of categorical factors, these designs can be used to answer slightly different questions. With continuous factors we are trying to estimate the influence that varying the level of the continuous factors has on the response.

Example 3.26: Carcinogenicity study in strain A/J mice

Nesnow *et al.* (1998) describe an experiment to assess the binary, ternary, quaternary and quinary interactions of a five-component mixture of carcinogenic environmental polycyclic aromatic hydrocarbons. The five hydrocarbons tested were benzo[a]pyrene, benzo[b]-flouranthene, dibenz[a,h]anthracene, 5-methylchrysene and cyclopenta[cd]pyrene.

To investigate these hydrocarbons, and how they relate and interact with each other, a full-factorial design was employed. The design consisted of five continuous factors, each factor at two levels corresponding to a low and high dose of the carcinogen. Either 20 or 24 mice were assigned to each combination of the levels of the five factors and the number of mice developing a lung adenoma was recorded (a discrete response). The experimental design employed, including the results of the experiment, are given in Nesnow *et al.* (1998). The analysis of the data generated involved estimating a response surface model, including interactions between the continuous factors. This statistical model

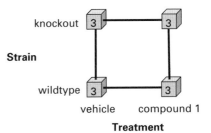

Figure 3.22. A two-factor factorial design with factors Strain and Treatment, $n = 3$ animals per combination of the two factors.

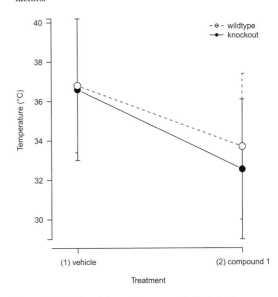

Figure 3.23. Plot of observed means with SEMs for the combinations of Treatment, Strain and Time for Example 3.25.

predicted, to a significant degree, the observed lung tumorigenic responses of the quinary mixtures and suggested that although interactions between polycyclic aromatic hydrocarbons do occur, they are limited in extent.

3.5.5.1 Strategies for setting up a new animal model

The strategies that can be used to investigate continuous factors are similar to those described in Section 3.5.4 for categorical factors. We highlight the differences with an example.

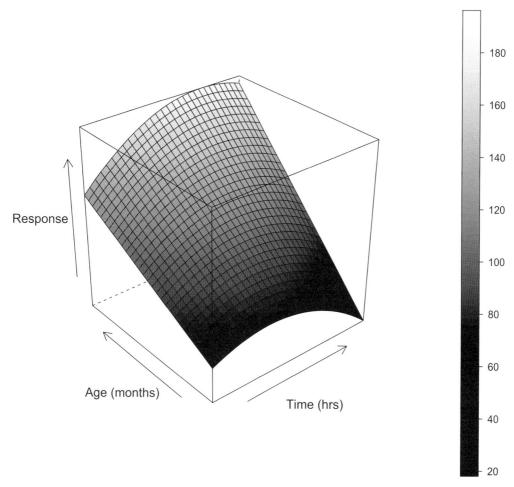

Figure 3.24. Three-dimensional surface plot illustrating the effect of the age of the mice and time of sample collection on a biomarker for Alzheimer's disease.

Example 3.27: Transgenic model for Alzheimer's disease

Consider the case where a scientist wants to set up a new transgenic mouse model for testing compounds to treat Alzheimer's disease. There are many factors that may influence the animal model, for example, the age of transgenic animals at the start of the study and when samples are collected after dosing with the compound. Initially a series of pilot studies are planned to identify a suitable age for the mice and the time of initial sample collection. Hopefully this should provide enough information so that the window of opportunity for identifying treatment-related effects can be maximised.

Let us assume the actual relationship is as follows. There is an interaction between Mouse age and Time of sample collection, so

that the maximum size of response can be achieved with 10-month-old mice and a time of sample collection of around 7.5 hours post-dose. The relationship between the two factors can perhaps best be described using a three-dimensional surface plot (see Figure 3.24). The first two dimensions are mouse age and time of sample collection, and the third dimension is the size of the response. We can also represent the data by a two-dimensional contour plot (see Figure 3.25).

How can we best uncover this complex relationship while using as few animals as possible? We shall describe three approaches for investigating this. The first is the one factor at a time approach, similar to the

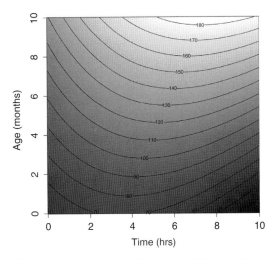

Figure 3.25. Two-dimensional contour plot illustrating the effect of the age of the mice and time of sample collection on a biomarker for Alzheimer's disease.

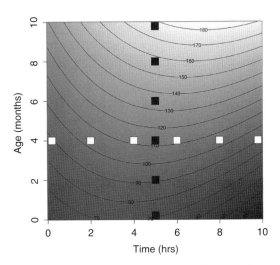

Figure 3.26. Two-dimensional contour plot illustrating the effect of the age of the mice and time of sample collection on a biomarker of Alzheimer's disease. White squares correspond to stage 1 experiments and black squares to stage 2 experiments.

one described above, the second uses an inefficient factorial design and the third uses a more powerful full-factorial design.

Approach 1: One factor at a time

This approach is a two-stage procedure. We begin by using mice of approximately the same age and vary the time of sample collection. This allows us to identify the time of sample collection that produces the maximal effect. Note the conclusion is only valid for mice of the same age as those used in this experiment. Having identified the time of sample collection that gives a maximal response, we then move onto the second stage. In stage 2 we fix the time of sample collection (at the time identified in stage 1) and vary the age of the transgenic mice.

Let us consider the above example. Assume the researcher begins by using mice that are four months old. The time of sample collection is now varied and it is found that the maximal response from the animal model is achieved when the sample is taken at approximately five hours (see Figure 3.26).

In stage 2 of the process the time of sample collection is fixed at five hours and the effect of age is assessed by

testing mice of different ages. From Figure 3.26, with the experimental points marked on, we can see that the maximal effect is achieved with mice that are 10 months old. The maximal effect of the response is concluded to be about 175. This testing procedure involved 12 groups of mice in total.

Unfortunately for the researcher the factors Age and Time interact with each other. The effect of the age of the animal varies depending on the time of sample collection. In other words the true maximum has been missed.

Approach 2: Varying combinations

The second approach involves testing in three stages:
1. at several sampling times (in mice of the same age);
2. in animals of varying ages (at the same early sampling time point);
3. at several combinations of increasing age and sampling time.

This is perhaps a more appealing approach than Approach 1 as it allows the researcher to investigate both factors separately. The combinations of the two factors are highlighted in Figure 3.27.

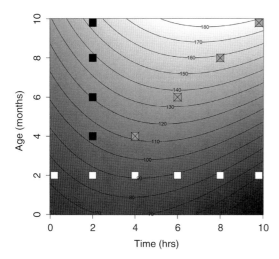

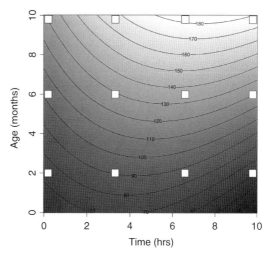

Figure 3.27. Two-dimensional contour plot illustrating the effect of the age of the mice and time of sample collection on a biomarker of Alzheimer's disease. White squares correspond to stage 1 experiments, black squares to stage 2 experiments and grey crossed squares to stage 3 experiments.

Figure 3.28. Two-dimensional contour plot illustrating the effect of the age of the mice and time of sample collection on a biomarker of Alzheimer's disease. White squares correspond to the experiments.

Using this approach the conclusion would be to use around 10-month-old mice with a time of collection of 10 hours to achieve a maximal response of magnitude around 180. This procedure requires 14 groups, three more than the previous approach.

The problem with this approach, while it is better than the first approach, is that there are large areas of the response surface some distance from the combinations of the factors tested in the experiment. The further we move from the positions where measurements were taken, the less certain we will be about predicting the shape of the surface. Unfortunately one of these areas included the maximal response.

Approach 3: The full-factorial design
The third approach involves using the methodology described in Section 3.5.4 to produce a full-factorial design with two factors. Each factor will be measured at either three or four levels. The more levels that can be included, depending on the practical constraints, the more accurate the estimation of the interaction between the factors will be. A possible design is illustrated in Figure 3.28.

The whole surface can now be estimated using this approach and we have covered the entire surface area with only 12 combinations. The maximum will be successfully identified (around 10-month-old mice and a sampling point of 7.5 hour post-dose).

A final technique to improve the reliability of the results generated would be to 'tilt' the design points slightly through, say ten degrees. In this case no mouse age or time of collection would be used more than once. We shall comment further on this principle in Section 3.6.2.1.

3.5.5.2 Drug combination studies

An interesting example of the use of two (or more) continuous factors in a factorial design setting is drug combination studies. This may be the case if the researcher is interested in seeing how two drugs act in combination. Effectively we are dealing with a situation where there are two crossed continuous factors, the dose of the first compound and the dose of the second.

Drug combination studies, and making assessments of drug synergies, are a subject in their own right and beyond the scope of this text. If the reader is interested

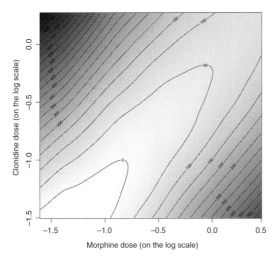

Figure 3.29. Two-dimensional plot of the interaction between morphine and clonidine, as described by Tallarida (2000, p. 169) for Example 3.28.

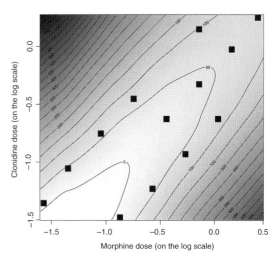

Figure 3.30. Two-dimensional plot of the interaction between morphine and clonidine, as described by Tallarida (2000, p. 169), including the original points where observations were made (black squares) for Example 3.28.

in reading about such studies and how to analyse them, then the text of Tallarida (2000) is recommended. We shall, however, give an example to highlight some of the design implications that should be considered when investigating how two drugs interact with each other.

Example 3.28: Synergism between morphine and clonidine

The following example is taken loosely from Tallarida (2000, pp. 163–4). An experiment was conducted to assess the synergistic effect of two drugs, morphine and clonidine, when given in combination to mice. Following administration of the drug combination, the mice were subjected to a nociceptive stimulus by immersing their tails in hot water (55°C). The latency of tail withdrawals, with an arbitrary cut-off of 20 seconds if an animal did not respond, was used as an animal model of antinociceptive effects.

Several combinations of the two drugs were administered to the mice, where the combinations of the two drugs administered were held at three fixed ratios. Figure 3.29 is a prediction of the relationship between morphine and clonidine. The results plotted are the average of at least ten animals, as given by Tallarida (2000, p. 169).

Although the purpose of the experiment was not to quantify the surface across all combinations of morphine and clonidine, it can be seen that the coverage of the design points is around the main diagonal (see Figure 3.30). The researcher has little information about the effect of the combination of the drugs in both the top left-hand corner and bottom right-hand corner of this plot. We suspect it is

highly unlikely that the effect really gets as high as 900, as predicted by the surface.

The purpose of the original experiment was to investigate the synergistic effect of morphine and clonidine. The design recommended by Tallarida is suitable for assessing this. However, let us assume the purpose of the experiment was to investigate the effect of the two compounds, and how they interact with each other. We can carry out this investigation using a factorial design with all combinations of four doses of morphine and four doses of clonidine.

The design is given in Figure 3.31 and the reader should note the similarities between this design and the full-factorial design discussed in previous sections. This design should allow the researcher to predict the effect of the combination of the two drugs at all drug combinations reliably.

In the example described in the previous section we highlighted the benefit that could be gained from including more factor levels in the experimental design. To achieve this we used the individual brain concentrations in the analysis rather than the nominal dose. We could achieve a similar effect in drug synergy studies by rotating the design suggested above slightly around the centre of the design. The design would now have 16 doses of each compound (with a sample size of one at each concentration) and it can be shown that this leads to more accurate estimates of the relationship between the two drugs. This design is given in Figure 3.32.

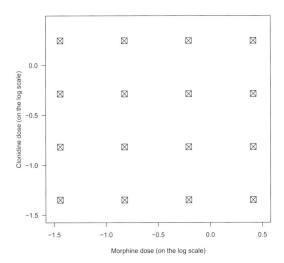

Figure 3.31. A full-factorial design for assessing the interaction between clonidine and morphine for Example 3.28.

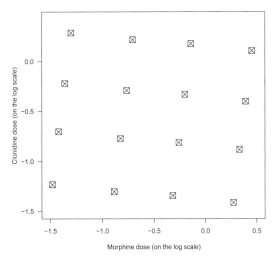

Figure 3.32. A full-factorial design for assessing the interaction between clonidine and morphine for Example 3.28.

3.5.5.3 Continuous vs. categorical factors

Sometimes a factor can be treated as either categorical or continuous. For example, assume that Age (of the animal) is to be used in the design and analysis. This factor could be assumed to be a categorical factor with two levels, young and old, say. We can then test to see if there is a difference between these two levels, or perhaps see if the effect of age interacts with other effects in the experiment. These tests could be used as an indication of whether the age of the animal was influencing the response. We could, however, take the actual numerical age of the animal when setting up the design. Age would then be treated as a continuous factor.

The difference between the way we deal with categorical and continuous factors is in the analysis. With a categorical factor we test, in some sense, to see if one level is different from the other. With continuous factors we are more interested in modelling how the response varies as the factor level varies numerically. We can model this relationship using a linear relationship or perhaps some more complicated curve.

3.5.6 Final thoughts on factorial designs

Regardless of whether factors are defined as categorical or continuous, in both cases the analysis allows the

researcher to assess how the effects quantified by the factors relate or interact with each other. Despite these similarities, the previous example highlights the different questions that can be answered by assuming the factors in a factorial design are continuous. With categorical factors we can investigate if the levels of each factor are different from each other. With continuous factors we are more interested in assessing how the response varies as we increase or decrease the level of the factor. By taking factors to be continuous we are effectively smoothing the response surface across the levels and this may mitigate the effect of the underlying variability in the responses themselves.

If there are more than two continuous factors, then estimating the surface becomes more difficult. However, there are certain statistical software packages that can deal with multiple continuous factors. Such packages allow the user to specify a range of responses that are of interest and then output which values of the continuous factors are required to satisfy this condition.

As a general rule, to obtain a more reliable estimate of the shape or nature of the relationship (between the continuous factor and the response) it is recommended that the researcher include more levels of the factor in the design, even if this implies there will be fewer animals at each individual level. Of course there are limits to this. We need to be careful that the sample size is sufficient to counteract the animal-to-animal variability. As mentioned above, as a rule of thumb we suggest including at least three animals per combination of the factor levels.

3.6 Dose-response designs

All of the designs considered so far in this chapter can be broadly described as comparative designs. The motivation for running experiments using these designs is to:
1. Investigate the overall effect of a factor.
2. Compare one level of a factor to another.
This corresponds to using experimental design within the hypothesis testing framework (Section 2.3). We can, however, construct and apply experimental designs within the estimation framework too (Section 2.5).

In the previous sections, whenever we have considered an experiment that involves increasing doses of a compound, we have assumed that the Dose factor is a categorical factor at a number of distinct levels (corresponding to the number of doses of compound in the experiment). We can then assess the differences between these levels in the statistical analysis. To ensure these hypothesis tests are sufficiently sensitive we require a suitably large sample size at each dose (see Section 3.7.2).

There is, however, an alternative. We could treat the Dose factor as a continuous numerical factor and then assess the effect on the response as the dose of compound varies. Some argue that this is a more appropriate way to investigate the effect of a compound as it more closely reflects the underlying biology. The effect of a compound will change steadily as the dose increases. Just because you only achieve statistical significance at 10 mg/kg (and not 1 mg/kg) does not imply that the compound has no effect at 9 mg/kg. In practice the purpose of most experiments is to investigate how the novel compound influences the response. Whether a specific dose is (statistically) significantly different from the control is of less interest. Such hypothesis tests are influenced by other things, such as sample size. The dose-response estimation approach described here is a creditable alternative to hypothesis testing.

Dose-response designs share many similarities with factorial designs consisting of continuous factors (see Section 3.5.5). However, the designs considered here usually consist of only one continuous factor (Dose) whereas factorial designs consist of two or more crossed factors. The same general principles apply to these designs as to the more complex factorial designs.

The purpose of these experiments is to estimate the dose-response relationship. This can be achieved by modelling the relationship using a linear line, the so-called *linear regression analysis* technique, or by a more complex non-linear curve. Commonly employed examples of the latter include the weighted and non-weighted four- and five-parameter logistic curves, or more complicated curves such as curves to quantify pharmacokinetic relationships. Many other types of curve can be used to quantify this type of data; see Slob (2002) for more details. In this section we assume the relationship can be estimated by fitting a logistic curve, although the general principles described apply to fitting any type of curve.

3.6.1 The four- and five-parameter logistic curves

When modelling the effect of a compound on a biological response, one of the models most commonly used in practice is the four-parameter logistic curve (Liao and Liu, 2009), sometimes defined as the Hill equation:

$$\text{Response} = D + \frac{(A-D)}{\left(1+\left(10^{\log_{10}(\text{Dose})-C}\right)^{B}\right)} \quad (3.3)$$

where A is the maximum, D is the minimum, C is the log D_{50} (an estimate of the dose that causes a 50% increase (or decrease) in response on the log scale) and B is the Hill slope. Note the definition of A and D are interchangeable, depending on the sign of the Hill slope parameter B.

We can fix any of the four parameters if we so choose. Sometimes this is necessary to achieve reliable results, especially if the minimum or maximum of the curve are not well defined. Even though we have fixed some of the parameters, the convention is still to call the fitted curve a four-parameter logistic curve.

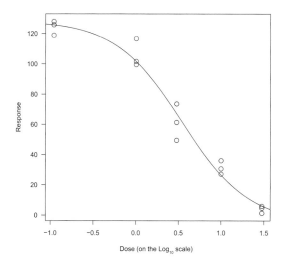

Figure 3.33. Example of a decreasing effect, with respect to the dose of compound, including a four-parameter logistic curve.

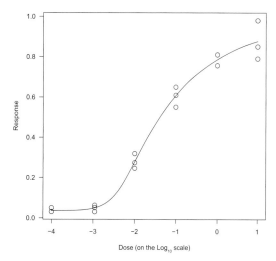

Figure 3.34. Example of an increasing effect, with respect to the dose of compound, including a five-parameter logistic curve.

This type of analysis is usually performed on the log-transformed concentration or dose scale as doses are usually equally spaced on the log scale. The D_{50} parameter is also usually log normally distributed and so modelling the log D_{50} simplifies the statistical analysis. An example of a four-parameter logistic curve is given in Figure 3.33.

The four-parameter logistic curve fit is symmetric around the point of inflection (log D_{50}). However, in certain cases the biological relationship is not symmetric and hence the four-parameter curve fit may not be appropriate. One option is to fit a five-parameter logistic curve to the data, where the fifth parameter (on top of the four in the four-parameter logistic curve) is an asymmetry parameter. The following equation, given by Liao and Liu (2009), is recommended as it is still possible to obtain an unbiased estimate of log D_{50} (the C parameter) directly from the analysis:

$$\text{Response} = D + \frac{(A-D)}{\left[1 + \left(2^{1/g} - 1\right)\left(10^{\log_{10}(\text{Dose})-C}\right)^{B}\right]^{g}} \quad (3.4)$$

where g is the asymmetry parameter. If $g = 1$ then the equation simplifies to the four-parameter logistic

curve described above. An example of such a curve, where the asymmetry parameter $g = 0.161$, is given in Figure 3.34.

3.6.2 Experimental design considerations

When constructing a dose-response experimental design there are several issues to consider:

- It is recommended that the number of doses included in the experiment is at least one more than the number of parameters to be estimated. So a design with at least five doses (and this can include the zero dose) is required if the scientist wishes to fit a four-parameter logistic curve to the data. Findlay and Dillard (2007) also comment that using more than eight doses does not improve the reliability of the curve fitting process.

- The purpose of this type of study is to estimate the dose-response relationship. It is not to compare individual treatment groups back to the control. So there is no need to have a large sample size at each dose to allow for reliable estimates of the group means. In fact it turns out that we get a more reliable estimate of the dose-response relationship if we include more doses in the experimental design (with fewer animals

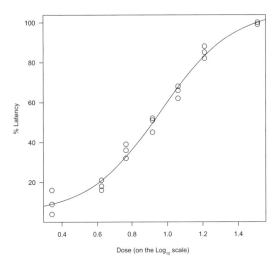

Figure 3.35. Plot of the analgesic action of morphine sulphate, as given by Tallarida (2000, p. 32), showing percentage latency vs. nominal dose of compound for Example 3.29.

at each dose if the total number of animals in the experiment is fixed).

- As with factorial designs with continuous factors, it is recommended to space the doses to be tested equally (on the log scale). This will produce an estimate of the dose-response curve that is as reliable as possible.
- When estimating the four- (or five-) parameter logistic curve we require a reliable estimate of both the minimum and maximum plateau of the curve. To achieve this it is a good idea to have a pair of anchor points at either end of the curve. This will allow the analysis to estimate the minimum and maximum of the curve best (Findlay and Dillard, 2007). It is also a good idea to have some doses around the point of inflection to estimate log D_{50} and the Hill slope.

3.6.2.1 Increasing the number of doses

As mentioned above, there is some benefit to increasing the number of doses included in a dose-response design, perhaps at the expense of the number of animals administered each dose. The following example, based on a study described in Tallarida (2000, p. 31), highlights the benefit that can be gained from including more doses in the dose-response design.

Example 3.29: Analgesic action of morphine sulphate

An experiment was conducted to assess the analgesic effect of morphine sulphate in rats. Rats were exposed to cold water, as a nociceptive stimulus, and the analgesic effect was assessed by measuring tail flick latency. There were seven doses and three rats were assigned to each. The dose-response relationship was estimated over these doses by fitting a four-parameter logistic curve to the data with the maximum of the curve fixed at 100%. The three parameters estimated were log D_{50}, the Hill slope and the curve minimum.

Figure 3.35 is a graphical display of the results using the dose of morphine sulphate in the analysis. The data are given by Tallarida (2000, p. 32). The estimate of D_{50} was 0.94 (on the log scale) or 8.53 on the original scale. The standard error of the log D_{50} estimate was 0.018.

Now assume that the researcher had been able to measure the actual concentration of morphine sulphate in the brain. It was hypothesised that these measurements may provide a better measure of compound exposure than the dose of morphine administered.

To investigate the benefit of using brain concentration (rather than nominal dose) in this type of analysis we added a random component to the dose variable to simulate actual brain concentration. It is interesting to note that we now have 21 individual concentrations within the experiment, with a sample size of one at each concentration, rather than seven doses. Figure 3.36 was obtained using the simulated brain concentration of morphine rather than morphine dose.

The estimate of D_{50} was still predicted to be 0.94 (on the log scale). The standard error of the estimate though fell from 0.018 to 0.016, an 11% decrease from before. It is interesting (although not unexpected, given that there are more distinct concentrations in the design) that there has been an improvement in precision when reducing the sample size from three to one.

3.6.2.2 Decreasing the number of animals

As mentioned above, if you plan to assume the Dose factor is a categorical factor, and then test the various doses back to the control, you will require a suitable sample size at each of the doses.

However, if you assume the Dose factor is a continuous factor, then the principles of efficient experimental design that were introduced for factorial designs (with continuous factors) can be applied in this scenario too. As discussed above, with factorial designs it is better to include more levels of the continuous factors. This results in a more reliable assessment of the change in the response variable as the experimental conditions change. The same is true when there is only a single continuous factor in the experimental design. It is better to

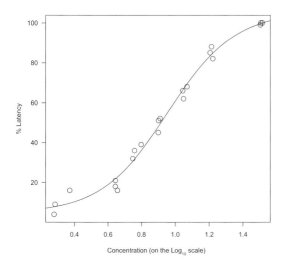

Figure 3.36. Plot of the analgesic action of morphine sulphate, based on data given by Tallarida (2000, p. 32) with an additional random component added to the nominal concentrations. Percentage latency vs. simulated brain concentration of the compound is shown rather than the nominal dose for Example 3.29.

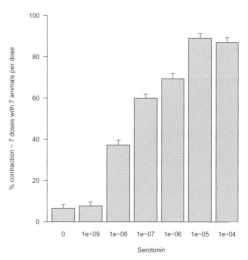

Figure 3.37. Plot of observed means with within-dose standard errors for Example 3.30. Results were calculated using the dataset with seven animals at each of the seven doses.

include more doses, but with fewer animals per dose. To highlight this consider the following, based loosely on an example described by Tallarida and Jacob (1979, p. 156).

Example 3.30: Assessing the effect of a compound on the rat fundus strip

An experiment was conducted to assess the effect of serotonin on the rat fundus strip. Increasing doses of serotonin were tested in the experiment using an experimental design where $d = 7$ doses of serotonin (including the control) and $n = 7$ animals per dose level. A plot of the observed means with within-dose standard errors for simulated data is given in Figure 3.37. The four-parameter logistic curve can be fitted to the data as in Figure 3.38.

But was it necessary to use $7 \times 7 = 49$ rats to get a reliable estimate of the dose-response relationship for serotonin? To investigate this question we randomly removed rats from each dose group and re-estimated D_{50} using the reduced dataset. Table 3.11 summarises the effect that randomly removing animals from the dataset has on the estimate of D_{50}. The top row in the table corresponds to the analysis on the full dataset involving 49 rats. The remaining rows correspond to using between two and six rats per dose group. Table 3.11 is summarised in Figure 3.39.

The experiment involving only 21 rats (seven doses, three animals per dose) gave a comparable estimate of the serotonin D_{50} (2.30×10^{-8}) to the experiment involving 49 animals (2.50×10^{-8}), with reasonably similar confidence intervals.

3.6.3 Including the control group

When fitting a logistic curve to assess the dose-response relationship, it is standard practice to conduct the analysis on either the $\log_{10}$ or $\log_e$ dose scale. Doses are usually selected to be equally spaced on the log scale (for example 0.01, 0.1, 1, 10 mg/kg).

A minor complication with this approach is how to deal with the control group. This group will necessarily have a zero concentration of compound, and yet $\log(0)$ does not exist. There are several strategies that can be taken to deal with this problem. We shall consider three of the more popular and their impact on the experimental design.

3.6.3.1 Analysing a change from the control response

A seemingly sensible approach is to use a change from the control response in the analysis. We calculate the mean control response and then divide (or subtract) this mean from the remaining data. The curve can then have one parameter fixed, either the minimum (at 0) or the maximum (at 100% perhaps), depending on the direction of the curve and the method of normalisation.

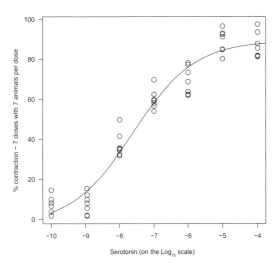

Figure 3.38. Scatterplot of all response vs. dose, including the four-parameter dose-response logistic curve for Example 3.30. Data includes seven animals at each of seven doses.

Table 3.11. D_{50} serotonin estimates for Example 3.30 calculated from datasets with reduced numbers of animals

	D_{50}	Lower 95% confidence interval	Upper 95% confidence interval
n=7, d=7	2.50×10^{-8}	1.27×10^{-8}	4.90×10^{-8}
n=6, d=7	2.36×10^{-8}	1.18×10^{-8}	4.70×10^{-8}
n=5, d=7	2.54×10^{-8}	1.07×10^{-8}	5.98×10^{-8}
n=4, d=7	2.35×10^{-8}	9.49×10^{-9}	5.80×10^{-8}
n=3 d=7	2.30×10^{-8}	8.09×10^{-9}	6.53×10^{-8}
n=2, d=7	1.48×10^{-8}	4.08×10^{-9}	5.31×10^{-8}

Unfortunately if we take this approach then we are effectively ignoring the variability in the control group when performing the statistical analysis. In effect we assume the control group mean is the true control group mean. If this were the case then it would justify subtracting (or dividing) the remaining data by this true value. However, the control group is only an estimate of the true control group mean and there will inevitably be some variability in the control group estimate. The adjustment to the remaining data and the subsequent analysis should reflect this.

3.6.3.2 Using a dual statistical model

There is a solution, applied at the statistical analysis stage, which allows the researcher to analyse the original data without having to manipulate the experimental design or response variable. This involves fitting a dual statistical model to the data. The statistical model fitted is either:

- A combination of the control group mean and the predicted minimum (or maximum) of the curve when the dose level is zero.
- The logistic curve if the dose level is greater than zero.

Effectively the predicted dose-response relationship, as the dose approaches zero (the control), is a weighted combination of the minimum (or maximum) of the curve and the control group mean.

This approach has many benefits but can produce awkward results if the predicted minimum (or maximum) of the curve is not similar to the control group mean due to the variability of the responses. It is also an approach that may require the help of a professional statistician to implement.

3.6.3.3 Adding an offset to the dose

It can be argued that we should use all the data to estimate the dose-response relationship. If we add a small offset to all the doses, then we can include the control group on the log dose scale.

The choice of offset is somewhat arbitrary, but if an offset is chosen so that the control group is situated on the plateau of the curve, then the choice of offset itself does not influence the curve fit or the results from the curve fit (at a practical level at least). We recommend using this approach.

Example 3.31: Varying the offset

In the following example the offset value has been varied so that the control group responses reside at –2, –4 and –6 on the log dose scale. With an offset of –2 the control group is not quite on the plateau of the curve, perhaps the offset was too large. Figure 3.40 and Table 3.12 illustrate the analysis if an offset of 0.01 is added to the levels of the Dose factor.

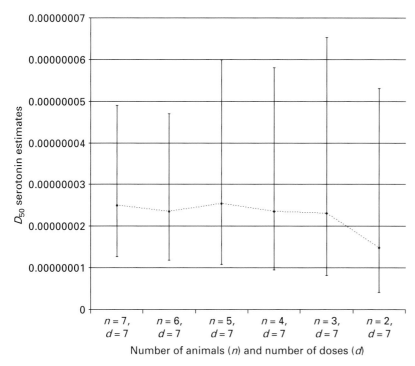

Figure 3.39. Plot of the D_{50} serotonin estimates, with 95% confidence intervals, for Example 3.30 calculated using data with between two and seven animals per dose.

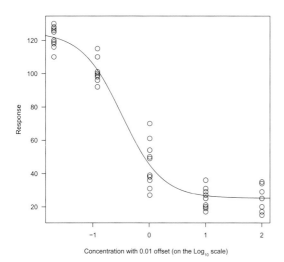

Figure 3.40. Scatterplot of response vs. dose, including the four-parameter dose-response logistic curve for Example 3.31, where the doses are plotted on the $\log_{10}$ scale. Analysis was performed using an offset of 0.01 to the levels of the Dose factor.

Table 3.12. Table of the four-parameter estimates for Example 3.31 calculated using an offset of 0.01 to the Dose factor levels

Parameter	Estimate	Std error	t-value	p-value
Max/Min	125.066	3.857	32.42	< 0.001
Slope	-1.215	0.146	-8.33	< 0.001
logD50	-0.485	0.063	-7.71	< 0.001
Min/Max	25.216	2.111	11.95	< 0.001

With an offset of −4 the control group is now on the plateau of the curve. The estimate of the log D_{50} and the Hill slope parameter have changed slightly, −0.51 vs. −0.49 and −1.14 vs. −1.17, respectively, but this is perhaps to be expected as the control group is now situated on the plateau of the curve. Figure 3.41 and Table 3.13 illustrate the analysis if an offset of 0.0001 is added to the levels of the Dose factor.

With an offset of −6 the control group is now further along the plateau of the curve (Figure 3.42). It is interesting to note that the log D_{50} and Hill slope parameter estimates have not changed between

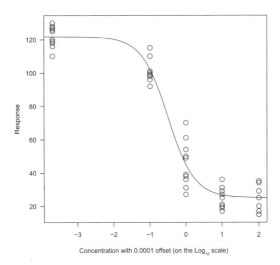

Figure 3.41. Scatterplot of response vs. dose, including the four-parameter dose-response logistic curve for Example 3.31, where the doses are plotted on the $\log_{10}$ scale. Analysis performed using an offset of 0.0001 to the levels of the Dose factor.

Table 3.13. Table of the four-parameter estimates for Example 3.31, calculated using an offset of 0.0001 to the Dose factor levels

Parameter	Estimate	Std error	t-value	p-value
Max/Min	121.854	2.705	45.05	< 0.001
Slope	-1.178	0.123	-9.55	< 0.001
logD50	-0.493	0.060	-8.16	< 0.001
Min/Max	25.153	2.114	11.90	< 0.001

the latter two analyses (where the control group was on the plateau of the curve in both cases); see Table 3.14. This highlights that the choice of offset does not influence the analysis as long as the control group resides on the plateau of the curve.

3.7 Nested designs

We now turn our attention to the fourth class of designs considered in this book, the nested designs. We define a design as nested if, within the experimental design, at least one factor is nested within another (Section 3.2.7.1). As mentioned earlier almost all experimental

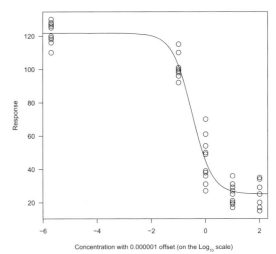

Figure 3.42. Scatterplot of all response vs. dose, including the four-parameter dose-response logistic curve for Example 3.31, where the doses are plotted on the $\log_{10}$ scale. Analysis performed using an offset of 0.000001 to the levels of the Dose factor.

Table 3.14. Table of the four-parameter estimates for Example 3.31 calculated using an offset of 0.000001 to the Dose factor levels

Parameter	Estimate	Std error	t-value	p-value
Max/Min	121.838	2.697	45.17	< 0.001
Slope	-1.177	0.123	-9.57	< 0.001
logD50	-0.493	0.060	-8.16	< 0.001
Min/Max	25.152	2.114	11.90	< 0.001

designs will contain at least one nested factor. Usually the Animal factor is nested within the Treatment factor. One set of animals is assigned to the treatment group and another set is assigned to the control group. So it is worth remembering that many designs can be defined as being nested. Perhaps the reason why the nested terminology is not more commonly known is that most statistical analysis packages automatically deal with designs with a single nested factor without requiring any user intervention. Hence the scientist need not be aware a nested design has been employed to run the statistical analysis.

Example 3.32: Testing fish-liver oil for vitamin D potency

A study was conducted to test a fish-liver oil additive in chick feed for its vitamin D potency (Mead *et al.*, 2003, p. 43). In the study 30 chicks were used. Each chick was fed a mash diet where 1% of the mash was made up of an additive: 20 animals received the fish-liver oil additive and as a control ten chicks received a standard cod-liver oil additive. The Treatment factor therefore had two levels (fish-liver oil additive and control). The chicks were divided into two groups, each of which was associated with one level of the Treatment factor; hence the Chick factor was nested within the Treatment factor. Animals numbered 1–20 were associated with the fish-liver oil additive level of the Treatment factor and animals numbered 21–30 were associated with the control level.

Chicks were randomly selected from the population of chicks, and then randomly assigned to the two treatments. Hence Chick is a random factor. It is usually the case that nested factors are random factors. We assume there are no systematic differences between the chicks (other than the chick-to-chick variability).

An informative way to understand a nested design is to visualise it. The design from Example 3.32 is illustrated in Figure 3.43.

The important point to make about the diagram, and this generalises to designs with more than one nested factor, is that the factor labels are unique (see Section 3.2.4.1). If two animals were labelled '1' in the diagram, then this would imply that animal '1' received both the control and the treatment at some point during the experiment. This idea is really useful when trying to identify if a factor is nested within another factor.

3.7.1 Types of nested designs

In this text we differentiate between two types of nested design: the single-order nested design and the higher-order nested design, although in reality the former is simply a special case of the latter.

3.7.1.1 Single-order nested design

In many animal experiments the only nested factor is the Animal factor, as was the case in Example 3.32. If a single measurement is taken on each animal, and each animal is assigned randomly to one of the treatment groups, then the Animal factor is nested within the Treatment factor. The animals are the experimental and observational units. This is true for one of the simplest designs where there are only two treatment groups and each

animal is allocated to one of them. Such an experiment could be analysed using a *t*-test. It is interesting to note at this stage that a nested design is required for one of the simplest and most commonly applied statistical tests.

3.7.1.2 Higher-order nested design

It may be the case that the scientist will be using a design where there is more than one nested factor. This can occur, for example, if there are multiple observations taken on each animal (this corresponds to Scenario 2 in Table 3.2). If the animals are measured repeatedly, but there is no between-animal structure to these measurements, then the design is a higher-order nested design.

Example 3.4 (continued): Assessing kidney lesions induced by p-aminophenol

Consider Example 3.4, where a histological technique was used to assess kidney lesions induced by p-aminophenol. Let us assume three sections of each rat's kidney were assessed and the number of lesions recorded. If the three sections were taken at specific positions for each animal, say the front, middle and back of the kidney, then there will be relationships between the sections across animals. If a factor (the Position factor) is constructed with levels 'front', 'middle' and 'back', then it will be crossed with the Animal factor. If, however, the three sections of each rat's kidney were taken at random positions across the kidney then there would be no relationship between the first result from the first animal and the first result from the second animal. In this case, as there are no relationships between the measurements made across animals, we say there is no between-animal structure to the measurements. The Section factor is therefore nested within the Animal factor.

Nested factors in a design are usually random factors. When there are multiple random factors in an experimental design, it can be useful to identify the amount of variability that can be attributed to each of these factors. If the amount of variability associated with each factor is quantified, then we can investigate the effect that changing the replication of the random factors has on the sensitivity of the statistical tests.

Replication is essential when performing an experiment for several reasons. To begin with we need replication of levels of the random factor(s) in order to estimate the variability of the responses. Without this

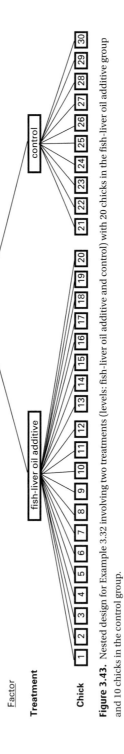

Figure 3.43. Nested design for Example 3.32 involving two treatments (levels: fish-liver oil additive and control) with 20 chicks in the fish-liver oil additive group and 10 chicks in the control group.

we would not be able to carry out the formal statistical tests described in Chapter 5. In certain situations, where there is more than one random factor present in the experimental design, it may be of interest to identify which factor is associated with the largest source of variability. The researcher can then concentrate resources on dealing with the variability associated with this factor. For example, consider an experiment involving a number of animals where four samples are taken from each animal. If the sample-to-sample variability proves to be larger than the animal-to-animal variability, then the researcher would be wise to investigate the cause of this first (and maybe increase the within-animal replication) rather than simply increasing animal numbers.

Before we consider these more complex questions we shall begin with the simpler case where there is only a single nested factor in the experimental design – namely the Animal (or more generally the factor whose levels correspond to the experimental units). In this case we may wish to investigate the replication of this factor, in other words how many animals do we need? This is perhaps one of the most important questions we should ask when designing animal experiments.

3.7.2 Sample size and power

Consider a design where the only nested factor is the Animal factor. It is important to consider the replication of the levels of the Animal factor to ensure that we use as few animals as possible without compromising the scientific validity of the study. This is perhaps the most important issue surrounding nested factors in animal experiments. It should be noted though that the method described in this section is the simplest example of the statistical investigation that can be performed when using higher-order nested designs involving multiple random factors.

If we assume that the animal-to-animal source of variability is the largest, then it is right to focus on the replication of the Animal factor ahead of all others. Historically much has been written about sample size calculation and it is generally recognised that sample sizes should be assessed before running a study. There are many software packages available to allow us to calculate suitable sample sizes.

3.7.2.1 Factors that influence sample size

Variability of the response
The variability of the response will influence the sample size. The greater the variability, the higher the sample size will be needed to achieve a suitable degree of statistical sensitivity. There are perhaps many factors within the control of the researcher that may increase the variability, for example the stress level of the animals, amount of handling and day of testing. The researcher should always look for ways to reduce the underlying variability of the data. For example, using a factorial design to investigate a number of factors in a pilot study will allow the researcher to identify which combination of factor levels gives the least variable responses. This combination can then be employed in future studies to help reduce the variability and hence the sample size.

Size of biological effect
The size of effect that is considered to be biologically relevant has a bearing on the sample size. If the researcher wants to identify subtle changes in the response, then relatively large sample sizes will be needed to achieve statistical significance. It may be difficult to decide in advance, but it is important to have some idea what constitutes a meaningful biological effect. The sample size can then be chosen so that only observed effects of this size (or greater) should be declared statistically significant. While it is not as likely to happen (due to the ethical constraints in animal experimentation) it is possible to use too many animals. If too many animals are used then the statistical tests become oversensitive and hence treatment effects may be declared statistically significant that are too small to be of any biological relevance. In reality though it is more likely that too few animals will be used rather than too many and hence the study will not be sensitive enough to detect meaningful biological effects (statistically). Choosing a sample size correctly so that biological relevance and statistical significance complement each other is vital if the conclusions from the study are to be scientifically valid.

Choice of experimental design
Experimental designs used correctly can help reduce the variability of the response. If we employ a suitable

experimental design, for example a block design, then we can control for nuisance sources of variability. By including a blocking factor in the experimental design (and then in the statistical analysis) we can reduce the underlying variability that we assess the treatment effects against. This can allow the researcher to reduce sample size.

Choice of statistical analysis

An appropriate statistical analysis, which uses all the relevant information recorded during the study, can help reduce sample size. For example, an analysis that includes baseline information as a covariate can account for animal differences that would otherwise inflate the variability of the response (see Section 5.4.6).

Significance level (Type I error)

The significance level, sometimes called the Type I error rate, is the probability (or chance) of finding a false positive result. It is the risk of declaring a result significant, and accepting the alternative hypothesis is true, when in fact the null hypothesis is true. Whenever we carry out an experiment there is always a risk that we may get an unusually positive set of results, just by chance. The significance level is the probability of this happening. It follows that the more certain you want to be that you are not reporting a false positive, the more animals you will require (all other things being equal). The usual convention is to set the risk of a false positive at 5%, although sometimes a 1% level may be selected. In other words we are prepared to accept the risk that five out of every hundred studies may result in a false positive conclusion. It is not possible to remove the risk of finding a false positive completely.

Statistical power

The statistical power of an experiment is the probability of rejecting the null hypothesis when it is false. It is the probability (or chance) of achieving a statistically significant result when conducting a study given that, in reality, there is a real effect (something we do not know before we begin the study of course!). A description of statistical power is given in Section 2.3.5.

The power of a study depends on the sample size. The larger the sample size the higher the statistical power and hence the greater the chance of identifying a genuine effect. The converse is also true, however. If there is a biologically relevant treatment effect but the sample size used is too small, say only two animals per group, then the chance of declaring the effect statistically significant is low. Usually a power of 70–90% is sufficient. This implies that if there is a genuine biologically relevant effect, then you have a 70–90% chance of identifying it when you conduct the study.

Before running a study it is always worthwhile investigating the power that the proposed experiment will have. If you discover that running a study with 12 animals per group gives only a 30% power for detecting a biologically relevant effect, and that to achieve 70% power 100 animals per group are required, then clearly it is not worth running the study. In such cases you should either:

• Find ways of reducing the variability before running experiments to test hypotheses.
• Increase the window of opportunity and hence the size of the biologically relevant effect.

Simply increasing the sample size to achieve the desired statistical power may not be the only answer, even though it is often the first thing a researcher will consider.

Type of response

When a researcher plans a study, one of the issues that will need to be considered is the type of response. The different types of response include continuous, discrete, ordinal, nominal and binary (see Section 3.2.1.1). As mentioned above, these responses contain differing amounts of information with continuous responses containing the most.

The type of response measured will also dictate the type of statistical analysis available to analyse the data. It is generally the case that the statistical tests routinely used by animal researchers for analysing continuous data are more powerful and more flexible than the tests employed when analysing binary data. It is also much easier to include extra information about the experimental design in the analysis of a continuous response, compared to the analysis of a more categorical one. As mentioned above this is of particular importance in animal experiments where we have almost total control over the experimental design. If at all possible, it is recommended that the scientist measures a continuous response. This way the sample size can be kept to a minimum (and the statistical analysis kept simple).

It may be the case that measuring a continuous response is more labour intensive than measuring a more categorical one. Perhaps we should accept this as a necessary compromise, if it achieves a reduction in total sample size.

Example 3.33: Dog socialisation study

A study was carried out to assess the benefits that can be gained from providing socialisation and training for laboratory dogs (Boxall *et al.*, 2004). Benefits include the dogs remaining calm during experimental procedures, which, it is contended, will lead to less variable results (and hence smaller group sizes). Several measures were taken including behavioural scores (ordinal measures) and two continuous responses: average behavioural score and heart rate. The animal behaviour score was measured on a ten-point numeric scale during several different activities. A score of eight was defined as the best score with higher scores indicating an over-excited dog, and lower scores indicating a nervous and timid dog.

The analysis of the data generated involved applying several statistical tests, due to the different types of response measured. It revealed that the socialisation programme had a significant effect on behaviour and welfare.

Care should be taken when comparing the results of statistical analyses as an analysis of continuous responses will be more powerful than an analysis of ordinal responses.

Hypothesis being tested

The hypothesis that is being tested can indirectly influence the sample size. Hypotheses that are tested can either be two-sided or one-sided (see Section 2.3.1). As described above, in a two-sided test the alternative hypothesis is that there is a difference between the two groups, in either direction. In a one-sided test we assume the difference between the two groups can only be in one direction, either negative or positive. If we assume that the direction of the treatment effect can only be in one direction, then in many statistical tests the *p*-value will be halved. Indirectly this implies that we can reduce the sample size. This approach is perhaps applied less often than it could be.

Uniformity of the animals

This is again linked strongly with the underlying variability of the response. The more uniform the animals are, the smaller the underlying variability of their responses will be, and hence the smaller the sample size will need to be. It is generally accepted that inbred strains are more heterogeneous than outbred strains and hence less variable. For a fuller discussion of these issues, see Festing *et al.* (2002, pp. 17–26).

3.7.2.2 Calculating sample sizes

There are many freeware packages available for the scientist who wants to investigate suitable sample sizes. Alternatively many of the commercial packages include power analysis techniques. A description of the power analysis module within InVivoStat is given in Section 6.8. For a description of some of the power analysis tools available if the responses measured are not numerical and continuous, see Cohen (1988, Chapters 3–7). In this section we will consider the power analysis that can be performed when the response is continuous and the assumptions of the parametric analysis are satisfied (see Section 5.4.1).

The sample size calculation procedure revolves around five variables: the power of the study, the Type I error rate, the underlying variability, the size of the relevant biological effect and the sample size itself. When assessing sample size and power we usually begin by fixing the Type I error rate at 5%. We then select or estimate a value for one of the other variables (normally the variability) and investigate the effect of changing the two remaining variables on the sample size.

Size of biological effect

Before starting the study the scientist should have some idea of the size of effect that is considered biologically relevant. This can be, for example, an actual effect size or a percentage change from control. If the scientist is interested in seeing a small change, say a 5% change from control, then a large sample size will be required. If, however, it is decided that the effect should be larger than, say 50%, for it to be considered biologically relevant, then a smaller sample size will be required. By selecting the biologically relevant effect size before running a study we can hopefully relate the statistical significance of the results obtained to the biological relevance. There is no point using too many animals, and hence achieving statistical significance, when the size of effect is too small to be of any biological relevance.

Statistical power

The scientist should try to conduct experiments that have a statistical power between 70% and 90%, although there is no fixed rule on the choice of these values. This power range implies that if the study were carried out repeatedly then, for a given biologically relevant effect, the experiment would be successful seven to nine times out of ten. If the power were 50% there is only an evens chance of achieving statistical success when running the study. This is the same chance as tossing a coin and getting heads. If we discover that the power of the study is even smaller, say 20%, then it is probably not worth running the study. With such a small chance of achieving statistical success (even if there is a real biologically relevant effect) then it is probably better to try to find ways to reduce the underlying variability first.

Variability

An initial estimate of the variability is required for most power analysis methodologies. This can be in the form of a variance or standard deviation estimate (see Section 5.2.2). The variability estimate calculated using data from a previous study can provide a good starting point, assuming the animal model and experimental procedures are the same. This variability estimate may be influenced by the experimental design employed. So if an influential blocking factor was used in a preliminary study, then this will have reduced the variability estimate. If future studies do not take into account this blocking factor, then the estimated sample sizes may be too small.

Other sources of information, such as those found in the literature, can provide an estimate of variability that the researcher can use before conducting any experiments. However, these sources will probably not provide a reliable estimate of the variability. It is usually better to use data generated from an experiment conducted by the scientist under their own laboratory

conditions. Another method that can be applied before any data has been collected is the resource equation, proposed by Mead (1988, p. 587) and discussed in Festing *et al.* (2002, p. 79).

Regardless of the method used, it should be remembered that the sample sizes calculated are only a guide to the final sample size. This is because the power analysis is based on an estimate of the underlying variability of the response. With animal studies this cannot always be a truly reliable estimate due to the small sample sizes that most studies employ.

The statistical test

We recommend powering the study under the assumption that the statistical analysis applied will be the *t*-test. The primary objective of many statistical analyses is comparing group means, so this seems a sensible test to consider. The *t*-test is probably less powerful than other tests available to the researcher, and so the power analysis will give a conservative sample size. We contend this is better than the alternative where the power analysis gives a sample size that is dangerously low. There are, however, many software tools now available for calculating sample sizes for various types of experimental design (Festing *et al.*, 2002, p. 77).

Example 3.34: Investigating mutations in transgenic mice

Festing *et al.* (2002, p. 55) describe a multi-laboratory study of mutations in transgenic mice. The study involved dosing 30 mice of a transgenic strain with either the vehicle or one of two doses of a mutagen, ten per treatment group. The DNA extracted was sent to five laboratories. Each laboratory estimated the number of mutations at a particular genetic locus in samples of DNA from two mice from each treatment group.

Unless accounted for in the design and analysis of the study, any differences between the five laboratories could artificially inflate the variability of the data generated. The researcher decided to replicate each of the treatments equally within the five laboratories, and hence block by laboratory in the statistical analysis to account for this.

In this discussion we shall analyse the data with and without the Laboratory blocking factor included. This highlights the benefit of accounting for differences between laboratories in the experimental design and then including the blocking factor in the statistical analysis.

To begin with the researcher needs to decide on what constitutes a biologically relevant effect. Assume that a 40% increase from control is required before the increase is considered biologically relevant. Assume also the significance level is fixed at 5%

Table 3.15. One-way ANOVA table for the analysis of Example 3.34

	Sums of squares	Degrees of freedom	Mean square	F-value	p-value
Dose	152.43	2	76.22	2.80	0.078
Residuals	734.09	27	27.19		

and the scientist intends to use a two-sided t-test to analyse the data generated.

Let us first consider the power analysis performed ignoring the Laboratory blocking factor. An estimate of the variability can be obtained from an ANOVA table (see Section 5.4.3.1). The residual mean square from the ANOVA table provides an estimate of the variance. The ANOVA table for the experiment, excluding the Laboratory blocking factor, is given in Table 3.15.

The variance estimate is 27.19 and hence the standard deviation is $\sqrt{27.19}$ = 5.21 (see Section 5.2.2.2). The mean of the vehicle group is 9.43. The power analysis module in InVivoStat reveals that a sample size of 8 achieves a power of 22%. Part of the output of the InVivoStat power analysis module is a power curve (see Figure 3.44). This plot shows the relationship between power and sample size for a given biologically relevant effect (40% change from control in this case).

We repeated the above calculation, but this time including the Laboratory blocking factor in the statistical analysis (see Section 6.3.3.3). The ANOVA table, with Laboratory included as a blocking factor, is given in Table 3.16.

By including the Laboratory blocking factor in the analysis the underlying variability is reduced. The new estimate of the variance is smaller than before. Including the Laboratory blocking factor in the analysis reduces the variability from 27.19 to 6.85. The new estimate of the standard deviation is $\sqrt{6.85}$ = 2.62

We now repeat the power analysis using this revised estimate of the variability. The result, taking into account the extra source of variability due to laboratories, is given in Figure 3.45.

A sample size of 15 gives a power of around 97%. This plot also suggests that a sample size of eight should provide sufficient power (around 75%). It can clearly be seen that by taking account of the experimental design in the statistical analysis, there was an increase in power and this will almost certainly allow the scientist to reduce the sample size in future studies.

3.7.2.3 When not to calculate the statistical power

Before we leave this section on calculating sample size and power, we highlight an issue with the power analysis methodology that is somewhat overlooked in the applied literature, namely the use of post-experiment power analysis as an analytical tool. This issue has

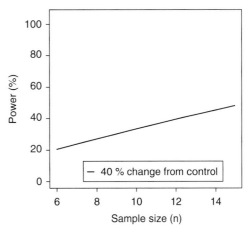

Figure 3.44. Power curve for a 40% change from control for Example 3.34 if the Laboratory blocking factor is ignored.

been considered in some detail by Hoenig and Heisey (2001).

We do not recommend using the post-experiment power analysis methodology when making analytical inferences about experimental results. In the power analyses described in the previous section, we did not assume the observed effect was the true effect. It was only an estimate of the true effect. Rather than conduct a power analysis using the observed effect, a predetermined biologically relevant effect was used and the sample size required to achieve statistical significance (when an effect of this magnitude occurs) was calculated. Power analysis methodology should therefore be used as a planning tool and not as an analytical device. If the reader is interested in understanding the reasoning behind this statement, then they should read either the following paragraphs or Hoenig and Heisey (2001).

The general principle, which may appear to be a sensible approach at first sight, is as follows: if a hypothesis test is performed and is found to be non-

Table 3.16. Two-way ANOVA table for the analysis of Example 3.34, including Laboratory as a blocking factor

	Sums of squares	Degrees of freedom	Mean square	F-value	p-value
Laboratory	576.45	4	144.11	21.03	< 0.001
Dose	152.43	2	76.22	11.12	< 0.001
Residuals	157.64	23	6.85		

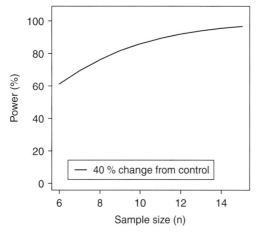

Figure 3.45. Power curve for a 40% change from control for Example 3.34 once the Laboratory blocking factor is taken into account.

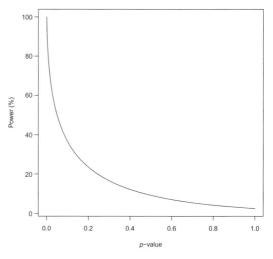

Figure 3.46. Relationship between observed power and statistical significance for a significance level of 5%.

significant, i.e. we accept the null hypothesis that there is no effect, then a power analysis is performed to aid in the interpretation of the non-significant result. If the observed power is low, then the argument follows that this shows weak evidence that the null hypothesis is true even if the hypothesis test was not significant (the p-value was greater than the significance level). In other words, we did not see a significant effect (hence the null hypothesis is accepted) but as we were not likely to find a significant effect (because the power was low) this does not imply the null hypothesis is necessarily true.

Unfortunately this argument is misleading. When performing a power analysis we suggest the researcher should identify the biologically relevant effect beforehand. This is a real effect that is assumed to be important and is not a data-driven

observed effect. The power analysis methodology described above relies on the assumption that the effect size used in the calculation is a true effect and not one that has been estimated (or observed) from experimental data.

When performing a power analysis using the observed effect (rather than the true effect) the observed significance level determines the observed power (they are mathematically linked): as one goes up the other goes down. So high p-values necessarily correspond to low observed power. If you have calculated one of these values you can immediately generate the other. Considering both does not add to your understanding of the experimental results. Figure 3.46 shows this relationship. From the argument described above if the power is low, then we would conclude there is weak evidence that the null hypothesis is true. But low power equates to high p-values, and most researchers accept that high p-values indicate the null hypothesis is likely to be true!

Figure 3.46 highlights another interesting feature of the observed power. When the p-value for the statistical test equals 0.05 (i.e., it is just statistically significant at the 5% level) then the observed power is only 50%. We may consider this power to be uncomfortably low, even if we have achieved statistical significance in our experiment. But again this is to confuse the observed effect with the biologically relevant true effect. The power analysis methodology is not being applied correctly. If we assume that the observed effect is actually the true effect, then if we repeat the experiment there is a 50% chance of finding a larger effect than the one observed in the first experiment and a 50% chance of finding a smaller effect (assuming the response is symmetrically distributed around the true effect). Now as we have achieved a significance level of 0.05 in the first experiment then (for the given variability and sample size) in the next experiment there is a 50% chance of getting a p-value smaller than 0.05 and a 50% chance of getting a p-value larger than 0.05. The power to detect a true effect is therefore only 50%. We have a 50% chance of achieving a significance result, assuming the effect is real.

3.7.3 Higher-order nested designs

It is often the case in animal experiments that treatment effects are tested against the animal-to-animal variability. Animals are randomly assigned to treatments and so we assess the significance of the treatment effect by comparing it to the underlying animal-to-animal variability. With only a few exceptions, the Animal factor will be nested within Treatment, Block and any other fixed factors within the study. This framework applies even if there are within-animal nested random factors within the design. So it is probably right that our attention, when investigating the random factors, should focus on the Animal factor. However, there are certain situations where more complex nested designs are employed. In these situations it is vital that we correctly identify the type of design that is being used; otherwise the statistical analysis may be invalid. Once identified

we can generalise the sample size calculations given in the previous section to investigate these more complex designs.

3.7.3.1 Identifying nested factors

When a scientist starts to plan an experiment the questions that need to be answered should be considered. This will influence the choice of design. However, there will also be practical and/or animal model-based constraints that dictate features of the experimental design. Such constraints may introduce nested factors and it is important that the scientist recognises this by considering the structure of the experimental design. For example, it may be the case that each blood sample taken from an animal is assayed in triplicate. If animals are allocated to different treatments, then there are (at least) two random factors: Animal is nested with Treatment and Assay is nested within Animal.

Example 3.35: Dietary study in white pekin ducklings

A study was conducted to assess the effect of cholecalciferol and phosphorus in the regulation of intestinal mucosa phytase in white pekin ducklings (Onyango and Adeola, 2011). There were 96 ducklings, group housed in six blocks of four cages, four ducklings per cage. The allocation to blocks was based on duckling body weight (see Section 4.2.1). Four corn-soya bean mash diets, consisting of all combinations of cholecalciferol at 0 μg/kg or 75 μg/kg and phosphorus at 3.6 g/kg or 7 g/kg were randomly assigned to the four cages within each block. As the original authors comment, the diets were administered to cages of ducklings, so the cages are the experimental units. For the purposes of this discussion we shall ignore the blocking factor. This (simplified) experimental design is described in Figure 3.47.

Ducklings 1 to 4 were housed in cage 1, ducklings 5 and 8 in cage 2 and so on. So Duckling is nested within Cage. Now the animals housed in cages 1 to 6 were administered the cholecalciferol at 0 μg/kg + phosphorus at 3.6 g/kg diet whereas the animals in cages 7 to 12 were given the cholecalciferol at 0 μg/kg + phosphorus at 7 g/kg diet. Hence Cage is nested within Diet. If we assume that the cages were selected at random from a large set of cages, and the animals were assigned to the cages (within block) at random, then Cage and Duckling will both be random factors.

Note the importance of the factor labels in the above diagram. Consider a (rather implausible) study that consisted of only six cages with 16 ducklings housed in each cage. If the animals were fed individually, where four animals per cage were given each diet, we would say that the Cage and Diet factors were crossed. Each level of Cage would be associated with all four levels of the Diet factor and

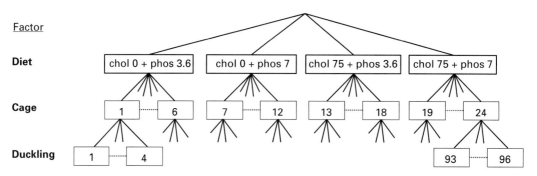

Figure 3.47. Nested design for Example 3.35 involving fixed factor Diet and two nested factors Cage and Duckling within Cage. In the design there were six cages per diet and four ducklings per cage.

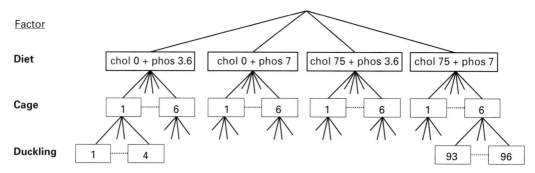

Figure 3.48. Nested design involving crossed factors Diet and Cage and nested factor Duckling. In the design there were six cages with four ducklings per cage per diet.

all levels of the Diet factor would be present in each cage (animals receiving all diets are housed in each cage). The diagrammatical representation of this design is similar to the one above, with the major difference being the labelling of the cages. The diagram is given in Figure 3.48.

In general if the factor labels are repeated, as the levels of the Cage factor are in Figure 3.48, then one of the factors is not nested within the other but the two factors are crossed with each other. A more appropriate way to visualise the data would be using a 2D diagram as given in Figure 3.49. The top of the structure consists of a 6 by 4 grid made up of all combinations of the levels of Cage and Diet. The individual ducklings are included underneath this structure to indicate the nesting relationship.

As a final comment, if the Cage label in Figure 3.49 is replaced by 'Block' and the grey boxes are used to

indicate the 24 cages, then the design structure presented is the same as that employed in the original paper.

In practice, the importance of the Cage factor depends on the length of the experiment and whether or not the cages are the experimental units. If the cages are not the experimental units, and the study is a short-term study, then there probably will not be differences between the cages and hence the Cage factor can be excluded from the analysis. In other words the cage-to-cage variability will not be influential and hence can be ignored. This will simplify the design and the analysis considerably. However, differences between cages may become more pronounced in long-term studies and hence cannot be ignored so easily. If the cages are the experimental units (i.e. treatments are administered to cages of animals rather than individual animals)

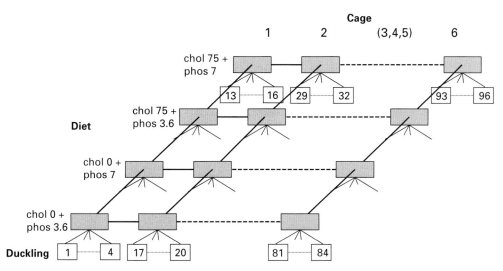

Figure 3.49. Nested design involving crossed factors Diet and Cage and nested factor Duckling. In the design there were six cages with four ducklings per cage per diet. If the Cage label is replaced by Block then the structure is that used by Onyango and Adeola (2011).

then we argue Cage should be included in the analysis regardless of its influence.

Identifying whether the experimental design has more than one nested factor is important, especially in animal research. Ask yourself, are you taking multiple random samples per animal? When this is the case we can generalise the question we asked in the previous section about sample sizes. Rather than consider the number of animals required, we can investigate the appropriate number of animals and also samples within animals. It may be the case, although not common, that increasing the replication of the samples taken from each animal will influence the statistical power more than simply increasing animal numbers.

3.7.3.2 Investigating the sources of variability in higher-order nested designs

In the following sections we shall describe some of the statistical investigations that can be carried out when using a higher-order nested design. We aim to do this without too much mathematical detail. The interested reader can find more technical derivations in

many texts, for example Snedecor and Cochran (1989, pp. 237–40) and Montgomery (1997, pp. 506–19). In this discussion we shall concentrate on issues pertinent to the non-statistician; see also Festing *et al.* (2002, p. 53).

There are two aspects of the design that we shall consider:

- The amount of variability (in the observations) that can be attributed to each of the random factors, the so-called *variance components*.
- The effect of replication (of the levels of the random factors) on the power of the statistical tests. For this we consider the variability of the experimental units, which is made up of a combination of the variance components.

For example, an experiment was conducted to assess the effectiveness of several types of anti-inflammatory skin cream, where cream is administered to several shaved areas of each animal. How much variability in the individual observations is due to animal-to-animal differences, and how much is due to the area-to-area differences within the animal? Should we apply cream to three areas of skin on each animal or four? More importantly, can we reduce the total number of animals required by testing on multiple areas on each animal (assuming there is no additional cost to the animal) and yet still assess the treatment effects with sufficient statistical power?

In the case where the design involves a single random factor (usually Animal), the questions around variance components and what replication to use simplify to performing a sample size and power analysis, as described in Section 3.7.2. As we have only one measurement per animal we can only get an overall estimate of the (animal-to-animal) variability. We cannot break this down into other within-animal sources of variability as there is no replication within-animal. However, this is not the case in higher-order nested designs. In this section we shall develop this power and sample size methodology to these types of experimental design.

3.7.3.3 Variance components: estimating the observational unit variability

Let us assume we only have random factors present in a higher-order nested design. The methodology described here can be generalised to more complex designs that also include fixed factors (such as the split-plot designs, see Section 3.9) but that is beyond the scope of this text (Montgomery, 1997, pp. 519–29).

As any researcher knows, there will always be variability associated with experimental data. Even though all the animals are housed in the same conditions, have the same body weight (within a given range) and are from the same inbred strain, there will always be differences in their responses. There may be many reasons why the results are different, and we call these the *sources of variability*. Some, such as the animal source, will probably be more influential than others but all contribute to the differences between the observations taken. In Section 2.1 we discussed trying to give a lecture when there are a number of alarms making noise in the room. These alarms are analogous to the sources of variability in an experiment. To get your message across in the lecture room, the key is to try to identify the loudest alarm and turn it down first. The same is true in an experimental setting. We need to identify which source of variability is the largest, and deal with that first. Nested designs provide a framework for doing this.

Consider a single-order nested design where there is only one random factor, namely Animal, where the animals are the observational units. The random Animal factor is used to quantify the variability associated with differences between the animals. The variability could be due to the animals, but it could be due to other sources, such as measurement variability. As we only have one measurement per animal, it is impossible to disentangle these other sources of variability as the replication within-animal is only one. To estimate the magnitude of any within-animal sources of variability we need to take multiple samples (holding the other factors constant) and quantify the differences (or variability) within these responses.

Now consider a higher-order nested design where we have more than one random factor nested within another. As we now have replication within-animal, the variability of each individual observation in the dataset can be broken down into a set of variance components. Each variance component corresponds to the proportion of the observational unit variability that is associated with that random factor. We can perform this breakdown because of the replication of the levels of the random factors within the nested design.

Variability of the observational units = Sum of the variance components

There is a mathematical way to calculate estimates of the variance components. An interested reader should consult Montgomery (1997, pp. 514–15) for details. However, conceptually we can derive an estimate for the within-animal variability by considering the spread of the observations within each animal. If we then average the within-animal measurements (i.e. generate one mean response per animal) then the variability of these means will give us a measure of the between-animal variability.

Example 3.36: Assessing joint pain using applied pressure

An experiment was conducted to assess the validity of using the pressure application measurement (PAM) device to quantify joint hypersensitivity in rats (Barton *et al.* 2007). It was hypothesised that readouts from this method would correlate with the established weight distribution readout obtained using an incapacitance tester and hence be a potential animal model for chronic joint pain in humans. The aim of the study was to determine if PAM was able to detect a Freund's complete adjuvant (FCA)-induced hypersensitivity in the knee joints of rats and compare the results obtained using PAM with the weight distribution approach. In the published paper several treatments were tested: prednisolone (1, 3 or 10 mg/kg), morphine (3 mg/kg) and celecoxib (15 mg/kg); however, we shall focus on the pilot study, which had two groups, FCA and control.

In the original experiment 16 rats were randomly assigned to one of two treatment groups, either the control or FCA treatment. Hypersensitivity was then assessed over 28 days using both the PAM and weight distribution approaches. We shall consider the responses measured on day 1; the repeated measures aspects of the experiment will be discussed in Section 3.8.1.3. On each day post-dose, three measurements were taken per animal per method. The design is illustrated in Figure 3.50.

The design consisted of several factors, related in a hierarchically nested way. These included Treatment, Animal (within Treatment) and Trial (within Animal). The two sources of variability were the animal-to-animal variability and the trial-to-trial variability.

The procedure used to assess of the sources of variability for the PAM response, using InVivoStat, is described in Section 6.14. From this analysis it was found that for the PAM response, the variance component for animals was 7542 (or 23% of the total variability) and for the trials was 25704 or (77% of the total variability).

This implied that much of the variability observed in the individual measurements was due to trial-to-trial differences rather than animal-to-animal differences. In other words the individual animals all behaved (on average) in a similar way, but the multiple measurements taken within an animal varied considerably. This is an interesting result; the researcher should investigate the cause of this variability and try to reduce it in future studies. However, if no obvious source is identified, then by taking multiple measurements per animal the effect of this variability can be taken into account in the statistical analysis.

3.7.3.4 Predicting the experimental unit variability

In the majority of statistical analyses of animal experiments the aim is to test the size of the effect of interest against the experimental unit variability, i.e. the animal-to-animal variability in most experiments. If a nested design has been employed then, as discussed above in Section 1.3.3, we first need to summarise all the within-animal measurements to obtain a single summary result per animal (this summary is usually the mean). We then compare the size of the effect of interest against the variability of these summary measures (the experimental unit variability), using a suitable statistical analysis procedure.

In higher-order nested designs, the variability of these summary measures (for example the mean result for each animal) is a linear combination of:

1. the variance component of the random factor that corresponds to the experimental unit (animals in this case);

2. any random factors that are nested within the factor that corresponds to the experimental unit.

The exact combination of variance components that are added together to produce the variability of the experimental units depends on the replication within the experimental design. So if we can estimate the individual variance components then we can predict the variability of the experimental units for any replication of the random factors within the nested design.

For example, consider a higher-order nested design involving Animal and Assay nested within Animal. Assume that the animals are the experimental units (i.e. treatments are tested against the animal-to-animal variability). Each sample from each animal is assayed multiple times. By calculating the variance components for Animal and Assay we can assess the effect that varying the number of animals and the number of assays within-animal has on the variability at the Animal level of the design. This is important because it is this variability that the treatments are tested against.

Example 3.37: Comet assay to assess genotoxicity

The comet assay is a test that assesses the genetic damage caused by novel compounds (Smith *et al.*, 2008). To begin with animals are assigned to one of the treatment groups. Following treatment, the animals are humanely killed and cells are harvested from the target organ. These cells are placed on a number of slides, normally three slides per animal, with 50 cells per animal tested on each slide. Each slide is placed on an electrophoresis plate for 20 minutes before electrophoresis (0.7 V/cm, 300 mA) for a further 20 minutes. If the cells have suffered genetic damage, then the DNA will unwind from the cell causing the cell to appear comet-like. For a general discussion of the design and analysis of the comet assay, see Wiklund and Agurell (2003) and Bright *et al.* (2011).

Assume that the experiment is conducted using a animals per treatment group, s slides per animal and c cells per slide. Also let VCa, VCs and VCc correspond to the variance components for Animal, Slide and Cell, respectively. It can be shown that the variability at each level of the nested design is given by:

$$\text{Animal-to-animal variability} = cs\, VC_a + c\, VC_s + VC_c \qquad (3.5)$$
$$\text{Slide-to-slide variability} = c\, VC_s + VC_c$$
$$\text{Cell-to-cell variability} = VC_c$$

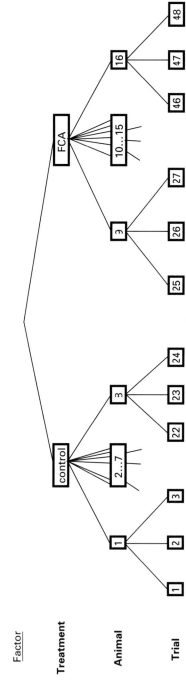

Figure 3.50. Nested design for Example 3.36, involving fixed factor Treatment and nested random factors Animal and Trial.

Notice how the linear combinations of variance components make up the variability observed at each level of the nested design. They are governed by the replication of the levels of the random factors within the design.

The individual animals are the experimental units in the comet assay, so the treatment effects will be tested against the animal-to-animal variability. When investigating the effect of varying the replication within the design, it is this level of variability that we need to focus on.

3.7.3.5 Investigating alternative nested designs

If you can estimate the variance components (using an existing dataset) then you can assess the effect that varying the replication of the random factors will have on the experimental unit variability. For example, in Example 3.37, if we have an estimate of the variance components, then we can use the above formulae to predict the magnitude of the animal-to-animal variability when c and s are varied. This estimate can then be used, in conjunction with the sample size a, to predict the statistical power of the tests that would be achieved using that replication of the random factors within the experimental design

So for a given biologically relevant difference, we can answer the following important question:

If I increase the replication of slides within-animal, can I reduce the total number of animals I require without compromising the statistical power?

While it is possible to investigate many types of design in this way, for complex designs involving multiple nested and crossed factors it is probably best to consult a professional statistician. For the higher-order nested designs described in this section, the scientist may want to attempt such an analysis themselves. A way of analysing these designs is available within InVivoStat's nested design analysis module (see Section 6.14).

Example 3.36 (continued): Assessing joint pain using applied pressure

Returning to Example 3.36, it was decided to investigate the effect of varying the number of animals within each group and also the number of trials per animal. Currently the design consists of eight animals per group with three trials per animal. It was decided to investigate the effect of varying the number of animals between

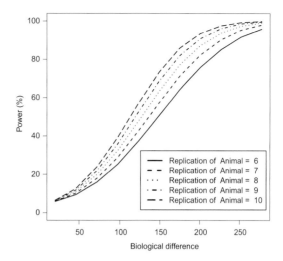

Figure 3.51. Plot of the power curves for Example 3.36 when increasing the replication of animals while holding the number of trials per animal at three.

six and ten while measuring each animal between one and six times.

For the PAM response, it was shown that there was a slight benefit when the number of animals in each treatment group was increased (approximately a 5% increase in power). Figure 3.51 shows the power curves for increasing the number of animals per group, where the number of trials per animal was fixed at three. Figure 3.52 shows the power curves for increasing the number of trials for each animal, where the number of animals per group was fixed at eight. This analysis revealed the benefit of increasing the number of trials per animal from three to six. There is approximately a 15% increase in power. Just to emphasise this result: *we have increased the power of the statistical test without increasing the number of animals required.* It also highlights that taking more than one measurement per animal (and averaging the within-animal measurements) is beneficial as the power when only one measurement is taken is much lower. In our experience this conclusion holds in most experimental situations. Taking more than one measurement per animal is usually beneficial.

The power curves in Figure 3.52 assume the number of animals within each group is eight. Note the large increase in statistical power that can be gained by increasing the number of trials per animal from one to three.

In the original paper it was found that by increasing the number of trials from three to five per animal per day, there was an improvement in the precision of the PAM method. This was in contrast to increasing the number of animals per group from eight to ten, which appeared to have little effect; see Barton *et al.* (2007) for more details. In contrast the weight distribution readout was improved by increasing the number of animals per group. Increasing the number

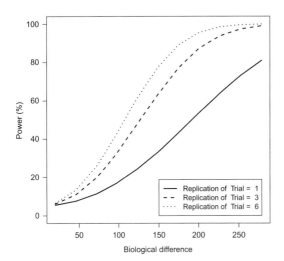

Figure 3.52. Plot of the power curves for Example 3.36 when increasing the replication of trials for each animal while holding the number of animals per group at eight.

of trials for each animal had little impact on the statistical power of this response as the triplicate measurements taken within each animal were all numerically similar.

3.7.3.6 Pseudo-replication

There is one pitfall that the unwary researcher may encounter if the correct nesting structure within the experimental design is not identified and that is pseudo-replication (Lazic, 2010). If the researcher does not identify and/or ignores the nesting structure, then the statistical analysis will be incorrect and the results potentially misleading. For a discussion of some of the more practical aspects of pseudo-replication, see Ruxton and Colegrave (2006, pp. 43–9) and Cumming *et al.* (2007).

Pseudo-replication occurs, more generally, when we think we have collected more information, using our experimental design, than we actually have. In many analyses, see Section 5.4.1.4, we assume that all the observations in the dataset are independent of each other. So if we analyse a dataset with ten observations, then we assume (by independence) that we have ten separate pieces of information. However, this may not be the case in certain practical situations. Failure to satisfy the

independence condition, or take the non-independence into account in the statistical analysis, results in pseudo-replication and hence incorrect statistical results.

Example 3.38: Atherosclerosis study

A long-term study was carried out to assess the effect of a novel compound on the build-up of atherosclerotic lesions within the aorta of rabbits. Such an experiment was discussed in Festing *et al.* (2002, p. 33). Three drug treatments were administered to the rabbits, one drug treatment per rabbit, with four animals receiving each treatment. Post mortem, the aorta was removed and cut into a number of *en face* sections. Five of the sections per animal were selected and the lesion area in each section measured, i.e. 60 sections were measured in total. The design consisted of Section nested within Animal and Animal nested within Treatment (Figure 3.53).

Assume the results from the 60 individual sections were used in the statistical analysis and the researcher ignored the nested structure of the experimental design. The treatment effects were assessed against the variability of the 60 sections using one-way ANOVA (see Section 5.4.3.1). The problem is that one of the assumptions of this statistical analysis is that the observations are independent (see Section 5.4.1.4), i.e. there are 60 separate pieces of information available for the analysis. Of course in reality the sections measured within each animal will be more related than those measured between-animal. The 20 measurements taken within each treatment group, using this design, were probably less variable than if they had been taken from 20 individual animals (one section per animal). This is because responses measured within-animal are likely to be more similar than responses taken from different animals. Hence if we ignore the nesting structure in the analysis, we may artificially lower the estimate of the variability. It is possible that this can result in false positive conclusions being drawn from the analysis.

As animals were dosed individually then the animals were the experimental units. The drug treatment effects should be assessed against the animal-to-animal variability. This implies we should begin the analysis by averaging the five observations for each animal before the statistical analysis begins. The analysis will then be made on the 12 average observations, one per animal, and not the individual 60 responses. Unfortunately it is almost certain that this correct analysis will not give as significant results as the incorrect analysis using the 60 observations.

Pseudo-replication and the hypothesis tested

While pseudo-replication can influence the statistical tests, through the variability estimate, it can also influence the underlying hypothesis that is being tested. If the scientist is not aware of this issue then the hypotheses actually tested may be different to the ones planned. We describe three related ways that this can happen.

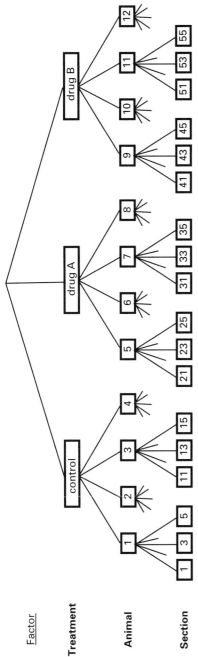

Figure 3.53. Nested design for Example 3.38, involving fixed factor Treatment and nested random factors Animal and Section.

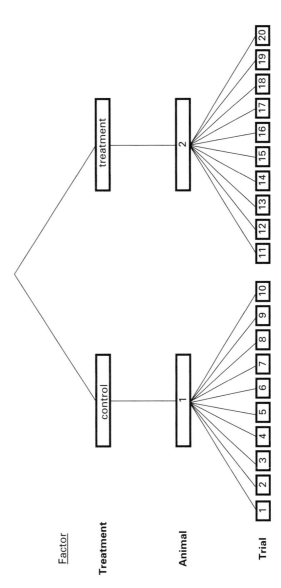

Figure 3.54. Nested design for Example 3.39 involving fixed factor Treatment and nested random factors Animal (with no replication) and Trial.

No replication of the experimental units This may appear a little extreme, but it may occasionally be the case that practical aspects of the experimental process imply that within the nested design the actual replication of the experimental units is one. This implies the hypothesis we are testing may be influenced (or completely confounded) with other factors.

Example 3.39: Odour span recognition

Consider a behavioural experiment, where rats are tested using the odour span recognition paradigm. The experimental designs described within this discussion are loosely based on the work of Dudchenko *et al.* (2000) although we stress the experimental designs we describe are not those used in the original paper.

During the acclimatisation phase, rats are trained to dig for food rewards in cups with novel scented sand. On a test day, the rats are first shown a cup of unscented sand with a food reward buried inside. Once the reward has been found the rat is removed from the test arena and a second cup (with a novel scented sand containing a food reward) is introduced. The rat is re-introduced and, in theory, if it remembers correctly, will dig for the food reward in the cup containing the novel scented sand. If the rat successfully finds the food reward, then it is removed from the test arena and a third cup with another novel scent is introduced. The test continues until the rat digs in a cup it has already investigated. The final response recorded is the number of trials successfully completed before the rat digs in a cup that it has already investigated. A set of 27 different scented sands was prepared in advance for the experiment.

Assume an experiment was conducted to compare two treatments. As the rats used in the experiment proved to be difficult to train, the researcher decided to use only two animals, one rat per treatment. Each animal was dosed individually and then assessed ten times over a period of time, each time with a random sequence of novel scents. The 20 observations, ten per animal, were then compared. An illustration of the design is given in Figure 3.54.

Clearly the results of this experiment will be misleading. The hypothesis that the researcher hoped to test was that the treatments were different, but the treatment effect is completely confounded with the animal effect. Is the treatment effect observed simply due to differences between the two animals? When conducting a statistical test such as this, we assume that we are sampling (randomly) from the wider population of rats. So any differences we observe experimentally reflect, in some sense, the wider population. Clearly this is not the case in this experiment. In reality we have answered the question: 'Are these two rats, each on a unique treatment, different?' We have not answered the wider question as to whether the treatments are different.

No replication of the experimental conditions The previous example may seem a little obvious; hopefully readers will appreciate the need to increase sample sizes beyond one. However, the issue may be more general than simply the level of replication of the animals.

Example 3.39 (continued): Odour span recognition

Assume the researcher now increases the number of rats to ten per group. It was also decided that the number of trials per animal should be reduced from ten to one. All rats were assessed using the same sequence of novel scents. While there is now replication of the experimental units, there is only a single replication of the experimental conditions. Only a single series of novel scents was used in the experiment (Figure 3.55).

So while the researcher believed the hypothesis: 'Are the treatments different?' was being assessed, in fact it was a more restrictive one: 'Are the treatments different when using this sequence of tests?' In practice, the former (more general) hypothesis is of interest and this can be tested if the series of scents is randomly generated for each rat. This was the approach taken by Dudchenko *et al.* (2000). Note by randomising the sequence of scents we have confounded the effects of Animal and Sequence, so the animal-to-animal variability that we test the treatments against will be inflated by any sequence differences (Figure 3.56). This is the price we pay for generalising the hypothesis. Alternatively, if the rats were tested multiple times, under different sequences, then we could separate the animal-to-animal variability and the sequence-to-sequence variability and see if the original confounding was a problem.

So in conclusion, replication allows us to answer more general questions. If we fail to replicate, and pseudo-replicate instead, then we can only answer more mundane questions that probably have obvious answers. For example, failing to replicate animals in the odour experiment left the scientist being able to answer the question: 'Are the two animals different?' It was perhaps not surprising that two animals gave different results (regardless of treatment). In the second version of the experiment described in this section it was the scent order that was not replicated, so again the hypothesis tested was not the one that the researcher had originally intended to evaluate. While we should randomly select multiple experimental units from a wider population, the same is also true of the experimental conditions, if we wish our hypotheses and hence conclusions to be valid in general.

Unreliable estimated results due to nesting relationship In the previous section we discussed how

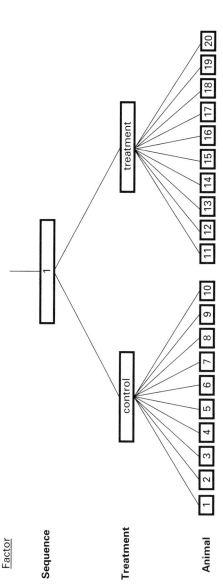

Figure 3.55. Nested design for Example 3.39, involving fixed factor Treatment and random factors Animal and Sequence. Treatments assessed using the same sequence of novel scents.

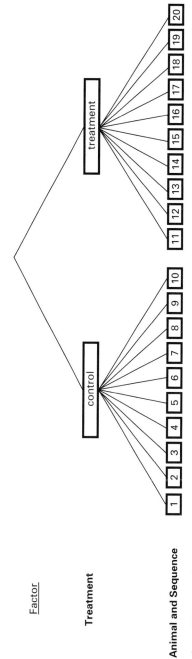

Figure 3.56. Nested design for Example 3.39, involving fixed factor Treatment and nested random confounded factors Animal, Sequence and Trial.

failure to identify the nesting relationships may result in an incorrect estimate of the variability being used in the statistical analysis. This will lead to unreliable test results. However, if the nesting relationship is not taken into account, then the estimated overall effects observed may not be reliable either.

Example 3.39 (continued): Odour span recognition

Returning to Example 3.39, assume that two rats were assigned to each group, with ten trials per animal. An illustration of the design is given in Figure 3.57.

Let us also assume that the two animals in the control group remembered more scents than those in the treatment group. This could be caused by the treatment itself or just natural variation in the rat population. If the nested relationships in the experimental design had not been identified, then the researcher may have compared the 20 treated results to the 20 control results. If 20 independently treated results are (on average) lower than 20 control results then, depending on the magnitude of the variability, this may be seen as clear evidence of an effect. However, in this example there are only four truly independent responses (corresponding to the four animals). The observed difference between the treatments is based on two pairs of observations. The difference is therefore less reliable. If another five rats per treatment were tested, giving a more reliable picture of the treatment effect on the population of rats, then this conclusion may change considerably.

With only two rats per treatment (even if we measured them at multiple occasions) we are effectively testing to see if the treatment varies between those two rats, and cannot generalise that to the wider population with any degree of certainty.

3.8 Repeated measures and dose-escalation designs

There are many ways we can repeatedly measure the animals in an experiment. Table 3.2 summarises seven different scenarios that lead to different families of experimental design. In this section we concentrate on the repeated measures designs (Scenario 1 in Table 3.2) and related dose-escalation designs (Scenario 6 in Table 3.2). We will then go on to consider some more complicated examples of repeated measures designs.

3.8.1 Repeated measures designs

The simplest and most common example of a repeated measures design involves randomly assigning the animals to treatments and then measuring them repeatedly over time. The experimental design involves three factors: Treatment, Animal and Time. Animal is nested within Treatment as each animal is assigned to only one group. Also Animal and Treatment are crossed with Time as each animal, and hence each treatment, is measured at multiple time points.

In general, we define a design as being a *repeated measures design* if it consists of:

1. A repeated factor that indexes the levels of the repeated measurements (for example the Time factor).
2. An experimental design, such as a block, nested or factorial design, that is assessed repeatedly across the levels of the repeated factor. We define this as the core design. The observational units of the core design are measured repeatedly at the levels of the repeated factor.

As well as these two properties, we define a repeated measures design as being a *nested repeated measures design* if there are also:

3. Additional factor(s) nested within the combination of the levels of the repeated factor and the factor that corresponds to the observational units of the core design.

We shall consider these properties in more detail in the next sections.

3.8.1.1 The repeated factor

The repeated factor is the factor that indexes the levels of the repeated measurements. Examples of repeated factors include: Time (when animals are measured over time at specific time points), Brain region (when effects are measured in different brain regions) and Task (when the animal model involves testing animals under a sequence of different conditions, for example the attentional set shifting task (Hatcher *et al.*, 2005)).

We usually assume that the repeated factor is a fixed categorical factor. It is normally crossed with all other experimental factors, including, crucially, the factor that corresponds to the experimental units. For example, the levels of the repeated factor are shared across the animals (all animals are measured at the same time points). This differentiates repeated measures designs from nested designs, discussed

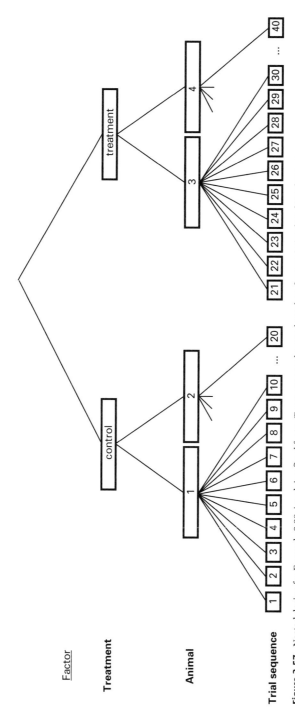

Figure 3.57. Nested design for Example 3.39, involving fixed factor Treatment and nested random factors Animal and Trial sequence.

in Section 3.7.3. In a nested design the factor that indexes the within-animal observations is random and nested within the Animal factor. Animals do not share the levels of the factor that indexes the within-animal measurements.

The levels of the repeated factor are not randomised and this differentiates a repeated factor from almost all other experimental factors. As the levels cannot be randomised (the hippocampus level of the Brain region factor cannot be randomly assigned to any other brain region, and day 1 must come before day 2) there will be spatial interrelationships between the repeatedly measured responses. In the statistical analysis we may need to take these interrelationships into account and this leads to the repeated measures analysis techniques (see Section 5.4.4).

Example 3.40: Assessing the effect of repeated stress on rat body weight

An experiment was conducted to assess the effect of repeated stress on rat body weight (see Harris *et al.*, 1998). Twelve adult male Sprague Dawley rats were randomly assigned to two groups based on body weight using a stratified randomisation (see Section 4.2.1). The first group was exposed to a moderate stressor by placing them in a plastic restraining tube for three hours on three consecutive days. A second non-restrained control group was housed in a shoebox cage for 3 hours. Following the three days of restraint the animals' body weights were measured daily for 40 days. The repeated factor was therefore Day (levels: days 1–40). The experiment revealed that stress had a permanent effect on adult rat body weight.

3.8.1.2 The core experimental design

The core experimental design is the design that is assessed repeatedly across the levels of the repeated factor. Any type of experimental design can be a core design, including block, nested, factorial, crossover, dose-escalation and even another repeated measures design.

We define a design as being a repeated measures design if the core experimental design is measured repeatedly while all factors that define the core design, and relationships between the core design factors, remain unchanged. Hence the core experimental design does not change across the levels of the repeated factor. Effectively the core experimental design at the first level of the repeated factor is assumed to be the same design at all other levels of the repeated factor. The repeated factor is therefore crossed with all the factors that define the core experimental design.

The experimental units of the repeated measures design are the same as the experimental units of the core design.

Example 3.40 (continued): Assessing the effect of repeated stress on rat body weight

The core experimental design for the experiment was a single-order nested design consisting of the factors Stress (levels: restrained and control) and Animal nested within Stress. The repeated measures design consisted of this core design with the repeated factor Day at 40 levels. Animals were the experimental units of both the core design and the repeated measures design and the animals on each day correspond to the observational units of the repeated measures design. The Day factor was taken as a fixed factor and was crossed with both Stress and Animal. The data generated were analysed using a repeated measures analysis approach to take account of spatial interrelationships between the within-animal measurements (see Section 5.4.4). An illustration of the core design and the repeated measures design (including only two days for clarity) is given in Figure 3.58 and contains both nested and crossed relationships.

3.8.1.3 Nested repeated measures designs

It is sometimes the case that an animal is measured multiple times at each level for the repeated factor. For example, blood samples are taken repeatedly over time, one per day for several days. The repeated factor would then be Day. If each of these samples is then assayed in triplicate, there will be an additional factor (Sample) that is nested within the combinations of the levels of Animal and Day. These designs are sometimes known as nested repeated measures designs.

As a rule of thumb, in cases where there are nested factors such as these it is recommended to average up to the experimental units at each level of the repeated factor (i.e. calculate the average result for each animal on each day) prior to conducting a statistical analysis. Once this averaging has been completed we may also want to generate suitable summary measures across time using these averages (see Section 5.4.4.2).

Example 3.36 (continued): Assessing joint pain using applied pressure

In Example 3.36, described in Section 3.7.3.3, we focused on estimating the sources of variability in the experimental material and investigating the replication of the random factors. To do this easily we only considered the data collected on day 1. However, results

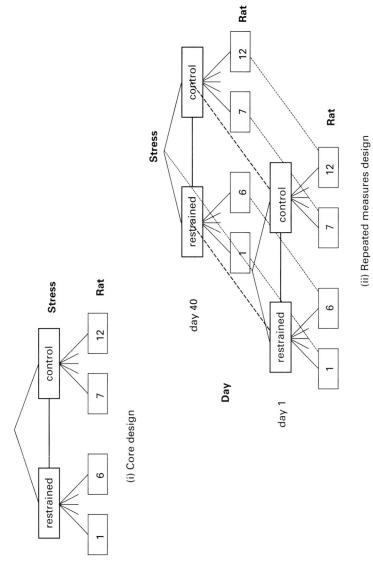

Figure 3.58. (i) The core design and (ii) the repeated measures design for Example 3.40. The dotted lines join the levels of the core design factors that are measured repeatedly across the levels of the repeated Day factor (only two levels are shown for clarity).

were taken repeatedly over time on days 1, 21, 24 and 28 post-administration of the test compound. We could, in a separate analysis to that described in Section 3.7.3.3, investigate the effect of treatments over time.

The core design involved Treatment and Animal nested within Treatment, where the animals were the experimental and observational units of the core design. The repeated factor was Day (at four levels) and this was crossed with Animal and Treatment (each animal was tested on each day).

As animals were tested three times per day, there was a further factor (Trial), which was nested within the combinations of the levels of Animal and Day. The observational units in the nested repeated measures design were therefore the individual measurements taken on the animals on each day.

An illustration of the core design and the repeated measures design is presented in Figure 3.59. Note only two levels of the repeated factor are included in the diagram for clarity.

To assess the change in response over time, the three measurements taken per animal per day were first averaged and then a repeated measures analysis (see Section 5.4.4) was performed on these averages. This analysis revealed that both the pressure application measurement and weight distribution approaches detected a reversal of hypersensitivity. It was also found that the two readouts were highly correlated.

Example 3.37 (continued): Comet assay to assess genotoxicity

In the description of the comet assay (Example 3.37) it was noted that the experimental design was a higher-order nested design. Cell is nested within Slide, Slide is nested within Animal and Animal is nested within Treatment. However, it may be the case that cells are taken from multiple organs rather than from just one target organ. If cells are taken from multiple organs then the design can also be viewed as a nested repeated measures design. The core design is a single-order nested design (involving Treatment and Animal) and the repeated factor is Organ (the levels of the Organ factor cannot be randomised). The factors Slide and Cell are now nested within the combinations of the levels of the Organ and Animal factors. The observational units of the core design are the organs from each animal. The observational units for the nested repeated measured design are the cells. The experimental units are still the animals regardless of the number of organs assessed.

In practice we may choose to analyse the data generated from each organ separately, the approach favoured by toxicologists, or conduct a repeated measures analysis. In either case we first need to summarise the individual observations taken on each animal; see Bright *et al.* (2011) for more details.

3.8.1.4 More complex repeated measures designs

In certain animal experiments some responses are measured repeatedly (i.e. over time) whereas others are only measured once. For example, in toxicology experiments animal body weight is measured repeatedly over time whereas organ weights are only measured once at the end of the study. In such cases the experimental design can be defined in terms of the core design itself (for certain responses such as organ weight) and as a repeated measures design for others (such as body weight). This should highlight to the reader that the term 'repeated measures design' is related to the nature of the responses as well as to the experimental design itself.

In this section examples of more complex repeated measures designs, where the core design is an example of one of the scenarios described in Table 3.2, are discussed. The first is an example of a double-repeated measures design whereas the latter is a crossover design and has been already discussed in Section 3.4.9. In practice it is common to measure the animals repeatedly in an animal experiment, regardless of the core experimental design used. So it is likely the reader will find themselves using these more complex repeated measures designs. As long as the structure of the experimental design has been identified, this should not be a problem.

Example 3.41: Double-repeated measures design involving time

McQuade *et al.* (1999) described an experiment to assess the effect of novel environmental stimuli on central noradrenaline function. The experiment involved placing rats in one of three test arenas, where each arena presented the animal with different stimuli. The three stimuli within the test arenas were dark (10 lx), light (2500 lx) and light (2500 lx) with an unfamiliar rat where two rats were placed in the test arena separated by a clear Perspex barrier. Rats were randomly assigned to one of the three arenas and hence the Animal factor was nested within the Arena factor. To measure noradrenaline, probes were implanted into both the frontal cortex and the lateral hypothalamus. As measurements were taken in both brain regions (and the Brain region factor levels could not be randomised within animal) the design was therefore a repeated measures design with repeated factor Brain region. Additionally, the animals were assessed every 20 minutes up to three hours after being placed in the test arena. Hence there were effectively two repeated factors in this experiment, Brain region and Time. If we considered the repeated measures design (with Brain region as the repeated factor) as a core design, then the Time factor was a second repeated measures factor. Hence the experimental design was a double-repeated measures design. The two repeated factors were crossed with each other.

Example 3.42: Double-repeated measures design involving three related end points

Double-repeated measures designs can be employed in many experimental situations, even when the animals are not measured

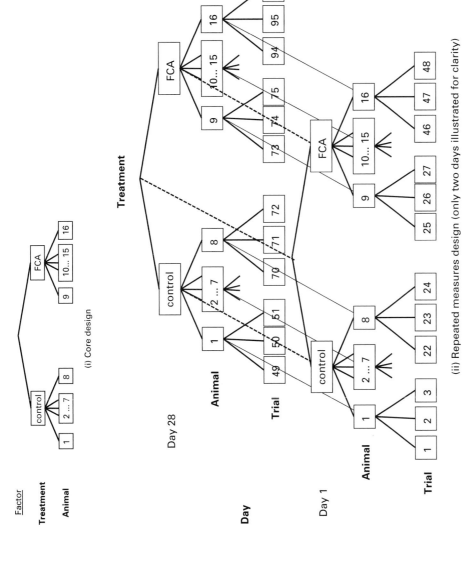

Figure 3.59. (i) The core experimental design and (ii) the nested repeated measures design for Example 3.36. The dotted lines join the levels of the core design factors that are measured repeatedly across the levels of the repeated factor.

repeatedly over time. For example, a study was conducted to assess the antidepressant efficacy of a synthetic pregnenolone-derivative MAP4343 (Bianchi and Baulieu, 2012). This drug is known to bind to MAP-2 *in vitro* and increase its ability to stimulate tubulin assembly. This is deemed important as evidence suggests that the pathogenesis of depressive disorders is associated with neuronal abnormalities, including α-tubulin isoforms, in brain microtubule function.

As part of the study rats reared in isolation were randomly assigned to six groups, receiving either MAP4343 (10 mg/kg), fluoxetine (10 mg/kg) or vehicle, by acute or sub-chronic administration. The α-tubulin isoforms (Tyr-Tub, Glu-Tub and Acet-Tub) were assessed in three brain regions (the hippocampus, amygdala and the prefrontal cortex). Now each isoform could be analysed separately, and hence the design would be a repeated measure design with Brain region as the repeated factor. However, we could alternatively assume that Isoform is also a repeated factor, and hence the design is a double-repeated measures design with repeated factors Isoform and Brain region.

Example 3.15 (continued): Five-choice serial reaction time task

Consider Example 3.15 described in Section 3.4.9.1, conducted to assess whether a 5-HT4 partial agonist was a candidate treatment for Alzheimer's disease (see Hille *et al.*, 2008). The design involved four treatments with each animal receiving all treatments, one per week over four weeks. Animals were tested on a baseline protocol over four days within each week (Monday to Thursday) and hence this can be considered a repeated measures crossover design, where the repeated factor was Day (of the week) and the core design was a crossover design.

The experimental units are still the animals within a test period as effectively the crossover design is measured repeatedly on four days. Day is therefore crossed with all other factors in the experimental design. The observational units are the measurements taken on each animal on each day. This approach allows the scientist to investigate changes in response during the working week.

3.8.2 Dose-escalation designs

Dose-escalation designs share many characteristics with repeated measures designs. When employing a dose-escalation design the animals are measured repeatedly over time, with one dose of the compound administered in each test period. The doses are administered in the same (non-random) order for all animals. Examples of dose-escalation designs are given in Brammer (2003) and include the guinea pig papillary muscle assay and the isolated lung assay.

However, according to our definition given in Section 3.8.1, we do not define dose-escalation designs as

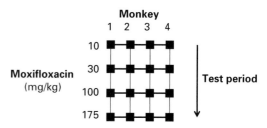

Figure 3.60. Dose-escalation design for Example 3.43. All animals receive the same sequence of doses of moxifloxacin across the test periods.

repeated measures designs. The dose of compound administered to each animal increases across the test periods, hence the levels of the Dose factor vary across the levels of the repeated factor. The experimental units in these designs are the animals in each test period and hence this also varies across the levels of the repeated factor. Note also that the Dose factor is completely confounded with the (repeated) Test period factor (see Brammer, 2003). This is a weakness of these designs as it is therefore not possible to separate the effects of these two factors.

As the doses of the compound are administered to each animal in a non-random order, there will still be spatial interrelationships between the responses measured for each animal. So a repeated measures analysis approach (sometimes called a within-animal analysis) is still appropriate due to the non-random allocation of the levels of the Dose factor (see Section 6.10).

Example 3.43: Cardiovascular telemetry in monkeys

An experiment was conducted to assess the sensitivity and validity of a cardiovascular monkey telemetry model as a predictor of QT interval prolongation in humans (Chaves *et al.*, 2006). We shall focus on the second study reported in the paper, a pharmacokinetic study. Moxifloxacin was administered orally by nasogastric gavage in 0.5% methylcellulose at 10, 30, 100 and 175 mg/kg using a dose-escalation design. All four monkeys received all doses of moxifloxacin in the same non-random order. Blood samples were taken predose and at 0.5, 2, 4, 8 and 24 hours postdose. The time to achieve maximal plasma concentration C_{max} was assessed for each dose in each animal. An illustration of the dose-escalation design is presented in Figure 3.60 and highlights that the Animal and Dose factors are crossed with each other.

The experimental units in this design are the animals in each test period. As the order of moxifloxacin dose allocation is non-random there will be spatial interrelationships between the results from

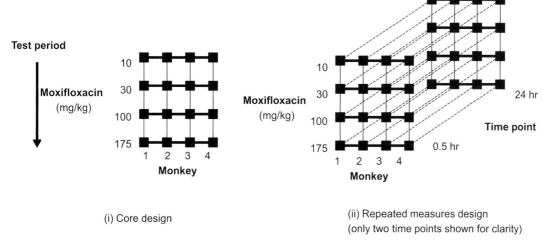

Figure 3.61. (i) The core design and (ii) the repeated measures dose-escalation design for Example 3.43. The dotted lines join the levels of the core design factors that are measured repeatedly across the levels of the repeated factor.

each animal and hence it may be appropriate to use a repeated measures analysis approach to analyse C_{max} to account for this. In the statistical analysis it was observed that the mean C_{max} values were less than dose proportional across the experimental groups.

3.8.2.1 More complex dose-escalation designs

It is possible for an experimental design to consist of both dose-escalation and repeated measures characteristics. We define these designs as repeated measures dose-escalation designs. Examples can be found in Ingram-Ross *et al.* (2012) and Aylott *et al.* (2011).

Example 3.43 (continued): Cardiovascular telemetry in monkeys

We return to Example 3.43 discussed in the previous section. To calculate the C_{max} response the animals were measured repeatedly at predose and then at 0.5, 2, 4, 8 and 24 hours post-dose in each of the four test periods. The design is therefore a repeated measures dose-escalation design. The core design is the dose-escalation design discussed above. This core design is then measured repeatedly over time. The experimental units are still the animals in each test period; however, the observational units are now the measurements taken on each animal in each test period at each time point. An illustration of the core dose-escalation design and the repeated measures dose-escalation design is presented in Figure 3.61 (where only the 0.5 hour and 24 hour time points are shown for clarity).

3.9 Split-plot designs

Split-plot designs (Scenario 4 in Table 3.2) have a long history in agricultural field trials but, in our experience, are not often employed by animal researchers. If the reader is interested in using such designs then more general texts, such as Montgomery (1997, pp. 521–6), should be consulted.

Traditionally these designs are said to consist of whole plots and subplots, where the factor that defines the subplot is nested within the factor that defines the whole plot. The whole plot treatments are randomly applied to the whole plots and the subplot treatments are randomly applied to the subplots within each whole plot. In other words these designs involve two sets of treatments, and each set is randomly assigned to a different unit in the experimental design. There are therefore two different types of experimental unit in a split-plot design.

3.9.1 Animals as whole plots

Consider a split-plot design that consists of two treatment factors (say A and B). The levels of Treatment A are randomly applied to the individual animal, one treatment per animal. In contrast all the levels of Treatment B are *randomly* applied to regions or areas within each animal. So the two types of experimental unit in this split-plot design are the animals and the regions within each animal. The effect of Treatment A is assessed against the between-animal variability whereas the effect of Treatment B is assessed against the within-animal variability. The design has both crossed and nested factors. For example, Animal is nested within Treatment A, but is crossed with Treatment B. Treatment A is also crossed with Treatment B.

The analysis of such designs may require the input of a statistician as the Animal factor will need to be defined as a random factor (most packages by default define all factors, other than the factor that corresponds to the observational units, as fixed). The scientist should ensure that the effect of Treatment A is tested against the between-animal variability whereas the effect of Treatment B is tested against the within-animal variability. It can also be shown that the interaction between the two treatments should be assessed against the within-animal variability.

There are some similarities between analyses of data generated using split-plot and repeated measures designs (the latter are discussed in Section 5.4.4). Both contain between-animal factor(s) and within-animal factor(s), hence both involve assessing factors against the appropriate within- or between-animal variability. However, we contend that the randomisation of the two designs is different. In a repeated measures design the levels of the repeated factor (such as Time) cannot be randomised whereas in a split-plot design the levels of the within-animal factors are randomised. This leads to different analysis strategies: an ANOVA-based analysis for split-plot designs and perhaps a repeated measures analysis for repeated measures designs (see Section 5.4.4).

Example 3.44: Coated implant assessment in rabbits

A study was performed to assess the effect of four coated implants on bone formation in New Zealand white rabbits (Hulshoff *et al.*, 1996). The four types of coating included in the study were a plasma-sprayed Ca-P coating, a heat-treated plasma-sprayed Ca-P coating, an amorphous magnetron-sputter coating and a crystalline magnetron-sputter coating. Four cylinders (one per coating type) were inserted into random positions in the lateral and medial femoral condyles of each of 18 rabbits. The rabbits were then humanely killed at three time points (three, six and nine weeks post-surgery) and the bone-implant interface evaluated histologically. As all four implants were administered to each rabbit, and post-mortem samples were taken at various time points, the design employed was a split-plot design. The rabbits were the whole plots and the positions within a rabbit the subplots. The time points (whole plot treatments) were randomly assigned to the rabbits and the types of implant (subplot treatments) were randomly assigned to positions within the rabbit. The results of the experiment revealed that the Ca-P coatings and the plasma-sprayed Ca-P coatings showed the same bone healing process.

3.9.2 Animals as subplots

While we envisage that the animals will correspond to the whole plots, this need not always be the case, as the following examples show.

Example 3.45: Developmental rat dietary study

Vitamin A deficiency is known to cause respiratory and mobility problems in neonate rats. An experiment was conducted to investigate whether a moderate deficiency of vitamin A plays a role in regulating key skeletal muscle regulatory pathways (Downie *et al.*, 2005). If there were effects observed, then this could be a major health concern as vitamin A deficiency is common in the developing world.

At the start of the study, 60 female Rowlett-hooded Lister rats were group housed. Let us assume they were housed in 12 cages, five animals per cage. These cages were randomly assigned to two groups, six cages per group. The first group were fed a vitamin A-moderate diet and the second group were fed a vitamin A-sufficient diet from weaning till the end of pregnancy. Prior to mating the rats were group housed but from mating to gestation the rats were singly housed. Rats were killed at various time points during and after pregnancy.

As the rats were group housed during the study, five per cage, and were killed at five time points post-mating, it would be sensible to kill one animal per cage per time point. The design used in this scenario would be a split-plot design. Cages correspond to the whole plots and animals correspond to the subplots. The diets (whole plot treatments) were randomly assigned to the cages of animals (whole plots) and the time points (subplot treatments) were randomly assigned to the animals within each cage (subplot treatments).

By running the experiment, the researchers were able to show that mothers fed the vitamin A-sufficient diet had reduced retinol concentrations and neonates had reduced relative lung weights.

Neonatal survival was lower in the vitamin A-sufficient group where neonates had increased relative heart weights.

Example 3.46: Environmental study using a split-plot design

An example of a split-plot design is described in Morris (1999, p. 67). An experiment was conducted to assess the effect of environmental temperature and dietary nutrition concentration on the egg-laying performance of hens. Of particular interest was whether putting more energy into the diet would reduce the adverse effect of heat stress. Hens were housed individually in six rooms (which were randomly assigned to a level of the Temperature factor). The four diets under consideration were then randomly assigned to the four hens within each room. Hence the rooms and the hens correspond to the two experimental units in this split-plot experiment. Temperature and Diet were defined as fixed factors and Room and Hen as random factors. Room was crossed with Diet but was nested within Temperature. Hence the Temperature factor was tested against the between-room variability, whereas Diet and the interaction between Temperature and Diet were tested against the within-room variability.

3.10 Experimental designs in practice

In this chapter we have considered the types of experimental designs that researchers require when performing animal experiments. This includes block designs, factorial designs, nested designs, etc. Each of the different design types has been introduced and their properties considered.

Although we have described each design type separately, in practice it is unlikely that an experiment will involve only one of these types. The experimental designs that are routinely employed may possess characteristics from many design types. Once recognised, this allows the researcher to design experiments more efficiently, perhaps performing different analyses to investigate different aspects of the same experimental design.

In Section 3.8.1.4 we considered more complex repeated measures designs. These involve designs where the core design (which is assessed repeatedly across the levels of the repeated factor) can be any type of design, such as a crossover, factorial or even a repeated measures design. Dose-escalation designs can also involve repeated measurements, as considered in Section 3.8.2.

However, in practice we can also combine different design types in non-repeated measures scenarios. For example, any experiment based on one of the designs considered in this chapter can also be blocked. In Example 3.34, an experiment to assess the effect of doses of a mutagen in transgenic mice, the design was a nested design with Mouse nested within Dose. However, the results were sent to five laboratories for testing, so the design was also a block design (blocked by Laboratory). Any type of design can also have multiple (crossed) factors of interest and hence be described as a small factorial design. For example, Example 3.17 consisted of a crossover trial conducted to assess marmoset preference for different types of nest boxes. The actual experiment involved two crossed factors of interest (Nest box and Camera) and hence was also a factorial design. This was an example of the multi-factor crossover designs discussed in Bate and Boxall (2008).

For the purposes of illustration, in this chapter we simplified the examples given so that only one of the characteristics was discussed. This hopefully makes it easier to understand the principles underlying each design type. However, considering the multiple features of a design can allow the researcher to obtain more information from the experiment, as the following example shows.

Example 3.10 (continued): Anti-microbial medication assessment

Example 3.10, described in Section 3.4.3, considered an experiment to assess whether spray-dried animal plasma (SDAP) in the diet could be used as an alternative to anti-microbial medication containing colistin sulphate in weanling pigs challenged with *Escherichia coli* K99 (Torrallardona *et al.*, 2003).

In this example it was stated that the design employed was a block design. However, the design itself was a little more complicated. The actual design involved blocks, a factorial treatment, structure nested factors and repeated measures, as described below.

Blocks

The 48 piglets were assigned to three blocks based on their pre-treatment body weight (blocking factor, levels: light, medium and heavy). The 16 animals in each block were then assigned to four pens, taking the litter into account, and the four treatments were randomly assigned to the four pens in each block. The design was therefore a complete block design with pens as the experimental units (dietary treatments were administered to the pen rather than the piglet). Note Litter may also have been a second blocking factor in this example.

Factorial treatments

The four treatments were actually all combinations of two factors: SDAP (levels: 0 and 7%) and colistin sulphate (levels: 0 mg/kg and 300 mg/kg). Hence the design was a small full-factorial design (see Section 3.5.4.3). The researcher could have assessed the differences between the group means, perhaps making use of the hidden replication (see Section 3.5.4). This design also allowed the researcher to see how the effects of the two factors interacted with each other.

Nested factors

For the growth rate and food intake end points the pens were the experimental units, and hence any results from the individual piglets within each pen were first averaged prior to analysis. However, the design could also be described as a nested design. The additional Piglet factor was nested within Pen (each animal was housed in only one pen). The researcher could therefore have considered the replication of the pens (using the power analysis technique described in Section 3.7.2) or perhaps investigated the interrelationship between the replication of piglets and pens (see Section 3.7.3). Would it be beneficial to house the piglets two per pen (rather than four) while increasing the number of pens (the experimental units)? Perhaps the researcher could use fewer piglets in future if fewer pigs are housed in the pens. In the actual experiment two of the four pigs were humanely killed (on days 7 and 14) so that samples of the small intestine could be taken to measure various disease end points over time. Hence the replication of piglets within pen may have been difficult to vary in this example.

Repeated measures

Finally, for some of the experimental end points, as discussed above, two animals per pen were humanely killed on days 7 and 14. These animals were not chosen at random (the second heaviest in each pen was selected on day 7 and the third heaviest on day 14). Hence for these end points the design was a repeated measures design. Intriguingly, if the animals within each pen that were humanely killed at each time point had been selected at random from each pen, then the design would have been a split-plot design with Time as the within-plot (or within-pen) treatment factor and SDAP and colistin sulphate as the two between-plot (or between-pen) treatment factors.

3.11 A good design should result in...

We have now discussed in detail some of the fundamentals of experimental design. Hopefully this will provide researchers with a theoretical framework when planning experiments. All of the methods discussed in this section will help the researcher make best use of the available resources and hopefully reduce animal use.

In practice many experimental designs consist of a combination of the types described above. For example, the researcher may want to use a blocked crossover design, or a factorial design with multiple nested factors. The principles though are the same for these more complicated designs as for the simpler cases. By seeing the way the designs are related to each other (using the ideas described above, such as crossing and nesting) the reader should now see how more complex designs can be constructed. We have hopefully also given sufficient examples of these more complex designs to show how they can be built up from the simpler examples.

Before we go on to consider the analysis of the data collected when using these designs, we summarise the properties of a good experimental design. A good experimental design should result in:

- An absence of systematic error: If the design is appropriate, then the researcher should be protected from the possibility that an unexpected or unplanned effect influences the experimental results. The design should reduce any treatment comparison bias.
- A wide range that the conclusions are valid: By including more levels of a factor in the design, for example using males and females rather than just one sex or using animals with a wide range of body weights, then the conclusions drawn from the study should be valid over a wider range of conditions. It may appear sensible to use animals from a narrow body weight range in a study. This may well reduce the animal-to-animal variability. However, the conclusions drawn from the study may only be valid for the limited body weight range included in the study. It may be better to use a wider range of body weights, but make sure that a body weight factor has been included in the design and analysis to account for the extra variability this may cause.
- Simplicity: Designs should be simple. Complex designs are more likely to be implemented incorrectly if conducted by a stressed-out animal technician working on a Sunday afternoon.

- A well-defined analysis strategy: The researcher should be able to investigate data generated from a well-designed experiment using a simple statistical analysis. If the design is planned properly the analysis should be straightforward to complete and follow on from the experimental design.

- Reliable estimates of variability: Good designs should allow the researcher to estimate the sources of variability. This will help reduce sample sizes by allowing the researcher to assess, and hopefully reduce, the various sources of variability in the study.

4

Randomisation

In the previous chapter we gave recommendations regarding the randomisation procedures that should be performed when employing factorial, block and cross-over designs. We also considered randomisation when differentiating between the various ways that an animal can be measured repeatedly. In this chapter we shall discuss some of the more general issues associated with randomisation and highlight how randomisation can influence the statistical analysis.

As a general rule it should be remembered that:

- Where possible, the levels of each factor should be randomly assigned to the labels of the experimental design. So, for example, if a design is constructed (or obtained from a textbook) and the labels within the design are given as '1', '2' and '3', then the actual treatments in the experiment (say drug X, drug Y and the control) should be randomly assigned to the labels '1', '2' and '3'.

- Randomisation should ensure that each animal has an equal chance of being allocated to any of the experimental groups.

- If a random factor is included in the statistical analysis, then we should always try to select the levels of the random factor randomly from a wider population of levels. For example, the study animals should be randomly selected from a larger population of animals. These study animals are then randomly assigned to the treatment groups. As we shall see, when we draw conclusions from the statistical analysis of an animal experiment, these conclusions can only be generalised to the wider population from which the animals were randomly taken. So, for example, the conclusions of an animal experiment

conducted using males will not necessarily generalise to females.

- Design first and randomise second. Leaving to chance the exact relationship between the factors in the design may be the easier option, especially if there are many effects that could influence the experimental results. However, we believe it is best to take into account as many effects as possible, by including corresponding factors in the experimental design, as this usually leads to a simpler analysis, more reliable results and more informed decisions.

This chapter, devoted to randomisation, is purposefully placed between the experimental design and statistical analysis sections of the book. This is to emphasise that randomisation provides a justification (it should be stressed not the only justification) for the statistical analysis. Randomisation can be seen as a link between the experimental design and the statistical analysis.

4.1 Practical reasons to randomise

There are many practical reasons why we should randomise the experimental material in an experiment. We describe some of the more important ones.

4.1.1 Bias reduction

Randomisation provides a way of reducing bias in the experimental outcomes. It can reduce or remove any systematic bias caused by procedural effects and also help ensure that the study is blinded, thus further reducing the risk of generating biased results. The effect

Table 4.1. Four types of bias affecting internal validity

Type of bias	Comment	Example
Selection bias	Bias caused by a non-random allocation of animals to treatment groups.	Do we try to avoid allocating the less healthy animals to the high-dose group?
Performance bias	Bias caused by differences, however subtle, in levels of husbandry care given to animals across treatment groups.	Are sick animals in the control group given the benefit of the doubt and kept alive longer than animals in the high-dose group?
Detection bias	Bias caused when the researcher assessing the effect of the treatment knows which treatment the animal received.	When assessing animal behaviour, it is human nature to want to see a positive effect in your experiment.
Attrition bias	Bias caused by unequal occurrence and handling of deviations from the protocol.	If many animals are excluded from the high-dose group, should we take this into account?

of randomisation (or lack of) was considered in a review of studies that assessed treatment interventions in multiple sclerosis (Vesterinen *et al.*, 2010). They found that of 1117 publications considered, only 106 reported using randomisation techniques. Interestingly, for the 36 interventions considered in greatest detail, the randomised studies revealed a smaller treatment effect (on average a 20.6% change from control) compared to the non-randomised studies (41.6% change from control).

Van der Worp *et al.* (2010) describe four ways that the result of an experiment may become biased, all of which can be addressed using a suitable randomisation. These biases will affect the internal validity of the experiment (see Table 4.1). It is recommended that the researcher not only consider these four sources of bias when planning the experiment, but also describe the strategies employed to reduce their influence when reporting experiments. We give two examples where a lack of randomisation may result in bias that reduces the internal validity of the experiment.

4.1.1.1 Removing unforeseen trends

When comparing treatments in a study, we aim to remove the influence of all nuisance effects that could bias the treatment comparisons. We do this by including blocking factors in the experimental design (such as Day of testing) or perhaps placing limits on the range of levels of an effect (such as body weight) that may

influence the results. However, no matter how well we achieve this, there is always a risk that certain effects (that we cannot control) may influence the responses. If we conduct a randomisation then, as mentioned by Festing *et al.* (2002, p. 35), we can assume that these nuisance effects (in theory) influence all treatment groups equally. Randomisation will therefore reduce or minimise the bias caused by these nuisance effects and hence we can assume treatment comparisons are unbiased.

In practice it may be the case that a scientist did not identify a potential source of bias when planning an experiment but may perceive its effect once the experiment has started. For example, if an experiment takes a whole working day to complete, it may be the case that a trend over time was observed that would then need to be taken into account. If the animals were randomly assigned to the order of testing during the day, or better still blocked by time of day, then the scientist may be able to account for the trend over time in the statistical analysis (or at least investigate it further). This would not be possible if, for example, all the control animals had been tested first during the morning.

4.1.1.2 Humans are systematic

While we think we are behaving in a random fashion, sadly it is well known that the human mind works systematically. For example, when assigning animals to groups, we may feel that we are performing a random allocation, but chances are we have introduced some underlying trends to the experimental material. 'Randomly' selecting animals from a cage is not random if the largest, slowest or easiest to catch animals are selected first. This may influence the results of the experiment. In practice it is best to leave the randomisation to either a computer or some other suitably independent mechanical device.

Consider the case of a lottery where punters are allowed to select their lottery numbers. While it is possible to select numbers at random, using a random pick, many people still use non-random strategies. For example, selecting numbers based on birthdays (implies that numbers greater than 31 will not be picked as often) or choosing to spread the selection across the card. How many other people are using the same approach? If there are other people using your strategy, then you are more likely to have to share any winnings with them because the set of numbers you are all selecting from is reduced.

So randomisation may help you keep the entire jackpot, assuming you do win. Unfortunately randomisation does not make you any more likely to choose the correct numbers.

4.1.2 Blinding

There appears to be growing evidence that the importance of blinding has been overlooked, or at least under-reported, in the animal research literature. Blinding is a crucial part of the experimental process and methods of blinding should be reported alongside the experimental results (see Kilkenny *et al.*, 2009). Randomisation is a useful tool to aid in the blinding of an experiment.

There are many ways that an animal experiment should be blinded. The treatment allocation should be blinded to the researcher administering the treatment and/or conducting any other interventions such as surgery or training. Technicians and/or veterinarians performing routine husbandry activities or making decisions about animal welfare should also be blinded to treatment allocation as such information may bias, however subtly, their decision-making process. Finally the researcher assessing the outcome of the experiment

should be blinded to the treatment allocation to avoid any research priorities influencing the results.

Rooke *et al.* (2011) reviewed 207 articles in peer-reviewed journals that describe animal experiments conducted to assess treatments for Parkinson's disease. They found that only 38 reported a blinded assessment of the outcome of the experiment. Intriguingly the authors found that treatment-related improvements in the neurobehavioural score (NBS) were smaller in blinded studies compared to the non-blinded studies (on average, 0.85 NBS vs. 1.18 NBS, respectively). Vesterinen *et al.* (2010) reported in a review of 1117 publications that only 178 described the assessment of the outcome of the experiment as being blinded. In the 36 interventions considered in greater detail, there was also an increase in observed efficacy in the studies that did not report blinding compared to those that did (on average an increase from the control of 41% vs. 29.8%, respectively). Both papers concluded that if the technicians involved in husbandry and the researchers that performed the treatment administration and assessed the outcome of the experiment were not blinded to the treatment allocation, then this probably had an impact on the size of the observed treatment effects.

When carrying out an experiment, it is difficult for a researcher to remain completely objective. This is particularly the case when the measurements taken are subjective. If possible some degree of blinding is useful to remove the risk of bias, and randomisation provides a tool for doing this.

If the researcher is trying to publish results, it is important to be fair and be seen to be fair. We argue that details of the randomisation employed should be given as part of the methods section in any journal submission. It will give the referee and reader alike more confidence that the results presented are unlikely to be influenced, however subtly, by the researcher's preconceptions or other unforeseen factors; see Macleod *et al.* (2009) and the ARRIVE guidelines (Kilkenny *et al.* 2010).

4.2 Statistical reasons to randomise

As well as the practical reasons described above, there are also important statistical reasons why we should randomise the experimental material. We shall describe some of them in this section.

4.2.1 Estimating the variability

When carrying out many statistical analyses, we compare the size of the factors of interest against a suitable estimate of the variability. If randomisation reduces the risk that unforeseen effects have biased the estimate of the factors of interest, then randomisation also implies that the estimate of the variability will be free of these effects. This is important if the results of the statistical analysis are to be reliable. However, using an appropriate randomisation can also increase the underlying variability of the data. This need not be a major problem, as long as an appropriate statistical analysis is used to analyse the data generated. We highlight this with an example.

Example 4.1: Stratified randomisation based on body weight

Assume the researcher needs to assign 15 animals to three treatment groups, five animals per group. There is a concern that larger animals will give higher responses. The effect of body weight could therefore:

1. increase the variability of the response;
2. bias any treatment comparisons if the animals in the control group were, on average, heavier than those in the treatment groups.

So, how should the animals be allocated to the treatment groups? We consider two scenarios.

Scenario 1

We could simply randomly assign the 15 animals to the three treatment groups. However, in doing this we run the risk that the largest animals will be assigned to the control group. It turns out there is approximately a 0.03% chance of the randomisation generating this allocation. If the researcher were unlucky enough to make such an allocation, then any treatment comparisons could be biased by the effect of body weight. In practice it is more likely that there will be a small difference between the group mean body weights and this may lead to a subtler bias caused by body weight differences.

Scenario 2

An alternative way to allocate animals to treatments is to block by body weight – the stratified randomisation. We first split the animals into five blocks, three animals per block, based on body weight. The largest three animals are assigned to block 1, the next largest three animals to block 2 and so on. We now randomly assign, separately for each block, the three treatments to the three animals within each block. We could then include the blocking factor in the analysis to account for any variability caused by differences in body weight.

It should be noted that while this approach reduces the overall bias to the group means caused by body weight differences (the average group body weights should now be similar) it may *increase* the variability of the data collected. The randomisation has guaranteed that each experimental group contains animals from a wide range of body weights (one from the largest three, one from the next largest three and so on). So we have artificially increased the range of body weights within each treatment group. The range of body weights within each group is now larger than what we would have expected to see if a completely random allocation had been made. Now assuming there is a relationship between the response and the body weight, then the stratified randomisation has not only artificially increased the range of the body weights within each group but also the range of the responses within each group, i.e. it has increased the variability. This could result in less sensitive statistical tests if the variability associated with the blocking factor is not accounted for in the statistical analysis.

So a stratified randomisation can increase the variability of the data, as well as reducing the bias. In this example we should account for this extra variability by either fitting body weight as a blocking factor in the analysis (see Section 6.3.3.3) or as a covariate (see Section 5.4.6). Either way the statistical analysis can remove the additional variability introduced by using a stratified randomisation. This is a good example where using the recommended experimental design does not necessarily guarantee that the most reliable results will be generated. The most accurate results are obtained by using an appropriate experimental design, a suitable randomisation and then a powerful statistical analysis.

4.2.2 Deciding upon the statistical analysis strategy

In certain situations the researcher may be confronted with more than one statistical analysis strategy. For example, a decision must be made about which factors and factor interactions to include in the statistical analysis. Which options should be chosen? It may not always be appropriate, but by considering the experimental design and randomisation the researcher can usually identify an analysis approach that is both theoretically valid and justifiable to a wider audience. While some may feel that the randomisation is not the most important part of the process, it does provide a useful aid in deciding which terms to include in the statistical analysis and which to exclude. Randomisation does not provide *the* answer, but it can provide *an* answer.

4.2.2.1 Including interactions in the statistical model

Consider the following two designs, both involving nine animals. The first is a full-factorial design with two factors, A and B, each at three levels. The second is a complete block design consisting of three blocks, with three treatments (a, b and c) randomly assigned to the three animals within each block. It can be seen, see Figure 4.1, that the two designs are structurally identical. In both cases the two factors (A and B for the factorial design, Treatment and Block for the block design) are fully crossed with each other. The designs are drawn in a non-randomised order.

While being structurally identical, the two designs serve markedly different purposes. When using the factorial design we are interested in the effects of both factors A and B and whether there is an interaction between them. In other words does the effect of factor A vary depending on the level of factor B? In contrast when using the block design, the researcher is only interested in the treatment effect. The second (Block) factor is simply a tool to account for the variability that can be associated with the levels of the blocking factor. In a blocked experiment we usually assume there is no interaction between the treatment and blocking factors, i.e. the effect of the treatment is the same within each of the blocks. If there is a blocking effect, then we assume this effect influences all responses measured within each block equally.

In the statistical analysis of the experiment employing the factorial design we fit an interaction between the two factors A and B (see Section 3.5.2). However, in the blocked experiment we do not normally include the Treatment by Block interaction. So what is the justification for two structurally identical designs being analysed differently? One answer is the randomisation. In the blocked experiment animals are assigned to blocks (usually non-randomly) and then, *separately for each block*, the treatments are randomly allocated to the animals within that block. In the factorial experiment the combinations of both treatment factors (that define the interaction) are randomly assigned to the animals. The latter randomisation provides a justification for including the interaction between factors A and B in the statistical analysis whereas the former randomisation

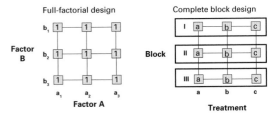

Figure 4.1. A comparison of a two-way full-factorial design and a complete block design. The number 1's within the boxes in the full-factorial design imply there is one animal at each combination of the two factors. The a, b and c labels within the complete block design correspond to the three treatments levels (one per animal within block) written in a non-random order.

implies we should exclude the Treatment by Block interaction.

There are exceptions to using the randomisation to justify the statistical analysis. For example, if the two crossed factors that define the factorial design were Gender and Treatment, then it would not be possible to randomise the combinations of the Gender and Treatment factors to the animals. However, in such experiments we may still want to test to see if the treatment effect varies between males and females (i.e. to investigate the interaction). Such tests can be performed, but their justification will not be based on the randomisation.

If the researcher believes there may be an interaction between the Treatment factor and the Block factor, then a factorial-type randomisation should be employed, where possible, as described above. When deciding whether the design is factorial or block, the following should be considered:

- What is the reason for including the additional factor in the experimental design? Is it a factor of interest or does it account for a nuisance effect?
- Is there a risk that the factors will interact with each other? What does this imply when making conclusions from the data? For example, if observed, is there a reason why a treatment effect is present in one room but not in another or is it a false positive result?
- What randomisation will be applied?

It may be the case that the researcher is actually employing a factorial design, and hence the interaction can be assessed if necessary.

4.2.2.2 Including blocking factors

From Example 4.1 we can see that animals were assigned to blocks based on their body weight. Animals (within each block) were then randomly assigned to the treatments. This randomisation implies that we can assess the treatment effects against the between-animal variability. However, there is no randomisation justification for testing the blocking. As animals were systematically assigned to blocks, rather than randomly assigned to them, we cannot use randomisation as a justification for testing the significance of the blocking factor. We argue that important blocking factors (factors that were deemed necessary when planning the experimental design) should be included in the analysis regardless of their calculated significance in a statistical analysis.

Example 4.1 (continued): Stratified randomisation based on body weight

Returning to Example 4.1, the randomisation implied that a blocking factor should be included in the analysis to deal with the additional source of variability introduced by the stratified randomisation process. As the three animals within each block were randomly assigned to the three treatments, so we should include the blocking factor in the analysis. However, we only test the statistical significance of the treatment factor.

4.2.3 Repeatedly measured responses

In Table 3.2 we describe seven different ways that the researcher can repeatedly measure an animal. These scenarios involve six types of experimental design. There are several different ways that we can differentiate between the scenarios, but perhaps the most important of these is the randomisation procedure applied. It is important the researcher understands not only what is being randomised but also the implications of the randomisation applied. This can affect:

- the type of experimental design;
- the statistical model that can be fitted when using the experimental design;
- the statistical analysis approaches that can be applied when analysing the data generated.

In Table 4.2 we summarise the different randomisations that are applied when the animals are repeatedly measured using one of the seven scenarios discussed in Section 3.2.8.

4.2.3.1 Repeated factors and randomised factors

With repeated measures designs (scenario 1, Table 4.2) we cannot randomise the levels of the factor that indexes the repeated measurements (the repeated factor). This lack of randomisation is in contrast to almost all other experimental factors, where some randomisation can be applied. Even factors such as Gender or Strain involve some degree of randomisation (animals within each strain or sex are randomly selected from a larger population of animals).

Randomisation allows the researcher to assume that observations are independent of each other (see Section 5.4.1). The lack of randomisation of the levels of the repeated factor implies we cannot assume that the within-animal results are independent. If possible we should take these spatial interrelationships (or correlations) into account in the statistical analysis. One way to achieve this is to perform a repeated measures analysis, as described in Section 5.4.4.

Example 4.2: Random allocation of treatments within-animal

The antidepressant bupropion is now prescribed for smoking cessation. A study was conducted to assess the hypothesis that bupropion's nicotine antagonist action contributes to its antidepressant effects (Shoaib *et al.*, 2003). Rats were trained to discriminate nicotine from saline, in a two-lever discrimination chamber, under a schedule of food reinforcement. In a randomised sequence of tests, the rats were dosed with either bupropion (1, 3 or 10 mg/kg, i.p.) or saline 30 min before injection of nicotine (0.025, 0.05, 0.1 or 0.2 mg/kg, s.c.). The percentage of nicotine-appropriate lever choices was analysed to assess the effect of bupropion on the nicotine-discriminative stimulus.

As the three doses of bupropion and saline were administered to each animal, the data could be analysed using a repeated measures analysis approach (see Section 5.4.4.3). This was the approach taken in the original paper. Alternatively, as the doses were administered in a random order, it could be assumed that there were no spatial interrelationships between the within-animal observations. Effectively the design was a block design with Rat as a blocking factor. This factor accounted for the between-rat variability and hence the treatment comparisons were within-animal tests.

4.2.3.2 Block and dose-escalation designs

The block designs (where Animal is a blocking factor) and dose-escalation designs (Sections 3.4 and 3.8.2,

Table 4.2. Seven different ways to measure an animal repeatedly – randomisation

Case	Description	Type of design	Randomisation
1	Animals measured repeatedly: levels of the factor that defines the repeated measurements are shared across animals	Repeated measures design	Randomisation of the levels of the repeated factor not possible – hence relationships exist between the within-animal measurements. Treatments randomised to Animals
2	Animal measured repeatedly: levels of the factor that defines the repeated measurements are not shared across animals	Nested design	In theory the levels of the random within-animal factor(s) are randomly selected from the wider population of levels
3	Treatments assessed at random positions within the animal	Block design	Treatments randomly assigned to positions in the animal – so we can assume that within-animal responses are not spatially interrelated
4	Two treatments: within-animal treatment levels are assessed at random positions within the animal and between-animal treatment levels are administered one per animal	Split-plot design	Between-animal treatments randomly assigned to animals and within-animal treatments randomly assigned to positions within the animal
5	Animals receive multiple treatments over time in a different order for each animal	Crossover design	Treatments are administered to animals in a pseudo-random order, hence we can assume results within-animal are not spatially interrelated
6	Animals receive multiple treatments over time in a non-random order	Dose-escalation design	Treatments are administered to animals in a non-random order, hence we should assume results within-animal are spatially interrelated
7	Multiple different responses measured on each animal	Any type of design	–

respectively) share many similar properties. They both involve administering multiple treatments to each animal. One of the differences between these scenarios is the randomisation applied. When using a block design we randomise the treatments within each animal separately and hence can assume the results generated within-animal are not spatially interrelated. In the dose-escalation designs, the treatments are administered in the same non-random order and hence results within-animal will be spatially interrelated. As we shall see in the next chapter, the techniques we recommend the researcher use to analyse data generated using these two designs are different and reflect the randomisation applied.

4.2.3.3 Crossover and dose-escalation designs

The crossover and dose-escalation designs (Sections 3.4.9 and 3.8.2, respectively) share many similar properties. They both involve repeatedly measuring the animals over a number of test periods, one treatment per test period. With crossover designs animals receive different sequences of treatments over time and hence multiple treatments are administered within each test period. The sequences are usually selected in advance and, when taken together, have certain beneficial properties (see Section 3.4.9). The animals are randomly allocated to the treatment sequences and the treatments are randomly assigned to the labels of the crossover design. In a dose-escalation design all animals receive the same sequence of treatments, normally in a non-random dose-related order. So although these two designs are structurally similar, they involve different randomisation strategies.

The benefit of the crossover design is that it allows the researcher to separate treatment effects from any test period effects (as different treatments are administered in each test period the factors Treatment and Test period are crossed with each other). However, if there are safety concerns about possible side effects associated with the higher doses of the compound, then it may be preferable to confound the treatment and test period effects rather than risk harming the animals and having multiple drop-outs.

The strategy for analysing data generated using these two designs will be different. The two randomisation strategies are different and it can be argued that these differences should be reflected in the statistical analysis. As the doses are administered to the animals in a non-random order (in the dose-escalation design), so there will be spatial interrelationships (or correlations) between the within-animal measurements. These can be accounted for in the analysis using a repeated measures analysis approach (see Section 6.10). This is not the case for the crossover designs where there is some degree of randomisation that, it can be argued, implies we can assume results within-animal are not spatially interrelated. This assumption simplifies the approach for the analysis of crossover studies to that of an experiment involving two blocking factors (Animal and Test period); see Section 6.3.3.3.

4.2.3.4 Including interactions involving the repeated factor

As discussed above, the lack of randomisation of the levels of a repeated factor implies that the responses (usually within-animal) will be interrelated, and so in certain circumstances it is recommended that a repeated measures analysis approach is used to account for these interrelationships (see Section 5.4.4.4). It is also recommended that all interactions involving the repeated factor are included in the analysis, so we can then investigate how the effect of the

factors change over the levels of the repeated factor. We do not require a randomisation-based justification for including these interactions in the statistical model because we are using a repeated measures analysis approach to analyse the data (which will account for any interdependencies). Of course such a decision on which interactions to include is also down to the researcher's discretion.

4.3 What to randomise

In general we advise the scientist to design first and randomise second. It is always best to remove the influence of nuisance effects by designing them into a study rather than leaving it to chance. Once a design is selected, you should then randomise where you can. Examples of randomisations are listed below.

Factor labels
While it may seem unnecessary, you should always randomise the experimental factor levels to the factor labels of the experimental design. So if an experimental design taken from a textbook is defined using the labels A, B, C and D, then the actual treatments (vehicle, low dose, mid dose and high dose) should be randomly allocated to these design labels. If you repeat an experiment and assign the vehicle group to label A both times, then you risk potentially biasing any conclusions drawn across both studies.

Animals to experimental groups
This is the standard randomisation most scientists usually perform. Be careful though, as noted by Macleod *et al.* (2009) picking animals 'at random' from a cage is unlikely to provide adequate randomisation.

Animals to cages
Animals should be randomly assigned to the cages and systematic patterns can occur if they are assigned in a non-random fashion. Consider the situation where animals newly arrived from the supplier are assigned to cages in the testing facility. The animal technician picks up the less active animals first and hence all the inactive animals end up in the first few cages. If treatments are

assigned to cages in a systematic way, then it is possible that all the inactive animals receive the same treatment. This could bias the treatment assessment, especially if locomotor activity is one of the end points of the study.

Treatments to cages

We have already seen that position of a cage in a room or rack may influence the experimental outcome (Gore and Stanley, 2005). Randomising treatments to cages across the racks would reduce the risk of bias, although using a row-column block design may be preferable (remember: design first, randomise second).

Order of testing

Randomising the order of testing should reduce the risk of trends across time influencing the results of the experiment. It should also help in the blinding of the study.

4.4 How to randomise

We now describe some methods that the researcher may employ to carry out a valid randomisation. While in practice a computer will probably be the safest option, there are some more traditional methods that can also be employed.

Mechanical methods

A straightforward way to carry out a randomisation is the 'balls out of a bag' method. This technique is often applied in public allocations, for example draws for cup competitions and national lotteries.

Computer software

Computer software can provide a quick and easy way of randomising experimental material. We present a simple yet flexible approach using Microsoft Excel. This approach can easily be generalised to more complicated experimental situations.

Example 4.3: A simple randomisation

Assume the researcher wants to randomise 15 animals to three treatments (A, B and C), five animals per treatment using Excel. The process consists of five stages:

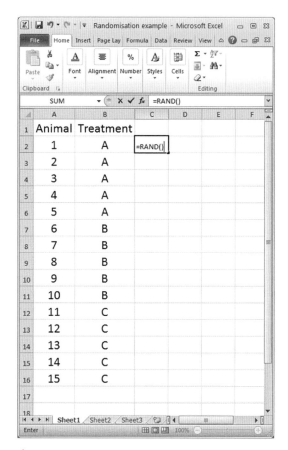

Figure 4.2. Microsoft Excel™ screenshot for randomising 15 animals to three treatment groups, including the first RAND() command required to perform the randomisation.

1. To begin with the experiment should be written out in a non-random order, with animal ID in column A and treatment group in column B (see Figure 4.2).
2. In the next column (in cell C2 in this case) we use Excel's random number generator to create a random number between 0 and 1 (see Figure 4.2). The formula required is:

= RAND()

3. Drag the formula in C2 down to fill the remaining cells C3 to C16. This creates a list of 15 random numbers between 0 and 1.
4. Highlight the treatment column (column B) and the column containing the random numbers (column C).
5. Use the Data → Sort command in Excel to sort column B (containing the treatment labels) by column C (containing the random numbers).

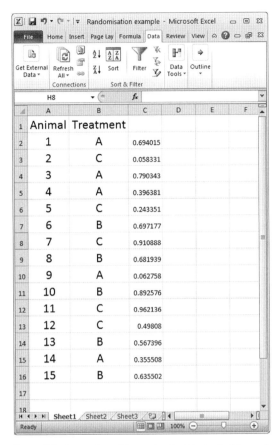

Figure 4.3. Screenshot of the randomised design in Microsoft Excel™.

We have now randomised the treatment labels of the design to the animals (Figure 4.3). Animal 1 will receive treatment A, Animal 2 treatment C and so on.

Note that the random numbers are regenerated by Excel whenever a change is made to the spreadsheet. So the entries in column C will have now changed. If you want to preserve the original random numbers, then copy and paste the random numbers:

Copy → Paste Special → As Numbers

before carrying out Stage 5.

With a little thought this approach (using the '= RAND()' function in Excel) can be applied to more complicated randomisations, such as the randomisation of block designs.

Statistical analysis

5.1 Introduction

For the remainder of this text we shall consider the statistical analysis of (hopefully) well-designed animal experiments. If a suitable experimental design has been employed then the statistical analysis should be relatively straightforward. It should be as concise as possible while making best use of all available information. We argue that to achieve this, the experimental design should direct the statistical analysis.

By this stage of the experimental process the researcher should have:
- identified all effects that may increase the variability of the data and attempted to account for them in the experimental design;
- selected a suitable sample size;
- measured a response that contains as much information as possible;
- attempted to ensure that other nuisance effects have not biased the experimental results.

With these criteria satisfied the analysis should be straightforward and hopefully give reliable and meaningful conclusions.

Before we describe in more detail some of the analyses available when analysing data generated from animal experiments, there are a number of general issues worth considering.

Use the experimental design to direct the analysis

As stated above, in animal experiments we have the luxury of having almost complete control over the experimental design. We should make the most of this in the statistical analysis. As we have seen in the previous chapter, difficult decisions regarding the analysis strategy can be solved, or at least a justifiable solution found, by recourse to the experimental design and randomisation (for example, see Section 4.2.3 for decisions on repeated measures status and Section 4.2.2 for model selection).

Get a feel for your data: make use of graphs

Before beginning any more formal statistical analysis it is highly recommended that the researcher investigate the data graphically using, for example, scatterplots or case profiles plots. These can highlight issues with the data that numerical analysis may not necessarily reveal, such as outliers, non-normality or the identification of a suitable summary measure of a repeatedly measured response.

Try to use parametric analyses

Many analyses can be carried out using a parametric approach (see Section 5.4). This family of tests, known as the general linear model family (or GLM for short) includes ANOVA, ANCOVA and t-tests. These tests allow you to make best use of the experimental design in the analysis since blocking factors, covariates and factor interactions can be included in the statistical model. Most packages now offer GLM analysis as an option. So why make life difficult for yourself? Rather than learn how to use multiple commands in your statistical package of choice it may be possible to use the general linear model command only.

Don't rely on *p*-values!

Finally do not rely on the *p*-values generated from a statistical analysis. Try to use the statistical techniques described in this chapter to get a better understanding of your data.

5.1.1 InVivoStat

Throughout this chapter we will generate results using the InVivoStat statistical software package (Clark *et al.*, 2012). This is a powerful package based on the R statistical language (R Development Core Team, 2012) and is designed specifically for animal researchers. It can be downloaded from www.invivostat.co.uk and is free to use. With the development of InVivoStat, researchers who do not have access to professional statistical support or commercially available statistical software can carry out complicated statistical analyses. A comparison of InVivoStat with other commonly used packages is described in Clark *et al.* (2012). Results from InVivoStat are presented throughout this chapter. Tutorials on how to obtain these results are given in Chapter 6.

5.1.2 A recommended five-stage parametric analysis procedure

Before we discuss in detail some of the methods for analysing data generated in animal experiments, we introduce a five-stage statistical analysis procedure that is easy to carry out and, in many cases, will generate reliable results. A professional statistician may be able to carry out a more powerful statistical analysis, but this text is aimed at the non-statistician who wishes to carry out reliable statistical analyses routinely.

If an experiment is well designed, including the choice of a suitable continuous response to measure, then the parametric analysis approach described here should be the researcher's first choice for the analysis. This approach includes *t*-tests, ANOVA and ANCOVA; see Sections 5.4.2, 5.4.3 and 5.4.6, respectively, for more details. This strategy can also be applied to experiments involving repeated factors, using a parametric repeated measures analysis approach (see Section 5.4.4).

Stage 1: Graphical plots of the data

Any statistical analysis should start with a graphical investigation of the data, preferably using the responses actually measured and not any derived responses. Such plots can reveal outliers and give the scientist a feel for the collected data. Plots should be categorised by the levels of the experimental factors, where possible.

Stage 2: Check the assumptions

Several assumptions are made when carrying out a parametric analysis. We assume the responses are continuous, independent and the residuals are normally distributed. We also assume that the variability of the response is similar among animals given different treatment regimes although prior transformation may be required to meet this assumption (the homogeneity of variance assumption). We shall consider each of these in more detail in Section 5.4.1. At this stage we note that the researcher should always check the assumptions *before* looking at the results of the analysis.

Stage 3: Tests of overall effects

The tests of the overall effects given in for example, the ANOVA table, are the gateway into the statistical analysis. They provide information on the statistical significance of the experimental factors and highlight how the factors interact with each other.

Stage 4: Predicted means

It is always worth reviewing, either in a table or a plot, the predicted means obtained as a consequence of fitting the statistical model to the data. The most common example is the least square (predicted) means. The predicted means can be more reliable than the observed means, which are obtained by calculating the arithmetic group averages. This is because the predicted means are adjusted for all the other terms included in the statistical model (such as blocking factors and covariates) whereas the observed means are not.

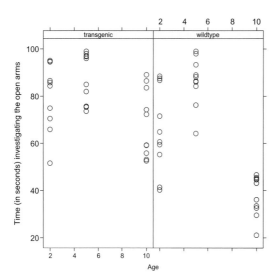

Figure 5.1. Scatterplot of the data for Example 5.1.

Stage 5: Comparisons between the predicted means

It is common practice in the statistical analysis of animal experiments to make comparisons between individual group means using a multiple comparison procedure (see Section 5.4.8). It could be argued that this is the primary purpose of many statistical analyses, although statisticians may prefer other ways of drawing conclusions. The subject of multiple comparison procedures is, however, a controversial one. There are nearly as many methods as there are statisticians! In this text we shall use the experimental design as our guide when navigating through this area.

Whichever multiple comparison procedure is used, when making comparisons between treatment groups, we should also make adjustments for underlying differences in, say, covariates like initial body weight. If comparisons are made using the least square (predicted) means, then the researcher can be surer that the analysis reflects the true differences between the treatments.

Example 5.1: Elevated plus maze

An experiment was conducted to assess the non-cognitive behaviour of a transgenic mouse strain. The strain was thought to be a possible animal model for Alzheimer's disease. To assess the suitability of

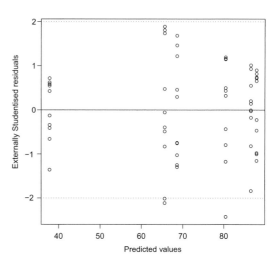

Figure 5.2. Predicted vs. residuals plot for Example 5.1.

the model, an experiment was conducted using an elevated plus maze (or X-maze). The X-maze had two open arms and two enclosed arms. Animals were placed in the centre of the maze and the total time spent investigating the open arms was recorded as a measure of anxiety. In the experiment, 2-, 5- and 10-month-old male wildtype and transgenic mice were tested, with ten mice per strain at each time point. In the following discussion, simulated data have been used.

Stage 1: Graphical plot

A scatterplot of the data revealed no obvious outliers (Figure 5.1). The variability (or spread) of the data in each group appeared to be similar across all groups (see Section 5.4.1.3).

Stage 2: Checking the assumptions

A plot of the residuals from the statistical model, given in Figure 5.2, revealed the assumption of homogeneity of variance was satisfied (as commented for stage 1 above, there was no obvious difference in the variability of the individual groups). See Section 5.4.1.3 for a more detailed description of this plot.

Stage 3: Tests of overall effects

The tests of overall effects, in this case presented in a two-way ANOVA table (Table 5.1), revealed significant overall effects of Strain and Age ($p < 0.001$) but more interestingly the effect of Strain varied with Age ($p = 0.003$). See Section 5.4.3 for more details.

Stage 4: Least square (predicted) means

A plot of the least square (predicted) means from the statistical analysis showed that the difference between the strains was largest in the 10-month-old mice (Figure 5.3).

Table 5.1. ANOVA table for Example 5.1

	Sums of squares	Degrees of freedom	Mean square	F-value	p-value
Age	11636.65	2	5818.32	34.12	< 0.001
Strain	3672.23	1	3672.23	21.54	< 0.001
Age:Strain	2166.94	2	1083.47	6.35	0.003
Residuals	9207.65	54	170.51		

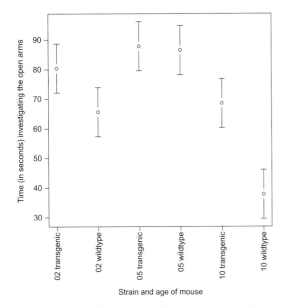

Figure 5.3. Plot of the least square (predicted) means of the combinations of strain and age for Example 5.1.

Stage 5: Comparisons between of the least square (predicted) means

Finally the planned comparisons of the predicted means (Table 5.2) revealed a significant difference between the strains at 2 and 10 months ($p = 0.014$ and $p < 0.001$, respectively) but not at 5 months ($p = 0.815$). See Section 5.4.8 for more details on multiple comparison procedures.

5.2 Summary statistics

In this section we shall consider some statistical tools for summarising data, the so-called summary statistics. This includes the measures of location (mean and median)

and the measures of spread (variance, standard deviation and interquartile range). It is always worth generating these measures as they provide useful information about the data. However, they may not necessarily reflect the results of the statistical (model-based) analysis. In many cases the mathematical methods that generate the summary statistics are different to the approaches used within the statistical analyses described later in this chapter. Summary statistics also (tacitly) make different assumptions about the characteristics of the responses. The parametric summary statistics assume the data are continuous and normally distributed, perhaps following a suitable transformation (see Section 5.4.1.3). The non-parametric summary statistics assume the data are continuous and uniformly distributed (see Section 5.5.1).

Example 5.2: Control group example

Consider the following set of responses from a control group. We shall use these data in the following discussion.

2.3, 4.3, 6.5, 3.2, 7.3, 4.4, 3.4, 5.6, 3.1, 2.6.

5.2.1 Parametric measures of location

Perhaps the simplest parametric measure of location is the mean of the data. There are, however, several different types of mean and the methods used to calculate them are different for each one. We shall consider here the true mean, the sample mean, the observed mean, the predicted mean and the geometric mean.

5.2.1.1 The true mean and the sample mean

The *true mean* is, as the name suggests, the true average value of the response. We try to obtain an accurate estimate of the true mean by running the experiment.

Table 5.2. Table of planned comparisons between the strains at each time point for Example 5.1

Comparison	Difference	Lower 95% CI	Upper 95% CI	Std error	p-value
02 wildtype vs. 02 transgenic	−14.785	−26.492	−3.077	5.840	0.014
05 wildtype vs. 05 transgenic	−1.376	−13.084	10.332	5.840	0.815
10 wildtype vs. 10 transgenic	−30.779	−42.487	−19.071	5.840	< 0.001

The true mean is a hypothetical measure that is the mean response of the whole population and is generally impossible to identify with 100% certainty.

So, for example, we may be interested in the body weight of a transgenic strain of mice at six weeks of age in a certain year. To discover the true mean we would have to measure every animal born in that year when they were 6 weeks old.

Instead of identifying the true mean we take a (random) sample of animals from the wider population and use the mean of the sample (the *sample mean*) to give us an *estimate* of the true mean. The purpose of running an experiment is to gather enough information so that we obtain a sufficiently accurate estimate of the true mean. It follows that the more animals that are sampled to calculate the sample mean, the more reliable it will be (as an estimate of the true mean).

5.2.1.2 The observed mean

The most commonly quoted sample mean, and perhaps the simplest to calculate, is the *observed mean*. This is simply an average of the data. Add together the responses and divide by the group size:

$$\bar{x}_{OM_i} = \frac{1}{n_i}(x_1 + x_2 + x_3 + \ldots + x_{n_i}), \tag{5.1}$$

where $\bar{x}_{OM_i}$ is the ith group observed mean, n_i is the ith group size and $x_1, x_2, \ldots, x_{n_i}$ are the n_i observations in the ith group.

Such calculations can easily be carried out using a hand-held calculator. These are the means usually plotted in the means with standard errors plot (Section 5.3.5).

Example 5.2 (continued): Control group example

The mean for the control group was estimated as:

$(1/10) \times (2.3 + 4.3 + 6.5 + 3.2 + 7.3 + 4.4 + 3.4 + 5.6 + 3.1 + 2.6)$
$= 4.27$.

One of the drawbacks of the observed mean is that it does not necessarily take into account the influence of any additional factors that may be present in the experimental design. The observed mean may therefore not be an accurate estimate of the true mean. A more reliable estimate can be calculated by taking these other factors into account (as we shall do in the statistical analysis). In a worst case scenario the observed means may contradict the results of the statistical analysis.

Example 3.13 (continued): Lamb dietary study

Consider Example 3.13 discussed in Section 3.4.6.3. The experimental design employed in the study was a balanced incomplete block design with all treatment pairs occurring once within the blocks (sibling lamb pairs). We will now analyse some simulated responses from the experiment (see Table 5.3).

Assume that the sibling lamb pair 1 gave higher results than the other pairs; as a result the observed means for treatments A and B will be higher than the observed means for treatment C and D. This is not a treatment effect; it is simply due to the overall differences between the sibling lamb pairs and the incomplete block design used.

The observed mean for treatment A is the average of the three observations from sibling lamb pairs 1, 2 and 3. It is not adjusted for differences between the sibling lamb pairs. Hence a comparison between the observed means of treatment A and treatment C will not be a true reflection of the treatment difference, it will be biased by differences between the lamb pairs.

The observed mean for:

treatment A $= (1/3) \times (15.4 + 7.2 + 2.1) = 8.23$

and

treatment C $= (1/3) \times (11.1 + 6.6 + 6.3) = 8.00$.

Table 5.3. Experimental design and simulated results for Example 3.13

Lamb	Sibling lamb pair					
	1	2	3	4	5	6
first	A (15.4)	A (7.2)	A (2.1)	B (4.5)	B (4.1)	C (6.3)
second	B (19.5)	C (11.1)	D (8.2)	C (6.6)	D (8.2)	D (8.4)

Table 5.4. Observed and predicted means for Example 3.13

Mean	Treatment			
	A	B	C	D
observed	8.23	9.37	8.00	8.27
predicted	4.94	7.94	9.44	11.54

5.2.1.3 The predicted mean

The predicted means are the sample means predicted by the statistical model that is fitted to the data. As the name suggests they will take into account all the effects included in the statistical analysis and hence are more reliable in complex situations. For example, in Section 5.4 the means discussed are predicted means as they take into account the additional effects included in the statistical analysis.

In many simple situations, for example where there is only a single factor of interest in the experiment, the predicted means will be the same as the observed means. However, as the experimental design and statistical analysis become more complex, with the addition of covariates or blocking factors (see Sections 5.4.6 and 3.4, respectively), the observed and predicted means will diverge. In such cases it is the predicted means that provide more reliable estimates of the true means.

Example 3.13 (continued): Lamb dietary study

The analysis of the data (assuming we included Sibling lamb pair as a blocking factor in the analysis) is adjusted for the fact that treatments C and D were not administered to sibling lamb pair 1. The predicted means for A and B were slightly lower than would be expected (compared to C and D) if the sibling lamb pair effects were ignored. This is because treatments A and B were present in sibling lamb pair 1 (which we know gave higher results). The predicted means took this into account as they were calculated using an analysis that fitted Treatment as a fixed factor and Sibling lamb pair as

a blocking factor. The observed and predicted means are given in Table 5.4.

Note the decrease in the treatment A and B means and the increase in the treatment C and D means (going from the observed mean to the predicted mean). This is because treatments A and B were allocated to the sibling lamb pairs that, on average, gave higher results whereas treatments C and D were allocated to those pairs that gave lower results. The predicted means adjusted for these sibling lamb pair effects and hence gave a more reliable estimate of the true treatment effects.

5.2.1.4 The geometric mean

There is one other type of sample mean that the animal researcher should be aware of, namely the *geometric mean*. These means are useful if there is a suspicion that the data are log-normally distributed (see Section 5.4.1.3).

The observed geometric mean for the ith group, $\bar{x}_{OGM_i}$, can be calculated in a similar way to the observed mean using the formula:

$$\bar{x}_{OGM_i} = (x_1 \times x_2 \times ... \times x_{n_i})^{(1/n_i)}. \tag{5.2}$$

Example 5.2 (continued): Control group example

The observed geometric mean for the control group was estimated as:

$(2.3 \times 4.3 \times 6.5 \times 3.2 \times 7.3 \times 4.4 \times 3.4 \times 5.6 \times 3.1 \times 2.6)^{(1/10)} = 3.99.$

We can also calculate a predicted geometric mean. If the data has been log-transformed prior to analysis (see Section 5.4.1.3), then the analysis is performed on the log scale and any predicted means generated within the analysis will also be on the log scale. To calculate the predicted geometric means we simply back-transform the predicted means onto the original scale. So if the data were transformed using the $\log_{10}$ transformation, then the ith predicted geometric mean $\bar{x}_{PGM_i}$ is calculated using the formula:

$$\bar{x}_{PGM_i} = 10^{\bar{x}_{PM_i}}, \tag{5.3}$$

where $\bar{x}_{PM_i}$ is the ith predicted mean on the $\log_{10}$ scale.

Note the observed geometric means (and the predicted geometric means) are usually numerically lower than the observed means as they are less influenced by high values.

5.2.2 Parametric measures of spread

5.2.2.1 Variance

The variance is a measure of the variability of the population. As with the mean there is a true variance (usually denoted by σ^2) and a sample variance (s^2). The sample variance is obtained from assessing the variability of a random sample taken from the wider population.

There are several ways to calculate an estimate of the variance. For example, the sample variance s_i^2 of a group i can be calculated using the formula:

$$s_i^2 = \frac{1}{n_i - 1} \left[(x_1 - \bar{x}_{OM_i})^2 + (x_2 - \bar{x}_{OM_i})^2 + \dots + (x_{n_i} - \bar{x}_{OM_i})^2 \right], \tag{5.4}$$

where $\bar{x}_{OM_i}$ is the observed mean of the ith group, and $x_1, x_2, \dots, x_{n_i}$ are the n_i observations in the ith group.

Example 5.2 (continued): Control group example

The sample variance of the control group was calculated as:

$(1/9) \times [(2.3 - 4.27)^2 + (4.3 - 4.27)^2 + (6.5 - 4.27)^2 + \dots + (2.6 - 4.27)^2] = 2.88.$

Unfortunately the estimate of the individual variances (the s_i^2's) may not be reliable. It was noted above that to get a more reliable estimate of the true mean we usually need to increase the sample size. The same is true of the estimate of variability. Each of the s_i^2's is calculated from only a subset of the total number of animals in the study. The most reliable (and reproducible) estimate of the variability is obtained using all the available animals. This estimate can be found in, for example, the residual mean square entry in the ANOVA table (see Section 5.4.3).

The residual mean square entry in the ANOVA table is a statistical model-based estimate of the variability that uses results from all animals. The estimate is, in some sense, a weighted average of the individual s_i^2's. This estimate is only a reliable estimate of the true variance if the variability is similar across all groups – and this leads to the homogeneity of variance assumption of the parametric analyses, as discussed in Section 5.4.1.3.

5.2.2.2 Standard deviation

The standard deviation is the square root of the variance. It is a measure of the spread of the responses on the original scale. The sample standard deviation (s) is given by:

$$s = \sqrt{s^2}. \tag{5.5}$$

Example 5.2 (continued): Control group example

The sample standard deviation of the control group was calculated as:

$s = \sqrt{2.88} = 1.70.$

5.2.2.3 Standard error of the mean

The standard error of the mean (SEM) is a measure of the variability (or reliability) of the estimate of the sample mean. The reliability of the sample mean estimate will depend on the variability of the responses but also the number of observations (sample size) used to estimate the sample mean. The more observations used to calculate the sample mean, the more reliable that estimate will be.

When calculating the SEM it is common practice to use a within-group estimate of the variability, i.e. for the ith group mean:

$$SEM_i = \sqrt{\frac{s_i^2}{n_i}}, \tag{5.6}$$

where n_i is the ith group sample size and s_i is an estimate of the standard deviation of the observations in the ith group.

It is this estimate of the SEM that is commonly used, along with the observed mean, in the popular means with SEM plot (see Section 5.3.5). It can be argued that this within-group estimate of the variability is an appropriate estimate of the standard error of the observed mean as both the variance estimate and the observed mean are calculated separately for each experimental group.

Example 5.2 (continued): Control group example

The estimate of the standard error of the mean of the control group mean was calculated as:

$$SEM_{control} = \sqrt{\frac{2.88}{10}} = 0.54.$$

5.2.2.4 Confidence intervals

Confidence intervals provide a useful range of values within which the parameter of interest would be expected to lie. For a sample mean:

$$\text{lower } (1-\alpha)\text{ \% confidence interval} = \bar{x} - t_{\alpha/2,n-1}\sqrt{\frac{s^2}{n}},$$

$$(5.7)$$

and

$$\text{upper } (1-\alpha)\text{ \% confidence interval} = \bar{x} + t_{\alpha/2,n-1}\sqrt{\frac{s^2}{n}},$$

$$(5.8)$$

where α is the significance level (see Section 2.3.3), s^2 is the sample variance and $t_{\alpha/2,n-1}$ is the critical value of the t-distribution with parameters $\alpha/2$ and $n-1$.

As it is standard convention to test at the 5% significance level, i.e. p-values less than 0.05 (5%) are declared statistically significant (Section 2.3.3), so the confidence interval usually quoted is the 95% confidence interval. These confidence intervals are also related to the p-values generated as part of the statistical analysis. If we calculate the difference between two group means and generate a 95% confidence interval around the difference, then the associated two-sided p-value will be significant as long as the confidence interval does not contain zero. If one of the 95% confidence limits lies exactly on zero, then the two sided p-value will be equal to 0.05.

The estimate of variability (s^2) in the above calculation is usually the overall estimate of variability (for example, the residual mean square in the ANOVA table). Confidence intervals are therefore normally presented around the predicted means from the statistical analysis.

Example 5.2 (continued): Control group example

The 95% confidence interval of the mean of the control group was estimated as:

$$\text{lower 95\% confidence interval } = 4.3 - 2.26 \times \sqrt{\frac{2.88}{10}} = 3.06,$$

$$\text{upper 95\% confidence interval } = 4.3 + 2.26 \times \sqrt{\frac{2.88}{10}} = 5.48.$$

As a rule of thumb the confidence interval is a range of values that contains the true mean. However, a more accurate definition of the confidence interval is that it is the range of values such that if the study is repeated multiple times, and multiple confidence intervals are produced, then the true mean will be contained within 100 $\times (1-\alpha)$% of these confidence intervals. So for example, if a study was repeated 100 times, then 95 of the 100 confidence intervals for the predicted control group mean would contain the true control group mean.

5.2.2.5 Coefficient of variation

The coefficient of variation represents the unexplained variability in the sample mean as a percentage of the sample mean, i.e.:

$$\text{coefficient of variation of a sample mean} = \frac{s}{\bar{x}} \times 100\%,$$

$$(5.9)$$

where $\bar{x}$ is a sample mean and s is an estimate of the standard deviation.

This number can be a useful measure of the spread of the responses when the variation in the response increases in proportion to an increase in the size of the response.

Example 5.2 (continued): Control group example

The coefficient of variation of the mean of the control group was estimated as:

$$1.70 / 4.27 \times 100\% = 40\%.$$

5.2.3 Non-parametric measures of location

There are several measures of location that make fewer assumptions about the response characteristics than those discussed so far. We shall concentrate on one that is most commonly quoted in animal research, namely the *median*.

If the observations are arranged in increasing order, then the median is the middle observation. If the number of observations is odd, then there will be a unique middle observation. If the number of observations is even, then the median is usually defined as the average of the middle two observations.

Example 5.2 (continued): Control group example

As there are ten observations in the control group, the median of the control group is estimated at the average of the fifth and sixth largest observations:

$(3.4 + 4.3) / 2 = 3.85.$

The median can be a useful summary measure, for example, when the responses measured are not continuous (see Section 5.4.1.1) or not normally distributed (see Section 5.4.1.2). In this case a mean may not be an appropriate measure to summarise the location of the responses. For example, these two statements are both correct, although the second is perhaps more reliable:

- An average dog has less than four legs.
- A median dog has four legs.

The first statement is true because, sadly, more dogs have less than four legs than have more than four. However, the second statement is perhaps the more informative. This is mainly because a dog can have 0, 1, 2, 3 or 4 legs and hence the number of legs observed is neither a continuous nor normally distributed response.

5.2.4 Non-parametric measures of spread

Alongside the median, there are measures of spread that do not make so many assumptions about the response characteristics. Assume that the observations are arranged in increasing order. The *lower quartile* (Q1) is defined as the response such that one-quarter of the observations are below Q1. The *upper quartile* (Q3) is the value such that one-quarter of the observations are greater than Q3. The distance between Q1 and Q3 is known as the *interquartile range*. Q2 corresponds to the median, as discussed in Section 5.2.3.

Example 5.2 (continued): Control group example

As there are ten observations in the control group, the Q1 of the control group corresponds to the third largest observation and Q3 corresponds to the eighth largest:

Q1: 3.1 = third largest observation,
Q3: 5.6 = eighth largest observation.

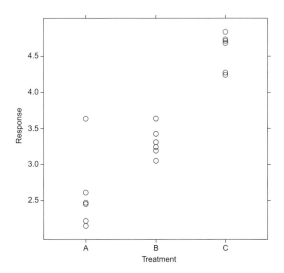

Figure 5.4. Scatterplot of the responses from an experiment involving three treatments.

5.3 Graphical tools

5.3.1 Scatterplots

When you begin the analysis of a dataset, we recommend you start by producing a scatterplot of the data. This plot provides a useful visual overview of the data and from it you can start to get a feel for your data. In its simplest form the scatterplot is merely a scatter of points in two directions (defined by the *X*-axis and the *Y*-axis). There are, however, many versions of the scatterplot, varying in complexity, which can be useful. We consider two different types that serve slightly different purposes.

In the first type of scatterplot the *X*-axis corresponds to a categorical factor and the *Y*-axis to the response. Each point on the graph corresponds to an individual observation in the dataset. For example, in Figure 5.4 the treatment factor has three levels (A, B and C) and the response ranges from about 2 to 5.

This plot allows us to get a feel for the size of the experimental effects, the spread (or variability) of the data (across all groups) and can also highlight any unusual observations. In Figure 5.4 there appears to be an unusually high response in treatment group A. We shall return to this plot in later sections, where it will be shown how it can help the researcher make certain

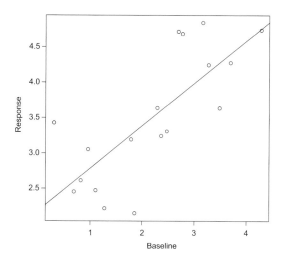

Figure 5.5. Scatterplot of the data assessing the relationship between the response and baseline variables including the best-fit linear line.

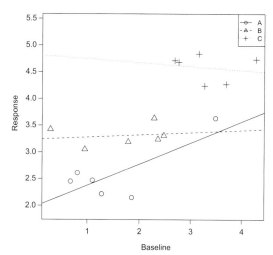

Figure 5.6. Scatterplot of the data assessing the relationship between the response and baseline variables including the best-fit linear line, categorised by treatment.

decisions about the statistical analysis, for example, by considering transformations (Section 5.4.1.3) and outliers (Section 5.4.1.5).

In the second type of scatterplot both the X-axis and Y-axis correspond to responses measured on the animal. These plots allow us to investigate the relationship between responses. In Figure 5.5 the response was measured at baseline and post-dose and this plot allows us to assess whether there is a relationship between them, i.e. if an animal is a high responder at baseline will it also be a high responder post-dose?

In many cases it is sensible to categorise such plots by a factor of interest. We can then investigate the within-group relationships between the two responses. This is particularly useful if the Y-axis corresponds to the response and the X-axis corresponds to a covariate (see Section 5.4.6.1). In Figure 5.5 we have ignored the Treatment factor. In the experiment the animals were administered one of three treatments and this may influence their responses. Such information may be important. Figure 5.6 includes this information.

The non-categorised plot revealed some evidence of an overall relationship between baseline and post-dose responses. By categorising the plot by the Treatment

factor we can see that there appears to be a relationship within each of the three treatment groups. The possible outlier in treatment group A (identified in the initial scatterplot) may have occurred because the animal has high responses before (as well as after) treatment. While this animal merits further investigation, it may not necessarily be an outlier if baseline information is used in the analysis (see also Example 5.17 in Section 5.4.6.4).

As the next example shows it can be dangerous to ignore the treatment factor categorisation when investigating the relationship between two responses.

Example 5.3: MRI quantification of the thymus

An experiment was conducted to see whether MRI could be used to assess glucocorticosteroid-related changes in thymus volume (Brooks *et al.*, 2005). This technique, the authors argued, provided many advantages over existing methods. It was non-invasive and allowed disease progression to be monitored over time within-animal. Animals were administered either the vehicle or increasing doses of the anti-inflammatory dexamethasone. The thymus volume was assessed pre and posttreatment using the MRI technique. To validate the approach the wet weight of the thymus was also measured post mortem.

A scatterplot of the resulting data, ignoring the treatment effects, was used to assess the overall relationship between the MRI and wet weight measures. This plot revealed there was evidence of an

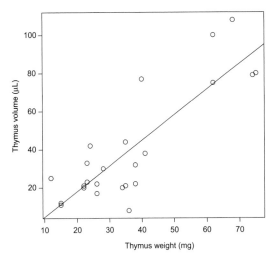

Figure 5.7. Scatterplot of the overall relationship between thymus volume and thymus wet weight, with best-fit linear line for Example 5.3.

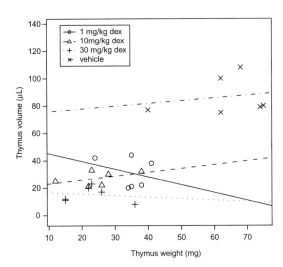

Figure 5.8. Scatterplot of the within-group relationships between thymus volume and thymus wet weight, with best-fit linear lines for Example 5.3.

overall relationship between the two measurement techniques. To investigate this relationship further, the within-group relationships were also assessed. If the within-group relationships were also strong, then this would be further evidence of a relationship between the two measurement techniques. If the within-group relationships were not strong, then it could be argued that the two measurement techniques were therefore not really related. Perhaps dexamethasone, acting independently on the thymus volume and wet weight, was causing the apparent strong overall relationship between them.

For example, consider the uncategorised scatterplot given in Figure 5.7 for some simulated data. There is strong evidence of an overall relationship. It is possible, however, that this relationship is caused by dexamethasone. It could be the case that there is no underlying relationship between the two responses but dexamethasone increases both thymus volume and wet weight (by different mechanisms). In other words, is the treatment effect causing the apparent correlation between the measures rather than there being an underlying relationship between them? If the same plot is categorised by treatment (and hence displays the within-group relationships) then the relationship is not quite so convincing (Figure 5.8). Of course, fewer observations are used to define the within-group relationships in Figure 5.8, hence it could be argued that these predicted lines are unreliable estimates of the true relationships.

5.3.2 Box-plots

Box-plots provide a useful way to summarise the data, particularly the within-group spread of the responses.

There are many ways to construct a box-plot, but the conventional way avoids certain tacit parametric assumptions that we shall describe below in Section 5.4.1. A box-plot is a series of boxes, one per group with lines (or whiskers) above and below the box. The following pieces of information can be displayed on a conventional box-plot:

- Median – see Section 5.2.3. Displayed as a dot within the boxes.
- Interquartile range – see Section 5.2.4. Displayed using boxes around the medians. The Q1 quartile defines the lower end of the boxes, the Q3 quartile defines the upper end of the boxes.
- Outlier range – usually a function of the size of the box. Displayed as the two whiskers above and below the boxes.
- Individual outliers – any observations that are outside the range of the whiskers are displayed as individual points on the plot.

An example of a box-plot involving three experimental groups is given in Figure 5.9. Note the unusual observation in treatment group A.

In many software packages it is possible to redefine these plotting options. For example, the central dot within the boxes can be the observed mean rather than

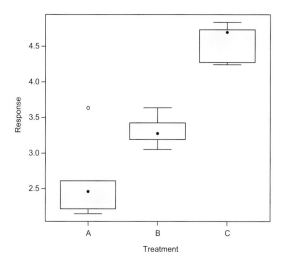

Figure 5.9. Box-plot of a response categorised by three treatment groups, including a possible outlier.

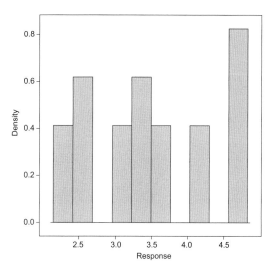

Figure 5.10. Density histogram of a response.

the median and the size of the boxes can be defined using the within-group variability rather than the inter-quartile range. However, if the scientist wants to produce a plot based on means and variances, certain assumptions about the nature of the response will be required. For example, the responses need to be continuous (see Section 5.4.1.1). We believe that one of the strengths of the box-plot (in its more conventional format) is that it is a plot of the data that does not rely on any parametric assumptions.

While it is usual to display possible outliers on box-plots we do not recommend using this approach to decide if an observation is an outlier; see Section 5.4.1.5 for more details. In the conventional box-plot, the method for defining an observation as an outlier is based on the within-group spread of the responses. These individual spreads can be unreliable if the group sizes are small.

5.3.3 Histograms

Histograms are a useful graphical tool for illustrating the distribution of the data. The *X*-axis corresponds to the response (and is usually broken up into a number of intervals) and the *Y*-axis corresponds to a measure

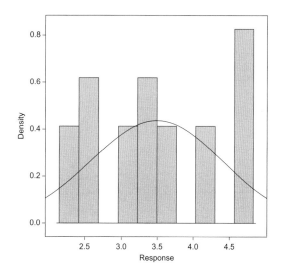

Figure 5.11. Density histogram of a response, including a normal distribution curve.

of the frequency of the response. The plot is then made up of a series of bars, where the area of each bar is proportional to the number of responses observed within that interval. An example of a histogram is given in Figure 5.10.

One assumption sometimes made when analysing experimental data is that the data are normally

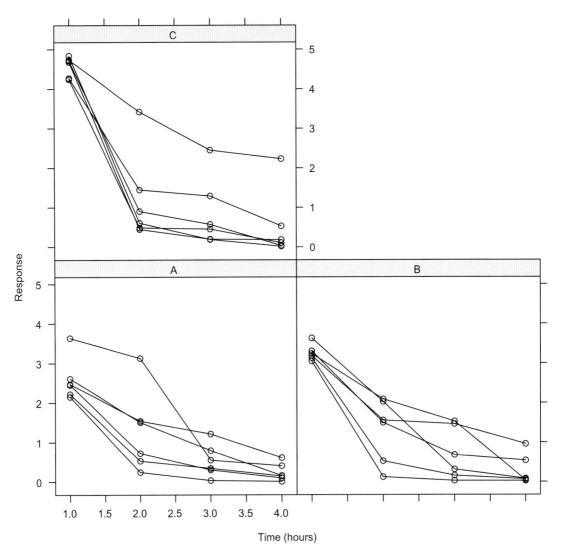

Figure 5.12. Categorised case profiles plot, categorised by a factor at three levels A, B and C.

distributed (see Section 2.2.4). This implies the distribution of the data follows a bell-shaped or Gaussian curve. The estimated normal curve can be superimposed on the histogram to give the scientist an idea of how normally distributed the response is. The bell-shaped curve is symmetrical about the central point, which indicates the location of the mean of the data. The shape of the curve gives an indication of the variability. The flatter

the curve the more variable the data. In Figure 5.11 a normal curve has been superimposed on top of the density histogram.

5.3.4 Categorised case profiles plot

If the response is measured repeatedly across the levels of a repeated factor, then the researcher should consider generating a categorised case profiles plot, an example of which is given in Figure 5.12.

A categorised case profiles plot is separated into a series of subplots, one per experimental group. For each subplot the Y-axis corresponds to the response and the X-axis corresponds to the levels of the repeated factor (usually time). The results for each animal are plotted in the relevant subplot, in a similar fashion to the scatterplot, except that the results for each animal are connected by a line. This gives an illustration of how each animal's response changes across the levels of the repeated factor.

These plots are useful for identifying the following.

Experimental group effects

The plot gives an overall view of the dataset. By comparing the profiles visually the researcher can start to identify any differences between the experimental groups.

Individual animal outliers

The plot allows the researcher to identify an animal that does not follow the overall group profile. In Figure 5.13 there appears to be one animal in group A with an unusual profile. When considering each time point separately none of the individual observations for this animal appears suspicious; however, the trend in the responses for this animal is in the opposite direction to the other group A animals. This may be worth investigating. By considering each of the time points separately we could have missed the unusual behaviour of this animal.

Individual observation outliers

While the profile of an individual animal follows the same general pattern as the rest of the group, there may be an individual measurement during the time course that is unusual. In the example in Figure 5.14 none of the individual responses in group A appears unusual, if each of the time points is considered separately; however, one of the animals in group A does appear to have a response at three hours that does not follow the overall trend for that group. If the three-hour data were

considered in isolation, this observation would not be considered an outlier as it is within the range of observations of the group A animals. In this case it *may* be better to remove the observation or replace it with the average of the neighbouring within-animal responses. This latter approach is, effectively, smoothing the data.

Choosing a suitable summary measure

If we can identify a summary measure that summarises the responses for each animal, then this will greatly simplify the statistical analysis. We describe some suitable measures in Section 5.4.4.2 and also discuss the benefits of using such a strategy in the statistical analysis.

For example, consider the example given in Figure 5.15 where there is no obvious trend across time. The average response per animal is perhaps a suitable summary measure that captures all the information recorded for each animal.

5.3.5 Means with SEMs plot

The observed means with standard errors plot (or means with SEMs plot for short) is perhaps the most popular plot produced by animal researchers. These plots are an established visual language that allows results to be communicated to others. They consist of a series of bars anchored at zero, where the height of the bars corresponds to the observed means (see Section 5.2.1.2) and the error bars on the plot correspond to the standard error of the means. SEMs are usually calculated using within-group estimates of the variability (see Section 5.2.2.1). An example of a means with SEMs plot, as produced by InVivoStat, is given in Figure 5.16.

5.3.5.1 Problems with the means with SEMs plot

While these plots are undeniably useful, they do have certain drawbacks that need to be recognised whenever they are produced. In this section we assume that the standard approach has been used to produce the means with SEMs plot, i.e. the means are observed means and the error bars are generated using the within-group variability estimates. Some of the criticisms described

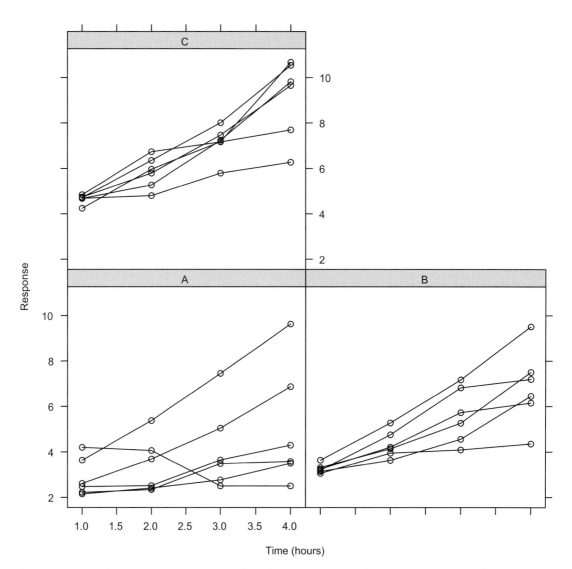

Figure 5.13. Categorised case profiles plot, categorised by a factor at three levels A, B and C, with an unusual profile for an animal in group A.

below can be avoided if the predicted means are included in the diagram and the variability estimate used to generate the standard errors is the single value calculated as part of the statistical analysis. However, this approach is not often taken by either scientists or statistical software packages and hence it would have to be carried out manually.

Reliability of the SEMs
If the sample size is small ($n = 3$, for example) then the standard errors may not be reliable. Each standard error relies on the estimate of the within-group variability. So if there are only three animals in a group, then these variability estimates will probably be unreliable. Cumming *et al.* (2007) suggest that in such cases

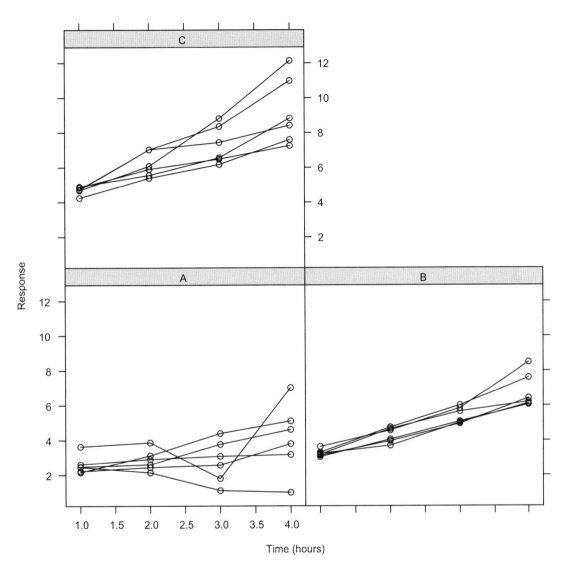

Figure 5.14. Categorised case profiles plot, categorised by a factor at three levels A, B and C, with an unusual result for one animal in group A at 3 hours.

it may be more appropriate to produce a scatterplot of the data rather than the means with SEMs plot.

SEMs depend on the sample size
The standard error is not only dependent on the within-group variability but also the sample size. So two error bars (on the same plot) are only comparable,

in some sense, if the sample sizes are approximately the same. The group with the largest sample size may appear to be less variable than the others simply because of the larger sample size. To avoid confusion the researcher should clearly state the sample sizes on the plot, especially if the sample sizes vary between the groups.

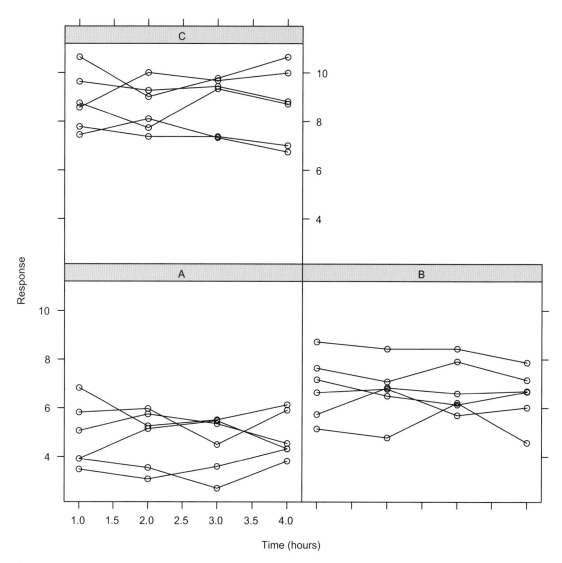

Figure 5.15. Categorised case profiles plot that suggests an average response for each animal may be a suitable summary measure to analyse.

No mathematical link between the means with SEMs plot and the statistical analysis

In many cases the plot is not linked (mathematically) to the statistical analysis and hence the plot can contradict the results of the statistical analysis. Consider the ANOVA-based analysis approaches, discussed in Section 5.4.3. One of the assumptions of many of these analyses, as we shall see, is that the variability

of the responses is the same across all groups. Now in the means with SEMs plot the variability is calculated separately for each group. While this has certain benefits, it does imply that when carrying out the ANOVA analysis we make assumptions that are not reflected on the means with SEMs plot. This can lead to contradictions! The authors have been asked many times:

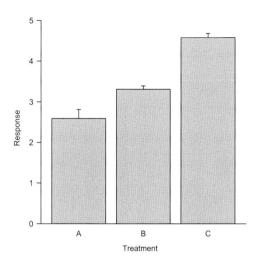

Figure 5.16. Observed means with standard errors plot.

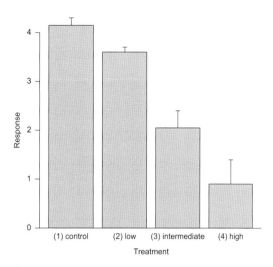

Figure 5.17. Observed means with standard errors plot where the variability varies across the four treatment groups.

Why was that comparison not statistically significant? It looks as if it should be.

As an example consider Figure 5.17. The statistical analysis revealed a non-significant difference between the lowest dose of the compound and the control (using a one-way ANOVA followed by planned comparisons, see Section 5.4.8.3). Perhaps the sample size was too low and the tests underpowered (Section 3.7.2). A visual inspection of the means with SEMs plot suggested that the comparison should be significant. However, as the statistical tests were based on the pooled estimate of variability (pooled across all groups) then due to the higher variability in the intermediate and high dose groups, it can be argued that the pooled estimate of the variability is overestimating the variability in the control and low dose groups. As the variability was slightly lower in the control and low dose group, compared to the variability in the other groups, the comparison appears significant on the means with SEMs plot when the statistical test was not significant.

In practice there may be biological reasons why these treatment groups are less variable than the others, or it may just be due to the random sample taken in this experiment and it does not represent true differences. Out of interest we used the pooled estimate of variability (from the one-way ANOVA analysis) when

calculating the SEMs on the above plot. In this plot the lack of significance in the control vs. low dose comparison is more apparent (Figure 5.18).

Non-applicability in more complex statistical models
When performing the statistical analysis, it may be the case that the variability of the data can be reduced by accounting for other nuisance effects in the statistical analysis. For example, if we can include a blocking factor in the analysis, then this will reduce the underlying variability. The (within-group) variance estimates used to calculate the SEMs do not take into account the reduction in the underlying variability achieved by fitting the blocking factor.

Consider an example where the experimental design for the study consists of a treatment factor and an influential blocking factor. The means with SEMs plot appears to show that there is not a significant treatment effect at the lowest dose (Figure 5.19).

However, if we plot the treatment means separately for each block (i.e. we take into account the reduction in variability achieved by including the blocking factor in the analysis) then the error bars become much tighter and the significant treatment effects are revealed. This plot is given in Figure 5.20.

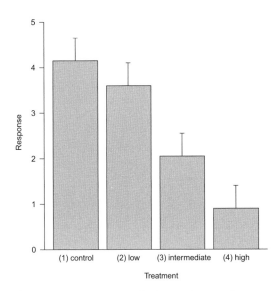

Figure 5.18. Means with standard errors plot using the pooled estimate of the variability to calculate the standard errors.

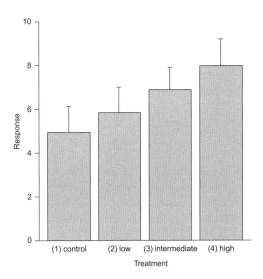

Figure 5.19. Means with standard errors plot from an experiment involving a blocking factor. The standard errors were calculated without taking into account the blocking factor.

Multiple sources of variability

Consider the case where there is more than one source of variability in the experiment, for example when

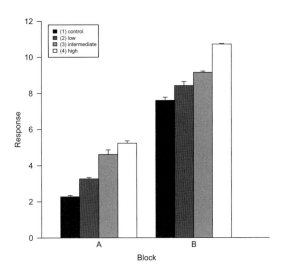

Figure 5.20. Means with standard errors plot from an experiment involving a blocking factor. Means and standard errors were calculated at each level of the blocking factor.

using repeated measures or split-plot designs. In such cases the level of variability that the experimental factors are tested against will vary depending on the factor. The means with SEMs plot does not reflect this.

For example, consider an experiment involving repeatedly measured responses. Each animal receives only one treatment and is then measured repeatedly over time. Comparisons between treatment groups (at a given time point) will be assessed against the between-animal variability, whereas comparisons made to investigate the change over time (within a treatment group) will be assessed against the within-animal variability. As the within-animal variability is usually smaller than the between-animal variability, the latter comparisons are more sensitive than the former. Nieuwenhuis *et al.* (2011) comment that the error bars on a means with SEMs plot should reflect the variability of the differences that are being tested. This is not apparent from the orthodox means with SEMs plot; see also Cumming *et al.* (2007).

In the following example, involving a repeated measures design, there was no evidence of a significant difference between the treatment and control groups at 1 hour ($p = 0.364$), but the change in the control group means between 1 and 2 hours was statistically

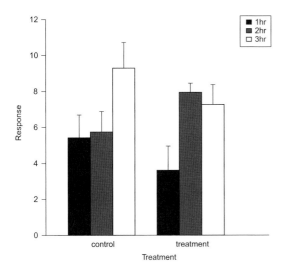

Figure 5.21. Observed means with standard errors plot from a repeated measures experiment.

Assessing the equal variance ANOVA assumption
As stated above, the error bars plotted are calculated separately for each group and this does have one advantage. By considering the size of the error bars, the scientist can get a feel for the validity of the assumption, required for the ANOVA analysis, that the variability is the same across all groups. If the error bars get bigger as the means get bigger then this may indicate that the response variable should be transformed prior to analysis (see Section 5.4.1.3). Note this approach only works if the sample size is approximately the same for all groups and there is no other factor, such as a blocking factor, present in the experimental design. If either of these conditions is not satisfied, then care must be taken when drawing conclusions using the plot. There is another plot that can be used that does not suffer from these constraints, as we shall see in Section 5.4.5. However, the means with SEMs plot does at least highlight that there may be a problem with the homogeneity of variance assumption.

significant ($p = 0.042$). This is not obvious from an examination of the error bars on the means with SEMs plot (Figure 5.21) and is due to the latter comparison being assessed against the much smaller within-animal variability, which is not shown on the plot.

5.3.5.2 Benefits of the means with SEMs plot

Given the issues highlighted above should we stop using this plot? Perhaps. However, there are two benefits that should be considered when using these plots that perhaps do endorse their use.

Universal graphical language
Plots of means with SEMs are a well-established visual way for scientists to communicate results. If the purpose of a graph is to summarise the results of an experiment so that others can draw their own conclusion about the study findings, then this plot provides a useful tool for doing so. It should be remembered that for simple experimental designs involving a single experimental factor, with equal sample sizes, the error bars plotted on the graph are a reasonable representation of the pooled variability estimate used in the analysis.

5.4 Parametric analysis

Once the data has been visually assessed the researcher should have a feel for the experimental results. Attention can now turn to performing a more formal statistical analysis. In this chapter we shall concentrate on parametric statistical analysis techniques.

Parametric analysis is an approach that relies on the assumption that the distribution of the responses we are measuring, once any fixed factors have been taken into account, follows a certain probability distribution. We then make statistical inferences about the parameters that define this distribution. For example, we may assume the response we are measuring is normally distributed (a distribution defined by the sample means and sample variance). Under this assumption we can then assess the differences between the sample means by comparing the size of these differences to the sample variance. We need not confine ourselves to the normal distribution though. For example, later in this chapter other parametric tests are considered that rely on the assumption that the responses are chi-squared distributed.

As well as making distributional assumptions, when performing a parametric analysis, we may also need to assume:

- the responses are numeric and continuous;
- the variability is the same across all groups (homogeneity of variance);
- the observations are independent;
- there are no outlying observations unduly influencing the results;
- the effects behave in an additive way.

The parametric family of statistical tests we consider in this section can take into account the experimental design employed and hence provides a flexible and powerful set of tools for analysing data. We argue that, where possible, the researcher should always aim to use a parametric test. These tests include the following.

t-test This test is appropriate if you have a single factor at two levels (for example you wish to compare a treatment and control). We do not recommend using the *t*-test in more complex situations.

One-way ANOVA This test should be used if your experiment consists of a single factor at more than two levels (for example three doses of a test compound and control). The ANOVA table provides an overall test to see if the experimental factor means are different. If you want to make pairwise comparisons between the individual factor means then you need to use *post hoc* tests, multiple comparison procedures or planned comparisons. Note that all of these tests (the overall test and any pairwise tests) use an estimate of the variability derived from all of the data. This estimate is a more reliable and reproducible estimate of the variability because all of the data have been used to calculate it.

Two- and higher-order ANOVA If the experiment was conducted using a factorial design, then the two- and higher-order ANOVA approaches allow the researcher to investigate these multiple factors of interest. The ANOVA table contains not only overall tests of the factors but also assessments of how the factors interact with each other. For example, the experiment may consist of testing several treatments in two strains of mice. Using a two-way ANOVA approach allows the researcher to assess not only the overall differences between the treatment and strain means, but also to investigate if the effects of the treatments vary between strains. As with the one-way ANOVA, pairwise comparisons between the predicted means can still be made using *post hoc* tests, multiple comparison procedures or planned comparisons.

Repeated measures analysis In many animal experiments the response of an animal to a stimulus is measured repeatedly, perhaps over time. In the analysis of these experiments we introduce a repeated factor into the analysis to assess how the response changes. As measurements recorded on the same animal are likely to be more related than those recorded on different animals, due to the lack of randomisation, we need to take these spatial interrelationships into account in the analysis. This can be achieved using repeated measures analysis techniques.

5.4.1 Parametric assumptions

Before we consider the parametric tests in detail, we shall look at some of the assumptions that are made when running these analyses. It should be remembered that these assumptions should hold, or at least be reasonably well satisfied, for the test results to be valid. When they do hold the parametric analysis is a (statistically) powerful analysis tool.

5.4.1.1 Numeric and continuous responses

There is a tacit assumption, made when carrying out a parametric analysis, that the response measured is numeric and continuous. As discussed above these responses should be the first choice for any animal researcher as they contain the most information (and hence will allow animal numbers to be reduced).

As well as being numeric and continuous, the response should not be bounded above or below and hence it should be possible to measure a response at any numerical value (positive or negative). Of course in practice many responses are bounded below by zero. An animal cannot have a negative body weight, although body weight change can be negative. It is also not uncommon for responses to be bounded above too. There may be a physical limit to the size an animal can grow to, and so any larger values are biologically impossible. There may also be practical constraints that produce an upper boundary. For example, in an experiment to assess the analgesic effect of a compound using the hotplate animal model, the response is bounded below by zero (a physical constraint) and above by 30 seconds (an ethical constraint). We discuss a strategy for analysing data with such limits in Section 5.5.3.

Sometimes this assumption can be relaxed. Discrete responses (Section 3.2.1.1) are numeric but not necessarily continuous. For example, the response measured could be a count response, such as the number of rearings observed in a five-minute time period. Such responses, while not necessarily being continuous, may behave in a quasi-continuous way if the number of counts recorded is relatively high and the range of counts sufficiently large. Count responses are (in theory) not bounded above; however, other types of discrete response are bounded. For example, in an animal model of arthritis each paw of the animal is given the clinical score of 0, 1, 2, 3 or 4. This gives the animal a maximum score of 16 (summing over all four paws).

So when should we be concerned that our data are not numeric and continuous? In practice it is difficult to define a formal rule. Almost all responses are bounded and so in theory few responses would pass if we strictly adhered to satisfying this assumption. It is our belief that:

- If the response is bounded, then as long as these boundaries are not attained by the majority of the animals within each experimental group, the researcher can proceed using a parametric analysis. If all the responses in a group (such as a positive control) are recorded at a boundary, then this group should be removed from the analysis. We contend this is one of the few justifications for removing a group from the analysis.
- For count and ordinal data, as long as there is a reasonably large range of responses observed within each group, and all the observations in a group do not consist of only one or two distinct values, then we feel we can assume the data are continuous.

In both of these cases a degree of common sense is required. If you feel that the data cannot be considered continuous, or you are worried about making assumptions that may not hold, then you should consider taking an alternative approach, such as performing a non-parametric test, a test of proportions or a survival analysis (see Sections 5.5.1, 5.5.2 and 5.5.3, respectively).

5.4.1.2 Normally distributed residuals

When we carry out most statistical analyses, we fit a statistical model to the data. This may involve, for example, simply calculating experimental group means, or estimating the non-linear relationship between response and the dose of the novel compound. Once a statistical model has been fitted to the data, for each observation in the dataset we can calculate a predicted value. This is the value that the statistical model predicts the individual observation should be. It can be a group mean or a specific point on the prediction curve. While there will be a spread of responses within each experimental group, the average or mean value is the value that we predict all the observations in that group should be. Of course in practice some observations will be observed above the predicted value and some below. The residual for an observation is a measure of the distance the observation is from the predicted value. So for the *i*th observation in the dataset:

$$observation_i = predicted_i + residual_i. \qquad (5.10)$$

When we perform a parametric analysis we assume that the residuals from the statistical analysis (and not the responses) are *normally distributed*. By saying normally distributed we imply that the distribution of the residuals follows a normal or bell-shaped curve (see Section 2.2.4). The majority of the residuals will cluster around the mean (zero in this case) but there will always be some high and some low residuals – these define the tails of the distribution. The easiest way to appreciate the distribution of the residuals is to plot a histogram of them. We can then superimpose a normal curve on the histogram to summarise the distribution.

To highlight that it is the residuals that need to be considered for normality and not the responses themselves, consider the following example.

Example 5.4: A simple drug study with non-normal residuals

A study was set up to test the effect of a novel compound. The experimental design consisted of two treatment groups (treatment and control) and it was decided in advance to measure a

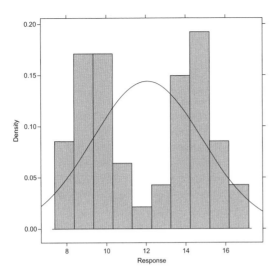

Figure 5.22. Histogram of the responses measured for Example 5.4.

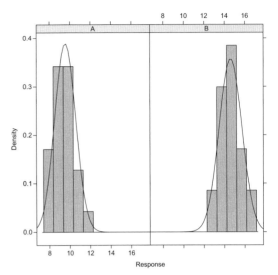

Figure 5.23. Histogram of the responses measured for Example 5.4, categorised by treatment group.

continuous numerical response. A histogram of the response, given in Figure 5.22, illustrated that the responses were not normally distributed; the distribution of the response appeared to have two peaks.

However, once the treatment effect was taken into account (which we achieved by fitting a statistical model to the data involving two groups) then the responses within each group did appear to be normally distributed. In Figure 5.23 we have categorised the histogram by treatment group. Note the heights of the bars are different in Figures 5.22 and 5.23 due to the differences in the number of bars included in the plots.

There are various ways to check the assumption that the residuals are normally distributed. To begin with there are several formal statistical tests, such as the Shapiro–Wilk (Shapiro and Wilk, 1965) and Kolmogorov–Smirnov tests (Kolmogorov, 1933; Smirnov, 1939). However, it can be argued that these tests are not powerful at detecting non-normality, especially if the sample sizes are small (as they invariably are in animal experiments). A second, and we believe more reliable approach, is to produce a normal probability plot of the residuals.

Normal probability plot
To produce a normal probability plot, the n residuals (corresponding to the n observations in the dataset) are ranked from the smallest to the largest. For each

residual R_i ($1 \leq i \leq n$) we then calculate the corresponding percentage point P_i from the standard-normal distribution. There are several ways to calculate the P_i's, for example:

$$P_i = \frac{(i-3/8)}{(n+1/4)} \text{ if } n \leq 10, \tag{5.11}$$

$$P_i = \frac{(i-1/3)}{n} \text{ if } n > 10, \tag{5.12}$$

where n is the total number of observations.

The P_i's are then plotted (on the X-axis) against the residuals (on the Y-axis). Effectively we are comparing the spread of the actual residuals against what they should be if normally distributed. If the residuals are normally distributed, then all the points on the plot should lie along a straight line. If the residuals are not normally distributed, then they will deviate from this line.

In the first of the following normal probability plots (Figure 5.24), the points do not lie on the line indicating that the residuals are not normally distributed. In the second plot (Figure 5.25), however, the points more closely follow the line, indicating the residuals are normally distributed.

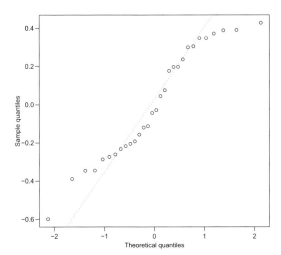

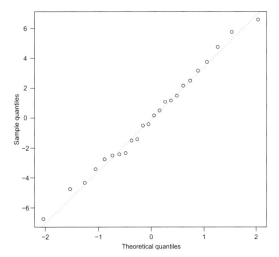

Figure 5.24. Normal probability plot showing the residuals are not normally distributed. The individual points do not follow the dotted line.

Figure 5.25. Normal probability plot showing the residuals are normally distributed. The individual points follow the dotted line reasonably well.

In practice certain types of response may not be normally distributed (and hence the residuals are not normally distributed either). For example, some continuous responses may be log-normally distributed (where the distribution is not a symmetrical bell-shaped curve but asymmetrical with a longer right-hand tail). We shall consider this situation later on in this section.

In conclusion it is worth noting that the parametric tests are fairly robust against some degree of departure from normality (Montgomery, 1997, p. 81). So perhaps in practice this is an assumption that we can afford to relax. As long as the points in the normal probability plot lie reasonably close to the straight line, then we should be justified in proceeding with the parametric analysis.

5.4.1.3 Homogeneity of variance

One of the key assumptions we make when performing most parametric analyses is the *homogeneity of variance* assumption. If the homogeneity of variance assumption holds then the variability of the response is not related to the size of the response. This implies that within-group variability is the same for all groups

and is not dependent on the size of the group means. In the authors' experience of biological experiments, this assumption may not hold and hence it should be checked prior to looking at the results of the parametric analysis.

It is often the case with biological responses that the variability increases as the response increases. Perhaps the response we are measuring increases exponentially, for example bacterial cell count. It may also be the case that there is a physical constraint on the response. For example, if the response cannot be negative then as the response measured approaches zero the variability tends to decrease. In both cases the homogeneity of variance assumption may not hold.

There are several statistical tests that can be used to assess the homogeneity of variance assumption. These include the Brown–Forsythe test (Brown and Forsythe, 1974), Levene's test (Levene, 1960) and Bartlett's test (Bartlett, 1937). The latter is suitable when there is only one experimental factor in the experimental design. However, care should be taken when using Bartlett's test as it is sensitive to non-normally distributed data.

We do not recommend using any of these tests to assess the homogeneity of variance assumption. For

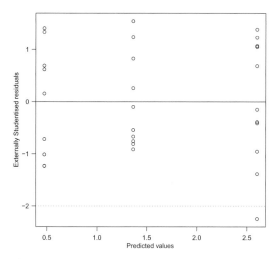

Figure 5.26. Predicted vs. residuals plot for an experiment involving three groups.

small sample sizes (as is invariably so in animal experiments) the power of these tests to identify heterogeneous variability is limited. Additionally, when these statistical tests suggest that the homogeneity of variance assumption does not hold, they do not offer a solution. It should also be noted that outliers can influence the results of these tests, especially when the sample size is small. As Box (1953) famously noted:

To make a preliminary test on variances is rather like putting to sea in a rowing boat to find out whether conditions are sufficiently calm for an ocean liner to leave port!

An alternative approach to these statistical tests is to use a *predicted vs. residuals plot* to assess the homogeneity of variance assumption. We recommend the researcher consider this plot before looking at the results of the analysis.

Predicted vs. residuals plot

As described above, each observation in a dataset can be broken down into two parts, the predicted part and the residual part. For the ith observation in the dataset,

$$\text{observation}_i = \text{predicted}_i + \text{residual}_i. \tag{5.13}$$

If the assumption of homogeneity of variance holds, then no matter how numerically large the observations

(and hence the predicted values) are, the residuals should all be approximately the same size. In other words, the spread of observations in a group with a high mean should be the same as the spread of observations in a group with a low mean.

To test the homogeneity of variance assumption we produce a scatterplot of the data where:

• The Y-axis corresponds to the residuals from the analysis.
• The X-axis corresponds to the predicted values from the analysis.
• Each observation in the dataset corresponds to one point on the scatterplot.

A typical example is given in Figure 5.26. The experiment involves three treatment groups; hence the predictions from the statistical model consist of three means, one per group. The lowest group mean is 0.5, the middle group mean is about 1.4 and the highest is 2.6. Hence the X-axis on the plot can only take three distinct values (corresponding to the three group means). The Y-axis corresponds to the residuals and has a range between +2 and –2 in this case.

Notice on this plot that the spread of the responses on the Y-axis is the same for each X-axis value. This implies the size of the residuals (Y-axis spread) is the same for each treatment group (distinct X-axis value). In general, assuming the assumption of homogeneity of variance holds, then the size of the residuals (or spread of the individual points in the vertical direction) should be the same for all the predicted values.

As mentioned above, usually in biological experiments the homogeneity of variance assumption does not hold because the variability increases as the response increases. Therefore, as the predicted values increase so the sizes of the residuals increase. If this is the case then you will observe a 'fanning effect' in the predicted vs. residuals plot.

Example 5.5: An experiment where the response needs transforming

The predicted vs. residuals plot given in Figure 5.27 was obtained as part of the analysis of a biological response. The plot displays the classic 'fanning effect'.

As mentioned above it should be possible in such cases to stabilise the variance by transforming the

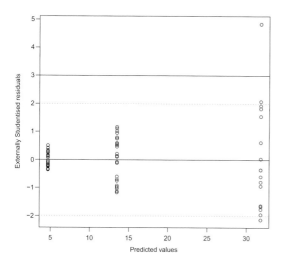

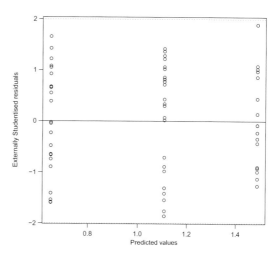

Figure 5.27. Predicted vs. residuals plot for Example 5.5, where the variability of the responses increases with the size of the response. The predicted vs. residuals plot displays a fanning effect.

Figure 5.28. Predicted vs. residuals plot for Example 5.5 (following a log transformation), with no evidence of a fanning effect.

data. By transforming the data we imply that all of the observations are transformed onto a new scale. For example, if the data are log-transformed then for the ith observation:

$$\text{transformed observation}_i = \log_{10}(\text{observation}_i),$$
$$\text{for } i = 1, ..., n. \tag{5.14}$$

Common transformations include:

Log transformation Useful for log-normally distributed data (where the within-group variability increases with the group mean) or when the response measured increases exponentially (such as bacterial cell counts). This is perhaps the most common transformation applied to biological data. It can be performed on either the $\log_{10}$ or $\log_e$ scale. $\log_{10}$ is favoured by researchers as certain types of response are often quoted on this scale. Statisticians tend to prefer $\log_e$ as it has some useful mathematical properties.

In the authors' experience many responses often require log-transforming, for example gene expression data, cytokine responses and triglyceride levels in blood plasma. Also a response that is bounded below by zero may need transforming if one or more of the experimental groups reduces the response so that the group means are close to zero. These groups often tend to be less variable due to the responses being close to the lower boundary and log-transforming may be required.

Example 5.5 (continued): An experiment where the response needs transforming

The analysis of the response above revealed a fanning effect in the predicted vs. residuals plot. Once the data was log-transformed this fanning effect was removed (Figure 5.28).

One of the disadvantages of the log transformation is that a zero response cannot be transformed ($\log(0)$ does not exist). So if you have zeros in the response being analysed, you will need to add a small offset onto all of the responses to avoid losing these data points. There is no correct value to use as an offset, but 10% of the lowest non-zero observation is a good starting point. In practice the offset chosen should not be too small because otherwise the zero responses (once transformed) will become unusually low results on the log scale and will look like outliers. These will show up on the predicted vs. residuals plot as points with unusually low Y-axis values.

We comment more on outliers below, but it is worth noting that an unusually large observation (with a correspondingly large residual) that appears to be an outlier on the original scale may not be an outlier on the transformed scale. For example, if the response is log normally distributed then this observation may appear

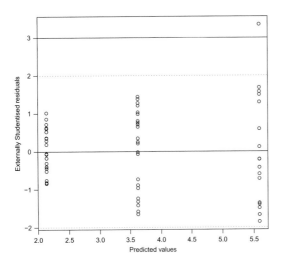

Figure 5.29. Predicted vs. residuals plot for Example 5.5, where the variability of the responses increases with the size of the response (following a square root transformation).

acceptable on the log scale. The response appears to be an outlier (on the original scale) simply because the variability is higher for the larger observations. An example of this can be seen in Example 5.5 where the largest observation in the dataset no longer appears to be an outlier when the responses are transformed onto the log scale (see Figure 5.28).

Alternatively you may find that an observation close to zero, which looks acceptable on the original scale, is an outlier on the log scale (see Example 5.7, Figure 5.32). Decisions on outliers should only be made after the transformation has been selected!

Square root transformation This transformation is not as strong as the log transformation and so can be used if the log transformation produces a fanning effect on the predicted vs. residuals plot that is the opposite of that observed in Figure 5.27.

Example 5.5 (continued): An experiment where the response needs transforming

The predicted vs. residuals plot for Example 5.5 following a square root transformation is given in Figure 5.29. We can see that the square root transformation has reduced the fanning effect seen in the predicted vs. residuals plot of the untransformed response (Figure 5.27), but it has not completely stabilised the variability across the groups. In this example the log transformation (Figure 5.28) is the most appropriate transformation to apply.

From a pragmatic point of view, square root transformations are useful if there are zeros in the dataset. There is no need to add an offset to the response as sqrt(0) = 0. If there is little to choose between the fanning effect observed in the predicted vs. residuals plot for the square root and log transformations, and there are zero responses, then the square root transformation may be preferable as it does not require an offset to be applied.

There is also theoretical justification for using the square root transformation if the response measured is a count response. It can be shown that the transformation

$$\text{transformed response} = \sqrt{(\text{count response} + 3/8)} \quad (5.15)$$

can be expected to satisfy both the homogeneity of variance assumption and the normality assumption discussed in the previous section.

Arcsine transformation For proportion responses (that are bounded above by 1 and below by 0), then the arcsine transformation may be appropriate:

$$\text{transformed response} = \arcsin(\sqrt{p}) \quad (5.16)$$

where $0 < p < 1$, p being the proportion response.

With responses bounded above and below there is a tendency for the variability of the response to decrease as it approaches these boundaries. The arcsine transformation increases the variability of the responses at the boundaries and decreases the variability of the responses in the middle of the range.

More generally any response that is bounded above and below can be transformed using the arcsine transformation. Of course they need to be normalised so that all responses lie between 0 and 1. An example of the use of an arcsine transformation can be found in the analysis of an attentional set shifting task experiment (Hatcher *et al.*, 2005). In this case one of the responses analysed was the proportion of the maximum number of trials performed (by one of the animals) within the experiment.

5.4.1.4 Independence of the responses

When carrying out a parametric analysis we assume that the responses are independent. So each response (and the procedures that were involved in generating that response) does not influence any other response in the dataset, once the experimental factors have been accounted for.

It can be argued that one of the purposes of the randomisation is to provide the scientist with a way of justifying the assumption that the responses are independent. If a suitable randomisation has been performed, as part of the experimental process, then this should remove the relationships between the responses that will not be accounted for by the experimental factors and hence we can assume the observations are independent.

It should be noted that the levels of the repeated factor in a repeated measures design (time points or brain regions, for example) cannot be randomised. This implies that the repeated measurements taken within an animal will probably not be independent of each other. This leads to the repeated measures analysis approach where we account for the interrelationships between observations taken on each animal within the statistical analysis.

5.4.1.5 Removal of outliers

While not strictly one of the assumptions of the parametric analysis, the presence of outliers may influence our decision to accept or reject the assumptions discussed above. So it is a good idea to see if any observations are possible outliers, and hence can be removed from the analysis, during the assessment of the parametric analysis assumptions.

An observation considered to be an outlier may be a genuinely unusual response, but it may also be identified because incorrect assumptions are made about the distribution of the responses. As we shall see below, it is possible that the responses are not normally distributed and hence observations that appear to be outliers (under the assumption that the responses are normally distributed) are not unusual when other distributional assumptions are considered.

There is no single rule that can be used to identify outliers, and even the definition of an outlier itself is a contentious one. Such decisions must come down to personal belief, type of response and the choice of statistical procedure. In this section we shall describe some of the statistical procedures that can be used

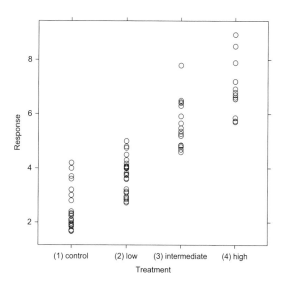

Figure 5.30. Scatterplot of the responses for Example 5.6 involving three treated groups and a control group.

when deciding whether an observation is an outlier or not. We emphasise, however, that this discussion should only be taken as a guide.

Use scatterplots to identify outliers
The scatterplot, described in Section 5.3.1, should be used as an initial tool for identifying possible outliers. This plot has the advantage that it allows the scientist to look at the distribution of the responses across the whole dataset when deciding on outliers.

Example 5.6: A drug study with an unusual observation

Consider the following example consisting of three treatment groups and a control. A scatterplot of the response data (Figure 5.30) reveals a possible high outlier in the intermediate dose group. But is this observation an outlier? While it may look unusually high (for that group) it does lie within the range of the responses observed in the high dose group. Perhaps it was an animal that responded well to the treatment? Crucially though if we look at the spread of data in the other three groups, we see that the spread in the intermediate dose group (including the suspicious observation) is not unusual. The observation looks unusual because the distribution of the observations within that group is not uniform. Perhaps if we repeated the experiment we would have measured responses in the gap between the 'outlier' and the rest of the intermediate dose group data. So in conclusion we would not exclude this observation.

Biological vs. statistical outliers

Some scientists feel that a biological (rather than statistical) argument is the *only* way to really justify the removal of an outlier from a dataset. For example, the animal was losing weight when the testing began or just looked unwell during the experiment. This would be a valid reason for excluding the subject's responses as they may have been influenced by other uncontrollable factors. If this is the case then it is a strong justification for exclusion.

Of course to be able to exclude observations using this approach detailed records of the conditions of the experiment must be kept to identify outliers after the data has been collected and assessed. However, even if there are no biological reasons to explain why an observation is unusual, we argue it is perhaps too strict a rule to always include it in the analysis. For example, the biological reason that would identify why the observation was unusual may not have been recorded. If the results of the statistical analysis are heavily influenced by an unusual observation, then we feel it should be excluded, or at least an analysis performed with and then without the observation present in the dataset.

The 2SD rule

Perhaps the most commonly employed rule to detect outliers is the two standard deviation rule (2SD). For each experimental group we first calculate the observed mean and the within-group standard deviation. If any observation is further than two standard deviations from the observed mean then it is declared an outlier. Effectively this approach involves looking at the residuals for each observation and rejecting observations that have residuals that are too large.

Although commonly applied, this approach can be problematic for several reasons:

Assumptions regarding the response Firstly it assumes the data are continuous and normally distributed. If they are not, and a non-parametric analysis is used to analyse the data, then the 2SD rule should not be applied. In these situations perhaps the median should be used rather than the observed mean when calculating the 'residual' for an observation. Also some function of the range of the data rather than the standard deviation should be used to quantify the spread of

the data (because the standard deviation is not a meaningful measure of the variability in such cases).

Transformations The 2SD rule should also not be applied if the response was transformed prior to analysis. An assessment of outliers should be made on the transformed scale and not the original scale. This is particularly true of log transformations where, as we have seen above, unusually high responses that appear to be outliers on the original scale are not outliers on the log scale.

Chance of finding an outlier It should be remembered that if the responses are normally distributed, then we would expect about 4.6% of the observations to lie beyond the 2SD boundaries. These are not outliers, they are just the observations we would expect to see in the tails of a normally distributed response. So by applying this rule we risk excluding valid data. If we apply the rule at the 3SD boundary, then only 0.3% of the observations from a normally distributed response would fall outside the boundary. Perhaps the 2SD boundary should therefore be seen as a warning limit and the 3SD as the action limit, as is the case in statistical process control.

Example 5.7: Outlier on the log scale

Consider the following experiment involving two doses of a compound and the vehicle. Let us assume the response being measured is known to be log-normally distributed. A scatterplot of the data on the original scale reveals a possible outlier in the 10 mg/kg dose group (Figure 5.31).

However, is this a true outlier, or is it an artefact of the response being log-normally distributed?

A plot of the data on the log scale, see Figure 5.32, reveals that it is the lowest observation in the vehicle group which is an unusual observation. The high response in the 10 mg/kg dose group is not an outlier. This result is high due to the increased variability of the larger responses. If the statistical analysis, perhaps using a one-way ANOVA, was performed on the log-transformed data, then it is the low observation in the vehicle group that would need to be removed.

Applicability of the variance estimate Finally (and perhaps most importantly) remember that most of the parametric analyses uses a pooled estimate of the variability, pooled over all groups. The 2SD test for outliers relies on the within-group estimates of variability and hence is not applicable if these parametric analyses are used. As many parametric analyses pool the variability

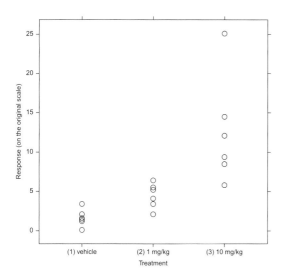

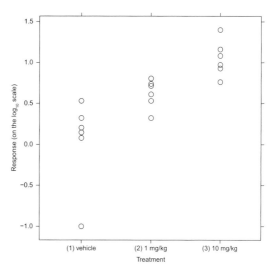

Figure 5.31. Scatterplot of the responses for Example 5.7, a drug study involving two treated groups and a control group. The response appears to be log-normally distributed (the variability increases with the size of the response). Note the unusually high observation in the 10 mg/kg treated group.

estimate across all groups, we should do the same when making an outlier assessment.

Example 5.6 (continued): A drug study with an unusual observation

Returning to Example 5.6, the group mean for the intermediate dose group was 5.62, the standard deviation for the group was 0.85 and hence the upper boundary for defining outliers (2SD) is 7.32. The unusually high observation was 7.79 and hence would be declared an outlier using the 2SD approach. We feel this is incorrect and is simply an artefact of the fact that the intermediate dose group happened to be slightly less variable than the other treatment groups in this experiment. If we repeated the experiment would we get a similar pattern in the within-group variability? If we think the variability of the response is different for each treatment group, then perhaps the parametric analysis is not an appropriate choice.

This also highlights one of the problems with animal experiments. When the sample sizes are small, the within-group variability estimates are never reliable and so should not be used when deciding on outliers.

The standardised and Studentised residuals

As mentioned above, the 2SD rule is effectively a test based on the size of the residuals, after having adjusted them for the within-group variability. Given that the within-group variability estimates may be unreliable,

Figure 5.32. Scatterplot of the responses on the $\log_{10}$ scale for Example 5.7, involving two treated groups and a control group. Note the unusually low observation in the vehicle group.

an alternative approach is to use the pooled estimate of variability from the parametric analysis. Hopefully this pooled estimate of variability will be a more reliable (and reproducible) estimate of variability than the individual within-group estimates. This is because, as discussed above, all of the data are used to calculate the single pooled estimate. It is this general approach that is taken when calculating the standardised and Studentised residuals.

The *standardised residuals* can be calculated by dividing the residuals by the pooled standard deviation. For observation i we calculate:

$$\text{Standardised residual}_i = \frac{\text{residual}_i}{\sqrt{MS_{\text{Residual}}}} \qquad (5.17)$$

where MS_{Residual} is the pooled estimate of variability (see Section 5.4.3.1).

Any observation with a corresponding standardised residual that is greater than two may be considered an outlier. This is a similar approach to that applied in the 2SD rule described above, except that in the 2SD approach the separate within-group estimates of variability were used rather than the more reliable pooled estimate of variability.

It can be shown that the predicted variability of each residual varies depending on the observation (Montgomery, 1997, p. 564). It turns out that some observations are more influential on the predicted (statistical) model than others. These observations will have smaller residuals than others because the model will be 'pulled' closer to them. We measure this by calculating the *leverage* (h) of each observation. It follows that we should take the leverage into account when making the adjustment to the residuals. These are the so-called *Studentised residuals*. For observation i we calculate:

$$\text{Studentised residual}_i = \frac{\text{residual}_i}{\sqrt{MS_{\text{Residual}}(1-h_i)}} \quad (5.18)$$

where MS_{Residual} is the pooled estimate of variability (see Section 5.4.3.1) and h_i is the leverage of the ith observation.

Many authors recommend using the Studentised residuals, rather than the standardised residuals, when making outlier assessments. Unfortunately an outlier may artificially inflate the pooled estimate of variability (the MS_E) and hence make the outlier assessment unreliable. This can be avoided, to some extent, by using *externally Studentised residuals*.

When calculating the Studentised residual for observation i, instead of dividing by the pooled estimate of variability (generated from the whole dataset) we calculate the pooled estimate of variability using a dataset where the ith observation has been excluded. If the ith observation is an outlier then the pooled estimate of variability will be artificially increased by including it. By removing the ith observation before calculating the pooled estimate of variability, this issue is avoided. This method is known as the deletion method by some authors. For observation i we calculate:

$$\text{Externally Studentised residual}_i = \frac{\text{residual}_i}{\sqrt{MS_{[\text{Residual}-i]}(1-h_i)}}$$
$$(5.19)$$

where $MS_{[\text{Residual}-i]}$ is the pooled estimate of variability from the dataset excluding observation i and h_i is the leverage of the ith observation.

It is recommended that the decision to exclude outliers should be carried out once and not iteratively, using a new variability estimate at each stage. Once outliers have been removed then the variability estimate will be reduced, hence other observations that were initially acceptable may now appear to be outliers (when compared to the new reduced variability estimate). This could be a vicious circle if the scientist is not careful. The variability estimate may become artificially reduced if too many observations are removed.

We recommend using externally Studentised residuals when trying to identify outliers. Our approach is as follows:

- If the externally Studentised residual for an observation lies outside the range +/–2, then it could be an outlier. The scientist must decide whether to exclude it.
- If the externally Studentised residual for an observation lies outside the range +/–3, then the scientist can be justified in removing it from the analysis.

A convenient way to carry out this test for outliers is to use the predicted vs. residuals plot. Rather than plot the residuals themselves on the Y-axis we plot the externally Studentised residuals. For example, InVivoStat produces a predicted vs. externally Studentised residuals plot by default for the single measure parametric analysis. The plot also includes dotted lines to help the scientist apply the outlier detection rules described here.

Example 5.5 (continued): An experiment where the response needs transforming

Returning to Example 5.5, assume a one-way ANOVA approach was used to analyse the data. The predicted vs. residuals plot, produced using InVivoStat, is given in Figure 5.33.

There is some evidence of an outlier in the top dose group, but as there is a fanning effect in the predicted vs. residuals plot we should consider transforming the data before making any final decisions about outliers. Log-transforming the response prior to analysis appears to remove the fanning effect and stabilises the variance in the higher dose groups. The suspicious observation has an externally Studentised residual that is less than two (on the log scale) and hence is not considered an outlier (Figure 5.34).

5.4.1.6 Additivity

When carrying out many parametric analyses we assume that the effects in the statistical model influence

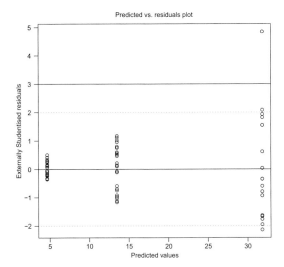

Figure 5.33. Predicted vs. residuals plot from the analysis of Example 5.5.

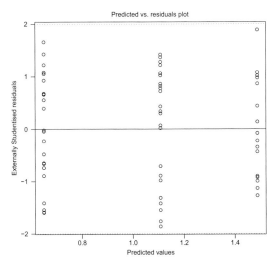

Figure 5.34. Predicted vs. residuals plot from the analysis of Example 5.5 following a $\log_{10}$ transformation of the response.

the response in an additive way. The effect of the factors present in the statistical model can be added together in a linear fashion (hence the terminology 'linear model').

For example, consider an experimental design that consisted of a single treatment factor (Drug) corresponding to different levels of the test compound.

Measurements were taken over two days and hence a blocking factor Day at two levels was included in the experimental design to account for any day-to-day differences. Assume the results were higher on day 2 than on day 1. A statistical model that could be fitted to the data was:

$$\text{response} = \text{overall mean} + \text{drug effect} + \\ \text{block effect} + \text{random error}. \quad (5.20)$$

We assumed that there was a fixed difference between the results on day 1 and day 2 and that this difference was the same regardless of the size of the response. We effectively accounted for this by *adding* on a fixed quantity to the results taken on day 2.

If we thought that the difference between the day 1 and day 2 results depended on the size of the response, i.e. the effect of day 1 was a percentage of the overall response, then it may have been better to analyse the data using a multiplicative statistical model instead. The multiplicative statistical model can be written as:

$$\text{response} = \text{overall mean} \times \text{drug effect} \times \\ \text{block effect} \times \text{random error}. \quad (5.21)$$

It is worth noting that such a model can be analysed using an additive approach if the response was log-transformed. This follows because:

$$\log(\text{response}) = \log(\text{overall mean}) + \log(\text{drug effect}) \\ + \log(\text{block effect}) + \log(\text{random error}). \quad (5.22)$$

5.4.2 The *t*-test

The *t*-test is one of the simplest parametric analyses to perform. As a test it requires little introduction, as it is perhaps the most popular of all statistical tests. Beware though: it is often applied in situations where other tests are more appropriate.

There are two types of *t*-test, the unpaired *t*-test and the paired *t*-test. We shall consider each separately. A description of how to perform the unpaired and paired *t*-tests using InVivoStat is given in Sections 6.9 and 6.10, respectively.

5.4.2.1 The unpaired *t*-test

The unpaired *t*-test, also known as Student's *t*-test, is applicable when the experiment consists of only two experimental groups and each animal is allocated to one of the groups. No other effects are thought to influence the response significantly. We can either say that the experimental design consists of two groups or alternatively that it involves one factor at two levels.

The assumptions made when carrying out the *t*-test are the standard parametric ones described in Section 5.4.1:

- The animals in the study are, in some sense, representative of the wider population of animals. They are randomly selected from that wider population. In animal experiments it is common practice to restrict the animal population to reduce the animal-to-animal variability. This can be achieved by using a transgenic strain or limiting the body weight range of the animals in the study. Remember, as discussed in Section 3.11, if the body weight range used in the experiment is narrow then the conclusions of the study are only valid over that narrow range.
- Each animal is selected independently and the observations generated should not be influenced by, or related to, any other observation. Choosing one animal from the population should not influence the chance of choosing any other.
- The variability of the two groups is the same, although this assumption can be relaxed if required (see Section 6.9 for details on how to perform Welch's *t*-test for unequal variances).
- The data should be normally distributed, although this condition can also be relaxed. In practice it is difficult to prove or disprove this assumption if the sample size is small.
- Animals are assigned to the two groups at random.

If these assumptions hold, and the animals are randomly allocated to the two groups, then the scientist can use the *t*-test to assess whether the difference between the two predicted means is statistically significant.

These experiments can be defined in terms of the experimental design characteristics described in Section 3.2:

- The experimental design consists of two factors: Group (a factor at two levels, perhaps treatment and control) and Animal (each animal is randomly assigned to one of the two groups).
- Animal is nested within Group, and hence the experimental design is a nested design (Section 3.7).

- Animal is a random factor and Group is a fixed factor.
- Individual animals are the experimental units and usually also the observational units.
- The Animal random factor corresponds to the variability (or noise) term we assess the size of the difference between the predicted means against.
- The *t*-statistic is an example of a signal-to-noise ratio. The signal is the difference between the two group means and the noise is the animal-to-animal variability.

Data generated from experiments based on this design can be analysed within InVivoStat using the Single Measure Parametric Analysis module (which assumes equal variance between the two groups) or the unpaired *t*-test module (where the equal variances assumption can be relaxed); see Sections 6.3 and 6.9, respectively.

When using an unpaired *t*-test we begin by assuming that there is no difference between the two group means. This is the null hypothesis. We then try to disprove the null hypothesis (and hence accept the alternative hypothesis) by collecting experimental data.

To test the alternative hypothesis we calculate the *t*-value, which is a signal-to-noise ratio:

$$t\text{-value} = \frac{(\bar{x}_1 - \bar{x}_2)}{\sqrt{s^2(1/n_1 + 1/n_2)}} \tag{5.23}$$

where $\bar{x}_1$ and $\bar{x}_2$ are the group 1 and group 2 means, n_1 and n_2 are the group 1 and group 2 sample sizes and s^2 is the sample variance.

Note in the above definition of a *t*-test the variance estimate s^2 is the variance estimated using the responses from those two groups *only*. In later sections we shall consider similar tests for comparing two group means where the variability estimate used is the pooled estimate across all the groups in the experiment. We do not define such tests as *t*-tests but rather as planned comparisons or the least significant difference test (see Section 5.4.8.3). We do this to differentiate between the relatively unreliable multiple *t*-tests, which use variance estimates calculated from animals in only two groups, and the more reliable planned comparisons, which use the more stable variance estimate calculated using data from all animals in the experiment.

It can be shown that the *t*-value is *t*-distributed with $n_1 + n_2 - 2$ degrees of freedom. Once we have calculated the *t*-value, we can calculate the probability of observing a *t*-value as large (or larger) than the one we have observed assuming, in reality, there is no difference between the two groups. We do this by calculating the area under the *t*-distribution curve (see Section 2.3.3) that lies beyond the calculated *t*-value. This calculated area corresponds to the *p*-value (for a one-sided test) or half the *p*-value (for a two-sided test).

Remember, the *p*-value is the probability (or chance) of observing a difference between the two groups at least as extreme as that measured, when in reality there is no difference between the two groups. The *p*-value is not the probability that there is no difference between the two groups! It is the risk of declaring a false positive (the probability of concluding there is a difference between the groups when in reality there is none). Usually we accept there is a significant difference between the groups if the *p*-value is less than 0.05 (or 5%). In other words, we are prepared to accept a 5% risk of finding a false positive. When we obtain a *p*-value as small as this we conclude that the evidence suggests the null hypothesis is probably not true.

Example 5.8: A study involving two groups

Consider an experiment that was carried out to compare a novel treatment to a vehicle. In total, 20 animals were available for the experiment and the scientist randomly assigned ten to each of the two treatment arms of the study. The design is illustrated in Figure 5.35.

The analysis was carried out using the unpaired *t*-test module in InVivoStat (see Section 6.9). A scatterplot of the data, see Figure 5.36, revealed some evidence of a treatment effect.

The unpaired *t*-test confirms this (Table 5.5). The *p*-value for the equal variance unpaired *t*-test is 0.016, indicating that there is a 1.6% chance of measuring a difference as large as the one observed if, in reality, there is no difference between the treatment and control.

5.4.2.2 When not to use an unpaired *t*-test

As has been mentioned above, the *t*-test is a popular test. This is perhaps because the analysis procedure is fairly transparent and the calculations can be carried out by hand if necessary. We should remember, however, that the *t*-test is not the most powerful statistical test available if:

- There is only one fixed factor but it has more than two levels. A *t*-test is only really appropriate if the experimental design consists of a single fixed factor at two levels. If the factor you are assessing has more than two levels, for example if you have multiple doses of the test compound then, as mentioned above, there are other more appropriate tests. If multiple *t*-tests are used to compare pairs of groups separately then:

  1. The individual tests are based on less accurate estimates of the variability. These variability estimates are calculated using data from only two groups of animals rather than all animals. Other more reliable estimates are available, which use all the data from all the animals.

  2. This approach cannot be so easily justified by the randomisation (assuming animals were randomised across all groups simultaneously).

- There are more than two factors of interest. The *t*-test is only appropriate if there is a single fixed factor in the experimental design. In many studies, however, there are multiple fixed factors in the design. For example, as well as testing the effect of a test compound you may have both male and female animals in the study (Gender factor) or perhaps wildtype and transgenic animals (Strain factor). In these situations it may be of interest to investigate how the two factors relate (or interact) with each other, i.e. is there a bigger treatment effect in males than in females? These questions can be best answered using ANOVA techniques, as discussed below in Section 5.4.3, and not using multiple *t*-tests.

- There are other blocking factors in the experimental design. For practical reasons you may have to introduce other blocking factors into the experimental design. Perhaps you have to carry out the experiment over multiple days. This is not necessarily a problem so long as you plan the experiment properly (using a block design) and then include the blocking factor in the analysis. It is difficult to analyse such data correctly using *t*-tests.

- Other information about the animals is recorded. When running the statistical analysis you should aim to make the best use of all the available information collected during the experiment. Have you recorded pretreatment body weight? Have you been given the

Factor

Treatment

Animal

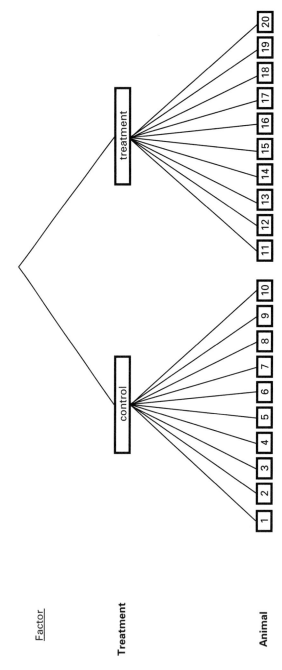

Figure 5.35. Nested design for Example 5.8.

Table 5.5. Unpaired t-test result for Example 5.8

	t-statistic	Degrees of freedom	p-value
Equal variance unpaired t-test	−2.649	18	0.016

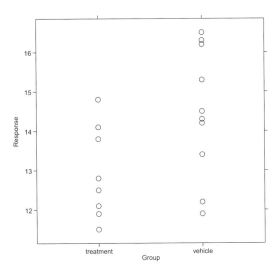

Figure 5.36. Scatterplot of the data for Example 5.8.

age of the animals? Have you taken baseline measurements of your response? There may be many additional pieces of information that could be used in the statistical analysis. However, it is difficult to use this information efficiently if you limit yourself to only using t-tests to analyse your data.

- The animals are measured repeatedly. If you have measured each animal repeatedly using a repeated measures design, then the individual observations taken on each animal will not be independent of each other. In these cases there are specific analysis techniques that can efficiently quantify the changes in response across the levels of the repeated factor, deal with the spatial interrelationships between responses measured within-animal and account for any missing data (see Section 5.4.4.3).

We contend that most animal experiments will possess one or more of the above properties. If this is so then the t-test is not the most appropriate test to use. It may of course be the case that once all other analysis options have been explored the researcher may decide to use a

t-test. For example, if a preliminary investigation was carried out to assess whether the responses recorded at baseline could be used in the statistical analysis. While this information was collected, the investigation revealed that it was not worthwhile including it in the final analysis. Before resorting to the t-test the researcher should always attempt to use other, more powerful, techniques. In the next few sections we shall discuss some of the analyses that are more appropriate in the scenarios described above.

5.4.2.3 The paired t-test

As has been discussed in the previous section there are two types of t-test. When using the unpaired t-test the size of the difference between the two groups is assessed against the between-animal variability. In practice this is usually the largest source of variability in any animal experiment. One way to reduce the variability that the groups are assessed against is to test both experimental conditions in all animals. This allows the difference between the two predicted means to be assessed against the within-animal variability. As this source of variability is usually smaller than the between-animal variability, such comparisons should be more sensitive. We use the terminology 'paired t-test' as we can pair up the observations from the two groups, one pair per animal.

This experiment can also be defined in terms of the experimental design characteristics described in Section 3.2:

- The experimental design consists of two factors: Group (the within-animal factor – a factor at two levels, perhaps treatment and control) and Animal (each animal receives both treatments).
- Animal is crossed with Group (in the unpaired t-test Animal is nested within Group).
- As Animal is crossed with Group we may think we can investigate the interaction between Animal and Group. However, each animal is associated with each

group only once, so there is no replication of the combinations of animals and groups. The interaction therefore cannot be separated from the underlying within-animal variability.

- Group is a fixed factor; Animal can be fitted as a random or fixed factor. There are some advantages to fitting it as a random factor, especially if some animals are allocated to only one of the groups or there is some data missing.
- The t-statistic that is generated when performing the paired t-test is an example of a signal-to-noise ratio, as discussed in Section 2.1. The signal is the difference between the two means, the noise is the within-animal variability.

To perform a paired t-test by hand we first calculate the difference between the two results for each animal. We then compare the average size of these differences to zero. If the average difference is significantly greater (or less than) zero, then this indicates a difference between the two groups. Note that as we are analysing the differences between the within-animal responses, rather than the responses themselves, any animal-to-animal differences are removed from the dataset (by the subtraction process) prior to analysis. The analysis is therefore performed using the within-animal variability.

The paired t-test can be performed easily within most statistical packages. The difficulty is recognising the pairing in the data beforehand!

5.4.2.4 Randomisation and the paired t-test

In general, the purpose of the paired t-test is to assess the size of difference between the two predicted means against the within-animal variability. There are at least three different analysis strategies that can be employed to do this, depending on the randomisation performed. Although the methods are different, in most scenarios they will give the same numerical results.

When randomising the experimental material we have to:

1. Randomly select the animals from the population of animals (as for the unpaired t-test).

We can then either:

2a. Separately for each animal, randomise the order the two groups are allocated to the animal.

2b. Allocate the two groups to each animal in a non-random order.

In practice it does not really matter which randomisation approach is taken; however, it can be argued that these two scenarios do lead to different designs.

If randomisation 2a is applied within the experimental process, then the design could be defined as a block design (blocked by animal) and corresponds to Scenario 3 in Table 3.2. The data can then be analysed using the ANOVA techniques (including Animal as a blocking factor) as described in Section 6.3.3.3.

If randomisation 2b is applied then the experimental design is comparable with the dose-escalation designs defined in Section 3.8.2 and corresponds to Scenario 6 in Table 3.2. In this case there are only two levels of the within-animal Group factor (where the Group factor does not necessarily correspond to the dose of a compound). Crucially in both the dose-escalation designs and the designs considered in this section the levels of the within-animal factor are not randomised. In this scenario a repeated measures analysis approach (see Section 5.4.4.3) can be used to analyse the data.

Regardless of which randomisation is applied, in practice the data can be analysed using either a paired t-test, an ANOVA with Animal as a blocking factor or a repeated measures approach. It can be shown that the results will be the same (in most cases) because there are only two levels of the within-animal factor. Differences may occur if there are any missing data in the dataset, in which case the repeated measures approach may be preferable. This approach is able to recover the information from animals that have only one of the two responses present. The repeated measures approach also generalises to cases where there are more than two levels of the within-subject factor. It is this approach that is implemented within the Paired t-test/within-subject Analysis module in InVivoStat.

5.4.3 Analysis of variance (ANOVA)

In this section we consider the parametric analysis of data generated using designs with two or more factors at two or more levels. This is known as the analysis of variance, or ANOVA, approach and was first developed by R. A. Fisher in the early part of the twentieth century.

Data generated using block, factorial and crossover designs can be successfully analysed using this approach. We shall consider experiments where each response is measured once per animal, as opposed to the repeatedly measured responses that are described in Section 5.4.4.

The ANOVA approach can be used to analyse datasets generated by many different animal experiments. This type of analysis includes the *t*-test but also generalises to include the analysis of experiments involving multiple factors of interest. This section describes the analysis process that generates the global overall tests of significance in the ANOVA table. It should be read in conjunction with later sections that describe other aspects of ANOVA-based analyses. For example, the parametric assumptions we make when performing an ANOVA analysis (Section 5.4.3) and the local pairwise comparisons of the predicted means that can be made post-ANOVA (Section 5.4.8). A description of how to perform an analysis of variance using InVivoStat is given in Section 6.3.

We shall begin by generalising the situation described in the previous section and consider experiments where the factor of interest has more than two levels. We shall then go on to consider the case where there are more than two factors of interest included in the experimental design.

5.4.3.1 One-way ANOVA

One-way ANOVA is a way of assessing the overall effect of the factor of interest by quantifying, in some sense, the amount of variability in the data that can be attributed to that factor. We use the terminology one-way ANOVA as there is a single factor of interest present in the experimental design.

This analysis involves, amongst other things, the formation of the one-way ANOVA table. This table contains an overall test of whether the levels of the factor of interest are different. This test does not take into account any structure that the levels of the factor may have. For example, assume the experimental design consists of a treatment factor that has four levels: control, low, intermediate and high dose of a novel treatment. The ANOVA table contains a test of whether the four levels of the Treatment factor are different

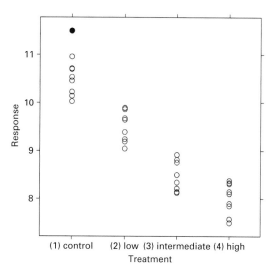

Figure 5.37. Scatterplot of the data from Example 5.9.

from each other. It does not take into account that one level of the Treatment factor is a control and that the researcher wants to compare each of the three treatments back to the control. We comment further on this later; however, we note at this stage that care should be taken if the overall test in the ANOVA table is used to decide whether or not specific pairwise tests between the means (that were planned in advance) can be made. This is sometimes defined as the gateway ANOVA test procedure (see Section 5.4.8.8).

Many statistical textbooks provide mathematical derivations of the analysis of variance, for example Clarke and Kempson (1997, pp. 32–8). The interested reader is invited to read such texts. In this section we shall avoid repeating such descriptions in favour of a more graphical explanation.

Example 5.9: A study involving three treatment groups and a control

Consider the following dataset involving three doses of a test compound and a control. A scatterplot of the data reveals evidence of a treatment effect. We shall focus our attention on the largest observation in the control group (the observation highlighted in Figure 5.37).

Why was the response of this animal approximately 11.5? Can we use a statistical model to predict why it was so high?

To begin with, and perhaps trivially, this animal's response will depend on many factors that influence all the responses obtained in the experiment. These include the type of response, the scale of

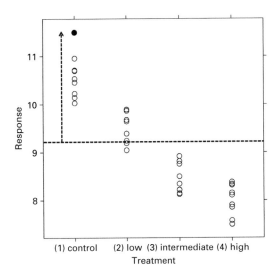

Figure 5.38. Scatterplot of the data from Example 5.9, including the grand mean of the data as a dotted line. The distance between the highlighted observation and the grand mean is illustrated with a dotted arrow.

measurement, the species of animal, the animal model itself and so on… We can capture the effect of all of these by calculating the overall average, or *grand mean* of the data. This grand mean (which equals 9.1) accounts for a lot of the variability in the data and to some extent explains why the response we have highlighted equals 11.5. The grand mean is added to the scatterplot as a dotted line and the distance between the selected observation and the grand mean is highlighted by an arrow (Figure 5.38).

But this is not the whole story. The highlighted observation (11.5) is higher than the overall average (9.1). This could be just chance, but it could also be related to the treatment that the animal received. Looking at the scatterplot it appears that all of the animals in the control group gave higher results than animals in the treatment groups. So this is an extra piece of information that can help to explain why the highlighted observation is 11.5. The control group mean equals 10.6. So the animal's response of 11.5 can be partly explained by the overall average of the data, but can also be explained by the treatment effect. Our new prediction for that observation (10.6) is obtained by including the Treatment factor in the statistical model and is closer to the animal's response than was achieved by simply using the overall average of the data (9.1). The predicted means are added to the scatterplot as dotted lines (Figure 5.39). Note the distance that the highlighted observation is from the new predicted value is now smaller, as denoted by the dotted arrow.

Our new prediction, in this case the control group mean (10.6), is still a little way from the observed response (11.5); however, without any other information this is the best that we can do. The bit that is left over (11.5 − 10.6 = 0.9) is called the residual for that response, as defined above in Section 5.4.1.3.

The bigger the residuals, the more spread the individual responses are around the predicted mean and hence the more variable the observed data. Obviously we want to reduce the residuals where possible by fitting the most appropriate statistical model to the data.

We can use these ideas to construct the ANOVA table. The one-way ANOVA table for this example is given in Table 5.6.

The one-way ANOVA table consists of two rows: the first corresponds to the Treatment factor (the signal) and the second corresponds to the residuals, or variability, of the data (the noise). The first column in the ANOVA table simply defines the source of variability, either treatment or residual in this case.

Sums of squares

To quantify the size of the treatment effect we consider the distance the Treatment factor predicted means are from the overall average of the data, i.e. for treatment i we calculate:

$$d_i = \bar{x}_i - \mu, \tag{5.24}$$

where $\bar{x}_i$ is the treatment i group mean and μ is the grand mean. The further the treatment means are from the grand mean of the data the bigger the treatment effect is. So if we add up all these distances, one per treatment group, we will get an overall measure of the size of the treatment effect. These individual treatment effects are illustrated with four arrows (Figure 5.40).

Inevitably some of the treatment means are above the grand mean and some are below, hence some of the distances will be positive and some negative. They will, in many cases, add up to zero. In this example the sum of the differences is:

$$1.44 + 0.39 - 0.70 - 1.13 = 0.$$

So the sum of the differences is of little use to us. One way around this mathematically is to square the calculated distances (i.e. making them all positive) before adding them together.

$$(1.44)^2 + (0.39)^2 + (-0.70)^2 + (-1.13)^2 = 3.99.$$

Effectively we are summing the squares, or calculating the sums of squares, and this forms the second column in the ANOVA table (once multiplied by the sample size 9, because there are effectively nine predicted results per group – one for each observation).

We can also add up the squared distances of the individual observations from their associated predicted

Table 5.6. One-way ANOVA table for Example 5.9

	Sums of squares	Degrees of freedom	Mean square	F-value	p-value
Treatment	35.92	3	11.97	92.96	< 0.001
Residuals	4.12	32	0.13		

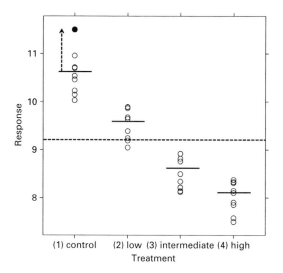

Figure 5.39. Scatterplot of the data from Example 5.9. The plot includes the grand mean of the data as a dotted line, the individual group means as solid lines and the distance of the highlighted observation from the statistical model prediction as an arrow.

means. This number is called the *residual sums of squares*. These values are highlighted in Table 5.7.

Degrees of freedom

The next column in the table is called *degrees of freedom* (*df*); see Table 5.8. There are many ways to describe this term. We prefer to consider it as the number of separate pieces of information available to estimate each effect.

Consider a Treatment factor at four levels (control, low, intermediate and high). We can compare the following treatments:

(i) control vs. low
(ii) control vs. intermediate
(iii) control vs. high

To make these comparisons, in the statistical analysis, we start off with the corresponding null hypotheses:

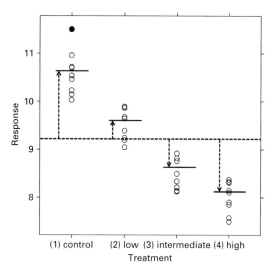

Figure 5.40. Scatterplot of the data from Example 5.9. The plot includes the grand mean of the data as a dotted line, the individual treatment means as solid lines and the distance of the treatment means from the grand mean as arrows.

$$
\begin{aligned}
&\text{(i)}\ \bar{x}_{\text{low}} - \bar{x}_{\text{control}} &&= 0 \\
&\text{(ii)}\ \bar{x}_{\text{intermediate}} - \bar{x}_{\text{control}} &&= 0 \\
&\text{(iii)}\ \bar{x}_{\text{high}} - \bar{x}_{\text{control}} &&= 0,
\end{aligned}
\tag{5.25}
$$

which we try to disprove using an appropriate statistical test.

Now any other comparison between the groups can be written down as a combination of these three group mean comparisons. So, for example, the low vs. high treatment comparison can be assessed using a linear combination of comparisons (i) and (iii). It can be written as (i) – (iii):

$$
\bar{x}_{low} - \bar{x}_{high} = (\bar{x}_{low} - \bar{x}_{control}) - (\bar{x}_{high} - \bar{x}_{control}) = \text{(i)} - \text{(iii)}.
\tag{5.26}
$$

The maximum number of separate, or *independent*, comparisons that can be made is three (note there

Table 5.7. ANOVA table for Example 5.9; sums of squares column highlighted

	Sums of squares	Degrees of freedom	Mean square	F-value	p-value
Treatment	35.92	3	11.97	92.96	< 0.001
Residuals	4.12	32	0.13		

Table 5.8. ANOVA table for Example 5.9; degrees of freedom column highlighted

	Sums of squares	Degrees of freedom	Mean square	F-value	p-value
Treatment	35.92	3	11.97	92.96	< 0.001
Residuals	4.12	32	0.13		

are many ways of finding three). Once you have found three, then any other comparison will be a combination of these three. Hence there are three degrees of freedom for the Treatment factor corresponding to the three independent comparisons that represent three independent pieces of information.

In practice degrees of freedom for a factor can easily be calculated. It is one less than the total number of levels of that factor in the experimental design.

If we think of degrees of freedom as pieces of information then calculating the *residual degrees of freedom* (the degrees of freedom for the term used to estimate the variability of the data) is straightforward too. If the dataset has 36 observations, then by running the study we have collected 36 separate pieces of information (assuming the observations are independent, as discussed in Section 5.4.1.4). We need one piece of information to estimate the grand mean of the data, and (in this case) three degrees of freedom, or three pieces of information, to estimate the differences between the levels of the Treatment factor. The remainder $36 - 1 - 3 = 32$ is the number of pieces of information available to estimate the underlying variability of the data, this is the so-called residual degrees of freedom.

Mean squares
Returning to the sums of squares, the observant reader will have noticed that as the number of factor levels increases so does the sums of squares for that factor. As all squared distances (between the predicted group means and the overall average of the data) are positive, the sums of squares will always increase as the number

of groups increase. So to get a true picture of the importance of the factor, we require a measure that is not influenced by the number of factor levels. To achieve this we divide the sums of squares by the degrees of freedom to effectively produce an average squared distance, the so-called *mean square*. The mean square column is highlighted in Table 5.9.

We do this for both the Treatment factor ($MS_{\text{Treatment}}$) and the residual (MS_{Residual}). In this case:

$$MS_{\text{Treatment}} = 35.92 / 3 = 11.97$$

and

$$MS_{\text{Residual}} = 4.12 / 32 = 0.13.$$

F-values
We are now in a position to test the significance of the Treatment factor. $MS_{\text{Treatment}}$ is a measure of the size of the effect or the signal. MS_{Residual} is a measure of the background variability or noise.

So we calculate the signal-to-noise ratio, as discussed in Section 2.1, by dividing one by the other. This value is highlighted in Table 5.10. This is called the *F-value*. It is a generalisation of the *t*-value (used in the *t*-test) but is still simply a signal-to-noise ratio. If the factor of interest only has two levels, then the *F*-value is also a *t*-value.

p-values
Finally (given the variability of the data and the sample size) we can use the statistical package to calculate the probability of observing a pattern in the treatment means as extreme (or more extreme) than that

Table 5.9. ANOVA table for Example 5.9; mean square column highlighted

	Sums of squares	Degrees of freedom	**Mean square**	F-value	p-value
Treatment	35.92	3	11.97	92.96	< 0.001
Residuals	4.12	32	0.13		

Table 5.10. ANOVA table for Example 5.9; F-value highlighted

	Sums of squares	Degrees of freedom	Mean square	**F-value**	p-value
Treatment	35.92	3	11.97	92.96	< 0.001
Residuals	4.12	32	0.13		

Table 5.11. ANOVA table for Example 5.9; p-value highlighted

	Sums of squares	Degrees of freedom	Mean square	F-value	**p-value**
Treatment	35.92	3	11.97	92.96	< 0.001
Residuals	4.12	32	0.13		

measured in the study given that in reality there was no treatment effect (Table 5.11).

The F-value is F-distributed with 3 and 32 degrees of freedom. This follows because (as discussed in Section 2.2.7):

1. Assuming the residuals are normally distributed, then the sums of squares in the ANOVA table are chi-squared distributed.
2. The ratio of two chi-squared distributed variables is F-distributed. Hence the Treatment sums of squares divided by residual sums of squares (adjusted for the Treatment and residual degrees of freedom) is F-distributed.

Once the F-value has been calculated we can use the assumption that it is F-distributed to calculate the probability of observing an F-value as large (or larger) than the one observed, assuming there is no difference between the treatments. This is achieved by calculating the area under the curve (of the F-distribution) for the region beyond the calculated F-value. This number is the p-value.

The p-value is dependent on the size of the F-value but also the Treatment and residual degrees of freedom. If you do quote ANOVA table p-values, then it is

advisable to include the degrees of freedom. For example, you should state:

The Treatment Factor was significant $(F_{(3,32)} = 11.97, p < 0.001)$.

In the following sections we shall present more complicated examples of the ANOVA table; however, the underlying principles are the same regardless of how large and complicated the ANOVA table is.

5.4.3.2 Including the positive control

An issue often faced by the researcher is which experimental groups to include in the statistical analysis. For example, if the experimental design includes a positive control group should this group be included in the statistical analysis when the primary purpose of the analysis is to compare the treatment groups back to the vehicle? This question can be answered by considering the quality of the variability estimate. As discussed above, a more reliable estimate is obtained if all the animals' responses are used to estimate the variability. The statistical power of the experiment may also be improved as the residual degrees of freedom will be higher if the positive control is included in the experiment.

We do not recommend this rule be strictly adhered to, however. If the variability of the positive control group is significantly different from the other treatment groups (which can often be the case), then it is advisable to remove the positive control group from the dataset prior to the statistical analysis. This ensures that the overall variability estimate reflects the variability of the control and treatment groups and the homogeneity of variance assumption holds (see Section 5.4.1.3).

Example 5.10: Anti-diabetic effects of epigallocatechin gallate

An experiment was conducted to assess the effect of epigallocate-chin gallate (EGCG), a catechin found in green tea, on type 2 diabetes in rodents (Wolfram *et al.*, 2006). The experiment consisted of five groups, with db/db mice randomly allocated to each group. The treatments were administered in the diet and included 2.5, 5.0 or 10.0 g/kg of EGCG in the diet ($n = 9$), a placebo control ($n = 9$) and a positive control of thiazolidinedione rosiglitazone at 72 mg/kg of diet ($n = 5$). After five weeks of treatment the animals were fasted and an oral glucose tolerance test performed. In this test, the animals were administered 1 g/kg of glucose orally and their blood glucose concentration measured over the following three hours. We shall concentrate on the area under the curve summary measure of the time course (see Section 5.4.4.2).

An observed means with SEMs plot, for a simulated AUC summary measure of the blood glucose concentration, is given in Figure 5.41. The data were analysed using a one-way ANOVA approach. The ANOVA table is given in Table 5.12.

As there were five treatments, the Treatment factor had four degrees of freedom. There were $4 \times 9 + 5 = 41$ observations in total, hence there were $41 - 1 - 4 = 36$ residual degrees of freedom.

The size of the treatment effect (quantified by $MS_{Treatment}$) was 1825.00 and the size of the animal-to-animal variability ($MS_{Residual}$) was 49.43. The signal-to-noise ratio was $1825.00/49.43 = 36.92$. This was a large ratio and hence the associated p-value was highly significant ($p < 0.001$), indicating that the null hypothesis was almost certainly not true. Hence we conclude there was an overall difference between the five treatments.

Table 5.12 shows 36 degrees of freedom were used to estimate the variability of the response. If, however, the positive control group is removed from the dataset prior to analysis, this figure decreases to $36 - 1 - 3 = 32$. While not a concern in this example, such a reduction in the residual degrees of freedom could affect the statistical power of the analysis and may also result in a less reliable estimate of the variability of the response.

From the method described in the original paper all groups were included in the statistical analysis. The data was analysed using a one-way ANOVA approach followed by Dunnett's test (see Section 5.4.8.5). We shall return to this example in Section 5.4.8.2.

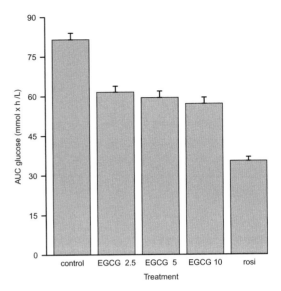

Figure 5.41. Plot of observed means with SEMs for Example 5.10.

5.4.3.3 Two-way ANOVA

Whilst one-way ANOVA is a simple generalisation of the *t*-test, we need not confine ourselves to experiments consisting of a single factor of interest. In fact we can have any number of factors of interest, at any number of levels, and still use an ANOVA approach to analyse the data. In this section we shall concentrate on the case where there are two factors of interest in the experimental design. Both factors are crossed with each other and the experimental design used is a full-factorial design. Such experiments are analysed using the two-way ANOVA approach. It should be noted, however, that the ideas discussed here could easily be generalised to experiments with more than two factors.

One of the main differences between one-way and two-way ANOVA is the presence of the interaction between the two factors. This interaction is a measure of how the effect of the first factor varies depending on the level of the second factor. One of the benefits of using the two-way (and higher-order) ANOVA approach is that we can test the significance of the interaction (Nieuwenhuis *et al.*, 2011).

Table 5.12. ANOVA table for Example 5.10

	Sums of squares	Degrees of freedom	Mean square	F-value	p-value
Treatment	7300.01	4	1825.00	36.92	< 0.001
Residuals	1779.56	36	49.43		

For example, consider an experiment carried out to test the effect of a novel compound in male and female rats. We could analyse the data from the two genders separately using a one-way ANOVA approach. Alternatively, we could analyse all the data together, with two factors Gender and Treatment in the statistical model. We could then include the Gender:Treatment interaction to see if the effect of treatment varies depending on the sex of the animals. Perhaps the treatment effect is more pronounced in males than in females.

Example 5.9 (continued): A study involving three treatment groups and a control

Returning to Example 5.9, we have seen that fitting the Treatment factor alone (along with the overall average of the data) explained most of the variability in the data. However, some of the residuals were still relatively large, as presented in Figure 5.39.

Let us assume that both male and female mice were used in the experiment. Half of the animals in each group were males and half were females. We can then include a second factor in the statistical model (Gender) to account for any differences between the sexes.

First we fit the Treatment factor as given above. We then calculate, separately for each treatment group, the mean of the male animals and the mean of the female animals. These are the new predicted means from the statistical model.

We can easily see from the scatterplot given in Figure 5.42 that the males gave consistently lower results than the females. If we omit the Gender factor from the statistical model, then this gender effect will inflate the between-animal variability. Hence fitting the Gender factor in the analysis should reduce the size of the individual residuals.

The observation we have discussed above is a female animal. By taking the Gender factor into account in the statistical model, the new predicted value for this response is 11.0. This is not too far away from the actual response (11.5). The predicted value is certainly closer to the actual value than was the case when the Gender factor was omitted from the statistical model (11.0 is closer to 11.5 than 10.6 was).

The two-way ANOVA table, given in Table 5.13, follows a similar structure to that described above for the one-way ANOVA. We now include extra rows in the table for the overall effect of Gender and also the Gender by Treatment interaction.

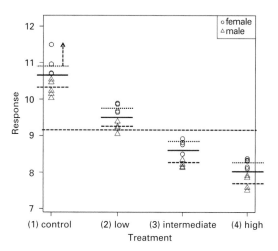

Figure 5.42. Scatterplot of the data from Example 5.9, categorised by gender. The plot includes the grand mean of the data as a dotted line, the overall individual group means as solid lines, the treatment group means for each sex as dotted lines and the distance of the highlighted observation from the predicted mean highlighted with an arrow.

The calculations follow in the same way as described above. The degrees of freedom for the interaction are calculated by multiplying together the degrees of freedom for the constituent factors (3 × 1 = 3 in this case).

We can see from the table that, as expected, there is a statistically significant overall difference between the levels of both Treatment and Gender. However, the interaction is not significant. This implies the size of the treatment effect is the same regardless of the sex of the animal. Another way to think of this result (as can be seen easily in Figure 5.42) is that the difference between the males and females is the same regardless of the treatment they receive.

It is also worth noting that $MS_{Residual}$, which was 0.13 in the one-way ANOVA table, is now 0.04. So fitting the second factor has reduced the underlying variability of the data considerably.

Example 5.11: Assessing strain effects

Consider the following experiment, discussed in Shaw *et al.* (2002), which used data taken from a larger experiment described in Festing *et al.* (2001). The experiment was carried out to assess the effect

Table 5.13. Two-way ANOVA table for Example 5.9

	Sums of squares	Degrees of freedom	Mean square	F-value	p-value
Gender	3.07	1	3.07	83.79	< 0.001
Treatment	36.75	3	12.25	334.90	< 0.001
Gender:Treatment	0.03	3	0.01	0.29	0.831
Residuals	1.02	28	0.04		

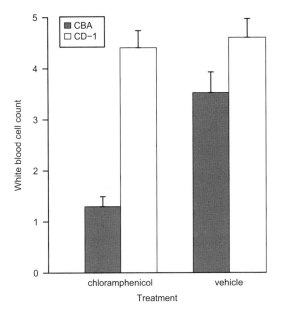

Figure 5.43. Plot of the observed means of the combinations of the Treatment and Strain factors, with SEMs, from Example 5.11.

of chloramphenicol (2500 mg/kg) on the white blood cell count in various strains of mice. Two different strains of mice (CD-1 and CBA) were given either chloramphenicol or the vehicle by gavage and their coded white blood cells counted.

The experimental design consists of two factors, Strain and Treatment, and hence the data generated from the experiment (the data here is simulated, see Figure 5.43) can be analysed using two-way ANOVA. The two-way ANOVA table provides a useful test to see if the effect of chloramphenicol varies between the strains.

From a table of the individual group means (Table 5.14) it can immediately be seen that the effect of chloramphenicol was greater in the CBA strain than in the CD-1 strain, but was this effect statistically significant? The two-way ANOVA table, see Table 5.15, confirms that the interaction between Strain and Treatment was

Table 5.14. Table of the treatment by strain means from Example 5.11

Level	Mean	Lower 95% CI	Upper 95% CI
chloramphenicol CBA	1.299	0.613	1.985
chloramphenicol CD-1	4.406	3.720	5.092
vehicle CBA	3.522	2.836	4.207
vehicle CD-1	4.603	3.917	5.288

significant ($F_{(1,28)}$ = 9.15, p = 0.005). In this case it would be unwise to investigate the overall effect of treatment, because the effect differs depending on the strain of the animal. In fact statisticians argue that the overall tests in the two-way ANOVA tables are meaningless in the presence of a significant interaction. If the interaction is significant you should stop there and not go on and consider the individual factor tests.

5.4.3.4 Two-way vs. one-way ANOVA

There are many similarities between the one-way and two-way ANOVA approaches. In fact it can be shown that many of the results from two-way ANOVA can be obtained using one-way ANOVA. To perform one-way ANOVA (if the experimental design consists of two experimental factors), all we need to do is manually generate a new factor whose levels are the combinations of the two original factors. We then analyse the data using this new combined factor using a one-way ANOVA approach.

Example 5.11 (continued): Assessing strain effects

Consider Example 5.11 again. Let us now manually combine the factors Strain and Treatment to create a new Group factor. If we include this new factor in the analysis, instead of Treatment and Strain, we

Table 5.15. Two-way ANOVA table for Example 5.11

	Sums of squares	Degrees of freedom	Mean square	F-value	p-value
Strain	35.08	1	35.08	39.11	< 0.001
Treatment	11.71	1	11.71	13.06	0.001
Strain:Treatment	8.21	1	8.21	9.15	0.005
Residuals	25.11	28	0.90		

Table 5.16. One-way ANOVA table for Example 5.11

	Sums of squares	Degrees of freedom	Mean square	F-value	p-value
Group	55.00	3	18.33	20.44	< 0.001
Residuals	25.11	28	0.90		

can analyse the data using a one-way ANOVA approach rather than the two-way ANOVA approach described above. In this case we produce the one-way ANOVA table given in Table 5.16.

The single degrees of freedom for the two factors and their interaction (in the two-way ANOVA table) have now been combined into a single source of variability with three degrees of freedom. Crucially though the residuals row is the same for both one- and two-way ANOVA tables ($MS_{Residual}$ = 0.90). Any statistical tests, such as the pairwise tests, that rely on this variance estimate will therefore be the same.

This raises the obvious question, why bother with the two-way ANOVA approach? There are two main reasons.

Firstly, two-way ANOVA provides a statistical test of the interaction between the two factors; one-way ANOVA does not. One-way ANOVA provides a test to see if the individual group means are different from each other. If the one-way ANOVA test is significant, then this could be because only one of the factors has an effect or the interaction between the factors is significant. We cannot separate out these effects by looking at the one-way ANOVA table. Two-way ANOVA can provide more information on what is causing a statistically significant test result.

If the interaction is not significant then the scientist can test to see if the levels of the factors are significantly different overall. This can be a more powerful test if there is no interaction between the factors and is an example of the hidden replication described in Section 3.5.4.3.

Example 5.9 (continued): A study involving three treatment groups and a control

Consider Example 5.9, where Gender and Treatment were two factors included in the experimental design. The Gender by Treatment interaction was not significant, see Table 5.13, implying that the effect of treatment is the same regardless of the gender of the animal. So why not compare the treatment effects back to control across both sexes together, rather than carrying out (effectively) the same test twice (once for each sex)? The latter approach is never a good idea. For example, see Section 5.4.8.1 for issues of multiple comparisons. The overall comparison is also likely to be more sensitive as the sample size, and hence the statistical power, is greater.

It seems sensible, looking at Table 5.13 and Figures 5.44 and 5.45, to compare the levels of the treatment factor back to the control ignoring the Gender factor (i.e. combining the two sexes). To perform this analysis you should remove the interaction from the statistical model and only fit the two factors, again using a two-way ANOVA approach. It is (in this case) still worth including the Gender factor in the statistical model as females appear to, on average, be giving higher results than males. If you do remove the Gender factor as well as the interaction, then you will increase the between-animal variability. This analysis will allow you to compare the effects of the treatments averaged over the sexes while still accounting for the influence of gender on the between-animal variability.

5.4.3.5 Dealing with missing factor combinations

It may be the case that there are two or more factors of interest in the experiment, but not all combinations of the levels of the factors are included in the experimental design, i.e. the design is not a full-factorial

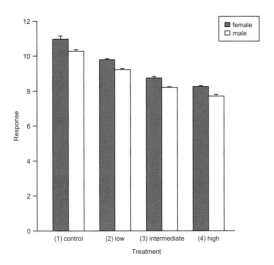

Figure 5.44. Plot of the treatment by gender observed means, with standard errors, from Example 5.9.

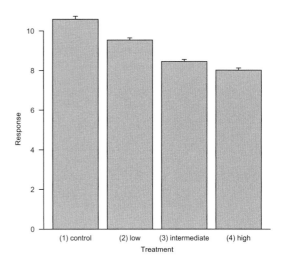

Figure 5.45. Plot of the overall treatment observed means, with standard errors, from Example 5.9.

design. Factor combinations are usually omitted from a design for practical and ethical reasons (for example, see Murphy *et al.*, 2003) although other more systematic design-based reasons are possible, such as those described in Section 3.5.4.4. The following discussion does not apply to designs such as the large fractional factorial designs, where the researcher has purposefully designed the experiment with missing combinations of the levels of the factors. Such designs would require a decision about which interactions to include in the statistical model as not all can be estimated.

While there are many practical arguments for omitting certain combinations of the factor levels from the experimental design, the researcher should be careful as it will weaken the overall power of the experimental design. The analysis options are also reduced as we may not benefit from the hidden replication that would have been present in a full-factorial experimental design (see Section 3.5.4.3).

When analysing data generated using designs with missing combinations of the levels of the factors, some care must be taken. To begin with the missing combinations will reduce the number of degrees of freedom, especially for the rows in the ANOVA table corresponding to the factor interactions. As a general rule each missing combination of the levels of two factors will

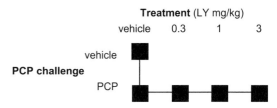

Figure 5.46. The incomplete factorial design for Example 3.21 involving two factors, PCP challenge (at two levels) and Treatment (at four levels).

reduce the degrees of freedom of the associated two-way interaction by one. Also, depending on how the statistical package carries out the analysis, there may be a reduction in the degrees of freedom associated with the factors. In extreme cases, this can reduce the degrees of freedom to zero. In such cases it is not possible to test for the effect. As a rule of thumb if the degrees of freedom in the ANOVA table are less than expected (and it is always advisable to check them) then a possible cause of this reduction is a missing combination of the levels of two or more of the factors.

Example 3.21 (continued): Antipsychotic activity in the mouse

Consider Example 3.21 described in Section 3.5.3. The study was conducted to investigate which of the mGlu2 and mGlu3 receptors

Table 5.17. Two-way ANOVA table for Example 3.21

	Sums of squares	Degrees of freedom	Mean square	F-value	p-value
PCP challenge	15276.63	1	15276.63	1848.91	< 0.001
Treatment	4337.67	3	1445.89	174.99	< 0.001
Residuals	123.94	15	8.26		

Table 5.18. One-way ANOVA table for Example 3.21

	Sums of squares	Degrees of freedom	Mean square	F-value	p-value
Group	19614.30	4	4903.58	593.47	< 0.001
Residuals	123.94	15	8.26		

mediate the effect of an mGluR2/3 agonist (Woolley *et al.*, 2008). Animals (C57Bl/6J mice) were placed in a test arena and the loco-motor activity measured. Prior to being placed in the arena for a habituation phase, the mice were administered either phencyclidine (PCP) or amphetamine (AMP) to produce what are effectively two different animal models. We shall consider the PCP challenge model in this section.

The test compound LY379268 (LY) was administered at one of three doses: 0.3, 1 or 3 mg/kg. There were five treatments in the study labelled as vehicle/vehicle, vehicle/PCP, LY0.3/PCP, LY1/PCP and LY3/PCP.

The design can be seen to be a factorial design involving two factors: PCP challenge (levels: vehicle and PCP) and Treatment (levels: 0, 0.3, 1 and 3 mg/kg). The design can be illustrated using a two-dimensional figure (Figure 5.46).

The degrees of freedom for PCP challenge and Treatment should be one and three respectively, as the PCP challenge factor has two levels and the Treatment factor has four. The interaction between PCP challenge and Treatment should therefore have $1 \times 3 = 3$ degrees of freedom. However, because there are three missing combinations of the levels of the two factors in the design this term has zero degrees of freedom and hence is omitted from the analysis. The ANOVA table (for some artificially generated data) created using the above experimental design is given in Table 5.17.

In the previous section we described the similarities between the one-way and two-way ANOVA tables. A similar approach can be applied here to address any complications caused by missing factor level combinations. To begin with the levels of the two factors are combined together to create a new factor (called Group) at five levels, where the levels are: veh/veh, veh/PCP, LY0.3/PCP, LY1/PCP and LY3/PCP. We can then we can carry out a one-way ANOVA on the new Group factor (see Table 5.18) and make comparisons between the levels of this new factor to investigate the effects of the two original factors (see Section 5.4.3.1).

5.4.4 Repeated measures analysis

In many experiments it is possible to measure the animals repeatedly, usually over time. This is important as we gain more information from each individual animal than would have been the case if we had only taken a single observation. Of course this benefit needs to be offset against the cost to the animal of taking repeated observations. As we shall see in this section, analysing responses that are repeatedly measured has its own challenges and pitfalls.

In Table 3.2 (Section 3.2.8) we described seven different scenarios that involved repeatedly measuring the animals. These scenarios can be subdivided into those that involve some level of within-animal randomisation and those that do not. If a within-animal randomisation can be performed, then the methods described above in Section 5.4.3 can be used to analyse the generated data. The randomisation allows the researcher to assume that there are no spatial inter-relationships between the within-animal responses. However, if there are no within-animal randomisations applied, then there may be spatial interrelationships between the within-animal responses that will need to be accounted for in the statistical analysis. We summarise the types of analysis that can be applied to the seven scenarios in Table 5.19.

In this section we shall focus on Scenarios 1 and 6 (repeated measures designs and dose-escalation designs). We shall describe two analysis strategies,

Table 5.19. Seven different ways to measure an animal repeatedly – statistical analysis

Case	Description	Type of design	Randomisation	Statistical analysis
1	Animals measured repeatedly: levels of the factor that defines the repeated measurements are shared across animals	Repeated measures design	Randomisation of levels of the repeated factor not possible – hence relationships exist between the within-animal measurements. Treatments randomised to Animals	Repeated measures ANOVA or repeated measures mixed-model
2	Animal measured repeatedly: levels of the factor that defines the repeated measurements are not shared across animals	Nested design	In theory the levels of the random within-animal factor(s) are randomly selected from the wider population of levels	Average up to the Animal level prior to ANOVA analysis and/or investigate the replication of the random factors
3	Treatments assessed are assessed at random positions within the animal	Block design	Treatments randomly assigned to positions in the animal – so we can assume that within-animal responses are not spatially related	Two-way ANOVA with blocking factor Animal. Animal can be a random or fixed factor
4	Two treatments: within-animal treatment levels assessed at random positions within the animal and between-animal treatment levels administered one per animal	Split-plot design	Between-animal treatments randomly assigned to animals and within-animal treatments randomly assigned to positions within the animal	Mixed-model approach or mixed effects ANOVA – Animal must be assumed to be a random factor to allow for within- and between-animal testing
5	Animals receive multiple treatments over time in a different order for each animal	Crossover design	Treatments are administered to animals in a pseudo-random order, hence we can assume results within-animal are not spatially related	Three-way ANOVA with factors Treatment, Animal and Test period
6	Animals receive multiple treatments over time in a non-random order	Dose-escalation design	Treatments are administered to animals in a non-random order, hence we must assume results within-animal are spatially related	Repeated measures ANOVA or repeated measures mixed-model with Dose as the repeated factor
7	Multiple different responses measured for each animal	Any type of design	–	–

although the researcher may prefer to use an alternative approach, depending on the experimental design employed and the hypotheses that are being assessed.

5.4.4.1 Categorised case profiles plot

As with any response, before making a decision about how to conduct the statistical analysis it is worth plotting the data. We can do this using a categorised case profiles plot, as described in Section 5.3.4.

The categorised case profiles plot is made up of a series of subplots, one per experimental group. Within each of the subplots, the Y-axis corresponds to the response and the X-axis corresponds to the repeated factor. The responses for each animal are then plotted as points within the appropriate subplot, with a line joining the repeated measurements for each animal.

As discussed in Section 5.3.4, there are several reasons why producing this plot is a useful first stage of any repeated measures analysis:

- It gives the researcher a useful overview of the whole dataset as an animal's responses can be tracked across the levels of the repeated factor. As we shall see in the following section, if we decide to analyse the data using a summary measure then we can use this plot to see if the chosen measure is a meaningful summary of each animal's responses.
- The plot provides a useful way to identify outliers. An example of such a plot is given in Figure 5.47, consisting of a response measured over four weeks. Note the unusual response in week two for one of the animals in the 30 mg/kg treated group.

5.4.4.2 Analysis of summary measures

Once the categorised case profiles plot has been generated, the scientist should then consider if a suitable summary measure can be found that encapsulates the information recorded for each animal. Examples include averaging all the animals' responses to produce a single average measure per animal or calculating the area under the curve for the responses from each animal (this is effectively a weighted average of the animal's responses). The latter could, in certain circumstances, be a measure of drug exposure. The aim of

a summary measure is to preserve as much of the information as possible that was gained by measuring the animal repeatedly.

The choice of summary measure will be influenced by the pattern of the animal's responses and also by the hypotheses that are being tested. The process (of considering if there is a suitable summary measure) is itself useful as it makes the scientist think about the questions that should be addressed by the statistical analysis.

One major benefit of using a summary measure, which should not be overlooked, is that it can lead to a much simpler analysis. A summary measure could be analysed using the ANOVA-based approach described in the previous section. This is usually more straightforward and involves making fewer assumptions than is the case when conducting a repeated measures analysis.

Using summary measures can also help avoid complications associated with the characteristics of the response. For example, assume that the individual responses are categorical and hence the assumptions of the parametric analysis do not hold. While there are specialist repeated measures analysis techniques that can be employed to analyse this type of response, if the scientist can use a suitable summary measure of the categorical response then this is likely to be more continuous and hence the analysis should be more straightforward. Even if the response is continuous, there are still certain assumptions that must be made when carrying out a repeated measures analysis, for example sphericity (see Section 5.4.4.4).

However, there are disadvantages when using summary measures and these should be weighed up against the benefits. To begin with the choice of summary measure will have an impact on the conclusions drawn from the statistical analysis. So care must be taken to choose a summary measure that is a meaningful summary of the animal profiles, but also answer the hypotheses that the researcher wishes to assess.

If there is a suitable summary measure, it should be remembered that this measure might not be on the same scale as the original response. For example, if the rate of decrease is used as a summary measure then it is not on the same scale as the original response. An overall average, however, is on the same scale. This may

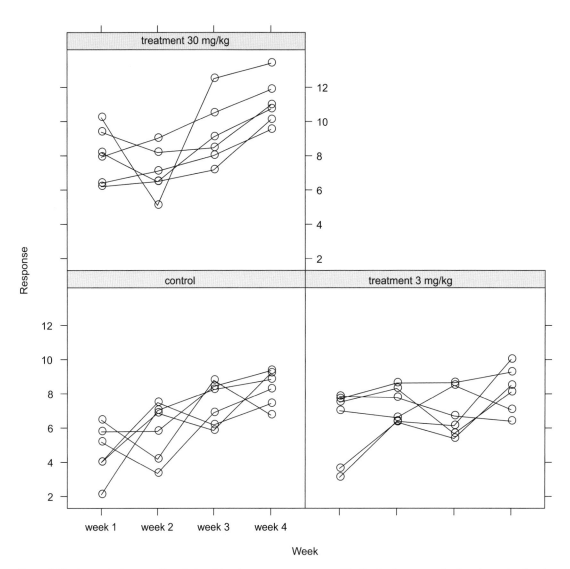

Figure 5.47. Categorised case profiles plot involving three treatment groups, with all animals measured at four time points (weeks 1, 2, 3 and 4). Note the unusual observation during week 2 in the 30 mg/kg treatment group.

influence the researcher's decision on which summary measure to use.

Examples of summary measure include the following.

Mean

In the example presented in Figure 5.48 each animal's response does not appear to vary over time, apart from random fluctuations, perhaps caused by the measurement-to-measurement variability. In this case a mean of each animal's responses should be a reasonable summary measure to analyse. The mean is on the same scale as the original data and hence has a biologically relevant meaning. If there is a reasonably small number of missing observations, then this can be accounted for within the averaging process.

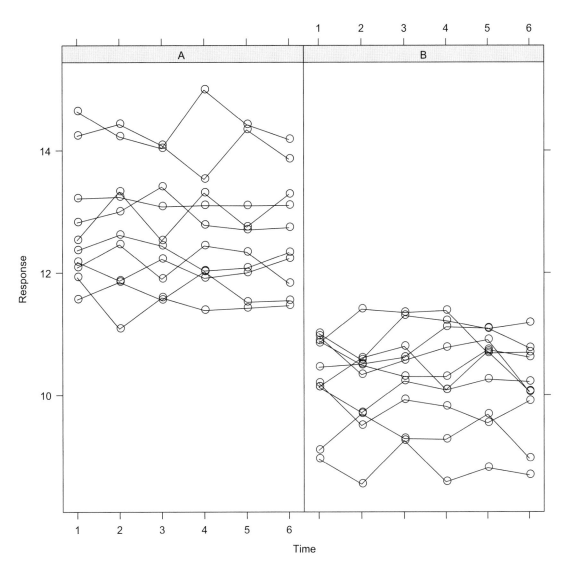

Figure 5.48. Categorised case profiles plot that indicates a mean response for each animal may be a suitable summary measure to analyse.

Area under the curve (AUC)

In Figure 5.49 the response profiles show a distinct curvature over time. A mean could still be taken over the time course, but this would not summarise the response profile as well as it did in the previous example. Perhaps a better way to summarise these profiles is to use the area under the curve (AUC). The AUC summary measure is effectively a weighted average of the individual responses, as opposed to the unweighted mean described above. It is not on the same scale as the original data, unless the AUC is divided through by time, but can be still be useful. For example, if the researcher wishes to investigate drug exposure, then the AUC provides a useful measure of this.

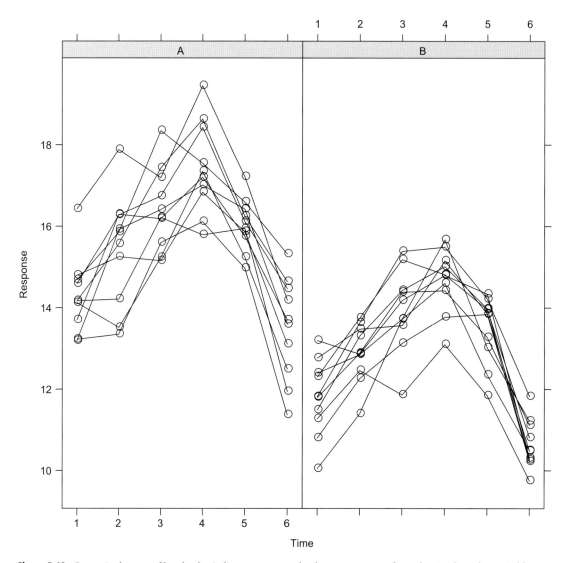

Figure 5.49. Categorised case profiles plot that indicates an area under the curve response for each animal may be a suitable summary measure to analyse.

There are several ways to calculate the AUC. Methods include the trapezium rule and Simpson's rule. Definitions and examples of these rules can be found in any good textbook on numerical integration; see for example Burden and Faires (2011, pp. 194–5).

The trapezium rule, which is an approximation to the true AUC, is defined as:

$$\text{AUC} \approx \frac{1}{2}\big[(x_1 - x_0)(y_1 + y_0) + \ldots + (x_i - x_{i-1})(y_i + y_{i-1}) \\ + \ldots + (x_N - x_{N-1})(y_N + y_{N-1})\big]$$

(5.27)

where N is the number of time intervals, x_i is the ith time point and y_i is the response at the ith time point ($0 \le i \le N$).

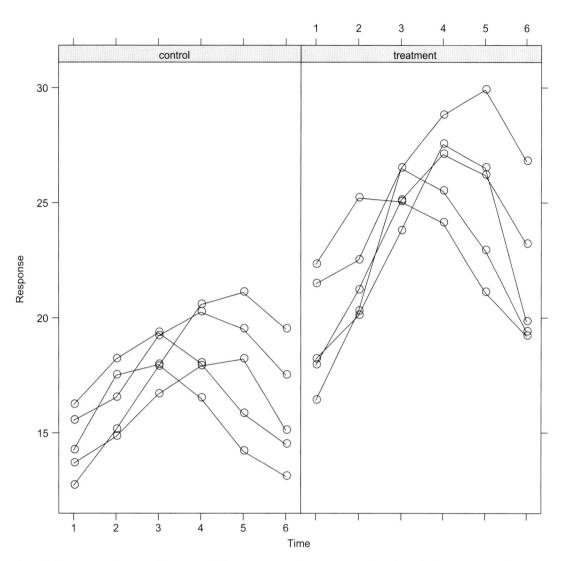

Figure 5.50. Categorised case profiles plot that indicates time to maximum response (T_{max}) for each animal may be a suitable summary measure to analyse.

Simpson's rule, for the case when the time intervals are equal (of size h) and N is even, can be written as:

$$\text{AUC} \approx \frac{h}{3}\left[y_0 + 4y_1 + 2y_2 + \ldots + 4y_{N-3} + 2y_{N-2} + 4y_{N-1} + y_N\right].$$

$$(5.28)$$

Although Simpson's rule may perform better than the trapezium rule under certain circumstances, and vice versa, for practical purposes both rules provide a sufficiently accurate estimate of the AUC for each animal.

Time to maximum response (T_{max})

It may be the case that an animal's time to maximum response is a suitable summary measure to investigate (Figure 5.50). If the effect of drug absorption varies between animals, then the researcher will not be able to control when the maximal response occurs. In such

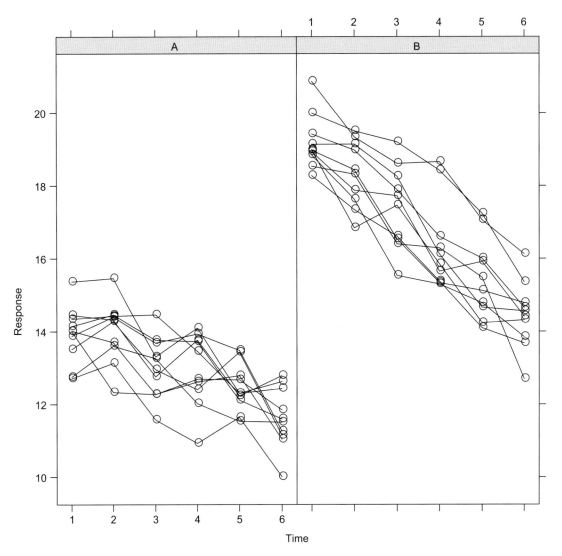

Figure 5.51. Categorised case profiles plot that indicates that the slope of the linear best-fit for each animal may be a suitable summary measure to analyse.

cases there will be an increase in variability of the data measured at each time point (caused by the different drug absorption rates). This will undermine the statistical power of any statistical comparisons made at a given time point.

Maximal effect (C_{max})
Linked to T_{max} is the maximal response for an individual animal. The decision on whether to consider

C_{max} or T_{max} will probably be governed by biological considerations.

Slope
It may be the case that it is not the actual responses that are of interest but the rate at which the responses change over time. For example, consider a behavioural test such as the Morris water maze, with data given in Figure 5.51. Animals are tested repeatedly

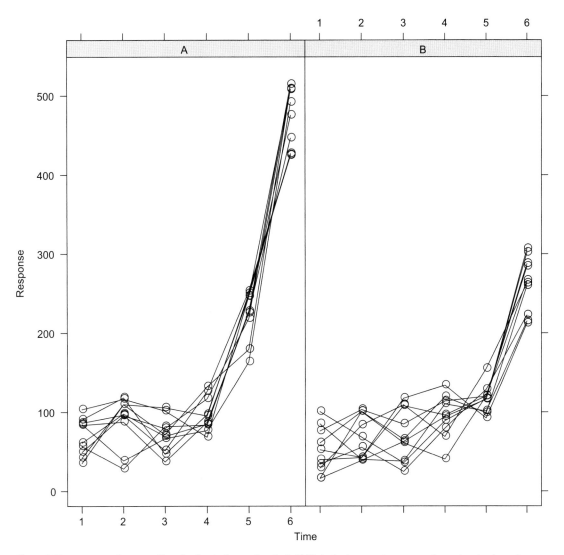

Figure 5.52. Categorised case profiles plot that indicates that the half-life in the increase in response for each animal may be a suitable summary measure to analyse.

over time and interest focuses on the decrease in time to complete the task. This gives an indication of an animal's learning ability. If this decrease occurs in a linear fashion, then perhaps the slope of the best-fit (or regression) line for each animal is a suitable summary measure that describes the animal's learning ability.

Half-life

It may be the case that the researcher is interested in the rate of change over time. Perhaps the change follows an exponential increase or decrease. In such cases an exponential curve can be fitted to each animal's responses. The half-life for each animal could then be used as a summary measure. Examples include

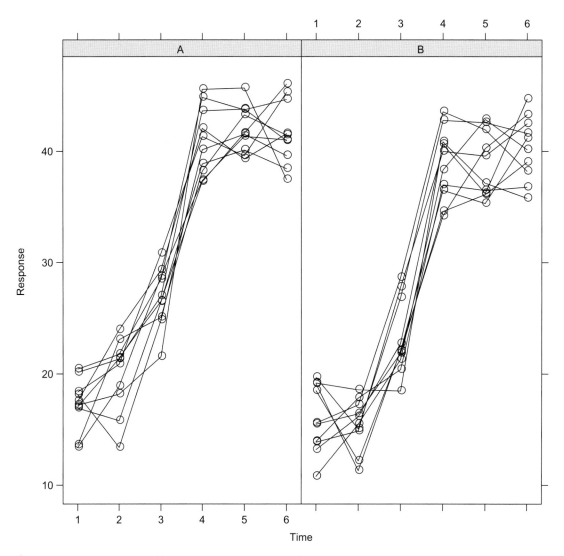

Figure 5.53. Categorised case profiles plot that indicates that the T_{50} for each animal may be a suitable summary measure to analyse.

bacterial cell counts (which grow exponentially) and responses that are known to need log-transforming prior to analysis to stabilise the variance. An example is given in Figure 5.52.

X_{50} of a response
The calculation of the X_{50} is usually carried out in experiments that do not involve repeated measures

(see Section 3.6.1). However, if the animal has been measured at a number of different concentrations or doses of compound, then it may be possible to calculate an X_{50} for each animal. Examples include the IC_{50} (half maximal inhibitory concentration), EC_{50} (half maximal effective concentration), T_{50} (time to 50% response) and ED_{50} (median effective dose). Regardless of the choice of summary statistic, we fit a logistic curve separately to each animal's responses (see Section 3.6.1). An example of such a response is given in Figure 5.53.

X_{50} of a summary response

Related to the previous example, it may be the case that animals are measured repeatedly over time within each of a number of test periods. For example, we may employ a repeated measures dose-escalation design, as described in Section 3.8.2.1. In such cases we could begin by calculating a summary statistic, perhaps an AUC, for each animal's responses in each test period. These AUC summary measures may increase or decrease across increasing doses of the test compound. In such cases we could then try to fit a logistic curve to the summary responses for each animal (across increasing doses) and hence obtain a single summary measure for each animal in the form of an ED_{50}.

Example 5.12: Measuring pain using the von Frey hairs

TRPA1 is a member of the transient receptor potential family of ion channels and is thought to have a role in sensing painful cold and irritating chemicals (Kwan *et al.*, 2006). To test the *in vivo* roles of TRPA1, a strain of mice with inactive TRPA1 was tested using von Frey hairs. In the model, the paw of the animal is pressed with a number of hairs of varying widths (ten times per animal per hair). Each hair exerts a different pressure on the paw. The response is a binary response, either yes or no, depending on whether the paw is withdrawn or not. Usually a number of hairs of different widths are applied to each animal's paw until a consistent 100% withdrawal rate is achieved.

This type of response, a binary repeatedly measured response, can be difficult to analyse. Ideally we would like to take into account the properties of the design, i.e. that each animal is measured repeatedly at different hair widths. This is not easy though as all animals will not necessarily be tested using hairs of the same width. This has the potential to leave gaps in the dataset.

Although not used in the original analysis, one method to analyse this type of data is to use a summary X_{50} measure. Defining 1 as a paw withdraw and 0 as no paw withdraw, we can fit a logistic curve to the binary repeated measures data for each animal to estimate the width of hair that would result in a 50% chance that the animal will withdraw its paw. For example, Figure 5.54 illustrates the data for an animal tested using 15 hairs.

The curve was fitted using InVivoStat's dose-response analysis module, with the curve maximum fixed at 1 and the curve minimum fixed at 0. The estimate of the X_{50}, back-transformed onto the original scale, is given in Table 5.20. Once the X_{50} has been calculated for each animal, then the analysis can be carried out on the X_{50} responses using, for example, an ANOVA technique.

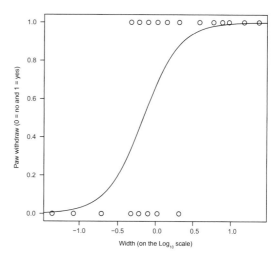

Figure 5.54. An animal's 10 (binary) responses at 15 different von Frey hairs, from Example 5.12. Multiple responses are overlaid and hence only a single point is visible when the same response is repeatedly observed at a given hair width.

It should be noted that this method will work if there is no separation in the responses for each animal. The response for an animal is defined as being separated if the animal does not withdraw its paw at all for the first few hairs but then removes its paw all ten times for the next width (and all others after that). In other words the hair widths can be separated into two distinct sets of all responders and all non-responders. In such a situation it is impossible to estimate where the X_{50} lies, except that it is somewhere between the two hair widths at the responder/non-responder interface.

5.4.4.3 Repeated measures analysis

In certain situations the researcher may not be able to find a suitable summary measure to use in the statistical analysis. Since the animals' responses were measured repeatedly, it may be of interest to know how the experimental groups change across the levels of the repeated factor. For example, does the difference between the treatment group and the control group vary over time?

As mentioned above, care must be taken when analysing repeated measures data in this way. The researcher should resist the temptation to include the repeated factor simply as an additional experimental factor in, say, a multi-way ANOVA analysis. This will lead to erroneous results and possibly false positive

Table 5.20. Table of the X_{50} estimate, with 95% confidence intervals, for one animal's responses to the von Frey hairs from Example 5.12

	ED50	Lower 95% CI	Upper 95% CI
Estimate	0.681	0.461	1.005

conclusions because the assumption of independence (see Section 5.4.1.1) does not hold in this case.

Two commonly applied techniques for performing a repeated measures analysis are the repeated measures ANOVA-based approach and the repeated measures mixed-model approach. Although the ANOVA-based approach is widely available in the statistical packages commonly used by animal researchers, we argue that it is the mixed-model approach that is more suitable for the analysis of animal experiments; see Brammer (2003), Clarke *et al.* (2012) and Smith (2012).

The ANOVA-based approach uses the least squares technique described in Section 5.4.3.1 to break down the variability into sources corresponding to the terms in the statistical model. The mixed-model approach uses restricted maximum likelihood (REML) to estimate the amount of information that can be attributed to each term in the statistical model. In this section we shall highlight some of the benefits of using the mixed-model approach to analyse data generated using repeated measures designs. A description of how to perform a repeated measures mixed-model analysis using InVivoStat is given in Section 6.4.

Repeated measures analyses

When performing a repeated measures analysis we need to test the factors against the correct source of variability. There are two sources of variability in these experiments, the between-animal variability and the within-animal variability. The levels of the treatments, in a repeated measured design, are applied to animals (animals are the experimental units) so these treatments are tested against the between-animal variability. The repeated factor and any interactions involving the repeated factor are assessed against the within-animal variability. Note that we include interactions involving the repeated factor (despite the lack of randomisation

of the levels of the repeated factor) because we have taken account of the spatial interrelationships between the repeatedly measured responses within the analysis. We do not therefore need to make the assumption that the observations are independent (using a randomisation-based argument).

For the mixed-model approach we can generate an ANOVA-like table that provides the researcher with overall tests of the significance of the fixed factors. The tests in the table are either within-animal or between-animal, depending on the effect being tested.

Example 5.13: Chronic stress model of depression in rats

An experiment was conducted to assess whether administration of nicotine to rats reverses anhedonic-like responses and cognitive impairment in the chronic mild stress (CMS) model of depression (Andreasen *et al.*, 2011). Following exposure to CMS, male Wistar rats were administered either the vehicle, nicotine (0.4 mg/kg/day), sertraline (5 mg/kg/day) or a combination of nicotine and sertraline. Animals were then assessed weekly using the sucrose preference test, with week 3 taken as a measure of stress prior to treatment and the average of the responses for weeks 8 and 9 providing a measure of the treatment effect. The design employed was a repeated measures design with a three-factor full-factorial core design, see Section 3.5.3, consisting of three between-animal factors: Nicotine (levels: nicotine or vehicle), Sertraline (levels: sertraline or vehicle) and Stress (levels: stress or non-stress), and repeated factor Week (levels: week 3 and 9). A baseline response was also measured and this was included in the analysis as a covariate (see Section 5.4.6).

The experiment revealed that the effect of nicotine in the CMS model was similar to the antidepressant drug sertraline. There was also some evidence that nicotine alleviated CMS-induced cognitive disturbance. Table 5.21 is a summary table containing the tests of the overall effects for Example 5.13.

Using this table we can perform (within-animal) tests of the interactions between the three treatment factors and time. These are tests to see if the differences between the treatments vary over time. They should be considered first. The interactions are assessed against the within-animal variability.

For the within-animal tests, assessed against the within-animal variability, the degrees of freedom for the within-animal variability is given by:

Table 5.21. Table of the tests of overall effects for Example 5.13

Source	Numerator degrees of freedom	Denominator degrees of freedom	Comment
Baseline	1	95	Tested against
Stress	1	95	between-animal
Nicotine	1	95	variability
Sertraline	1	95	
Stress*Nicotine	1	95	
Stress*Sertraline	1	95	
Nicotine*Sertraline	1	95	
Stress*Nicotine*Sertraline	1	95	
Week	1	95	Tested against
Week*Baseline	1	95	within-animal
Week*Stress	1	95	variability
Week*Nicotine	1	95	
Week*Sertraline	1	95	
Week*Stress*Nicotine	1	95	
Week*Stress*Sertraline	1	95	
Week*Nicotine*Sertraline	1	95	
Week*Stress*Nicotine*Sertraline	1	95	

df_{within} = No. of animals × (No. of repeated levels – 1)
   – df (for all within-animal terms).   (5.29)

To appreciate Eq. (5.29), consider the following derivation.

The number of separate comparisons we can make *within an individual animal* is, using the arguments given in previous sections, one less than the number of levels of the repeated factor. The total number of comparisons we can make within *all* the animals is therefore:

No. of animals × (No. of repeated levels – 1).   (5.30)

To calculate the within-animal degrees of freedom we take the number of levels of the repeated factor (minus one) multiplied by the number of animals and then subtract the degrees of freedom required to estimate the within-animal terms. In Example 5.13 we have 104 animals in total, two levels of the repeated factor and nine degrees of freedom for the within-animal terms, hence:

df_{within} = 104 × (2 – 1) – 9 = 95.

It is also relatively easy to check that the degrees of freedom for the between-animal test(s) ($df_{between}$) in Table 5.21 are correct. For the between-animal variability, the denominator degrees of freedom for the between-animal tests is:

$df_{between}$ = No. of animals – 1 – df (for all between-animal terms).   (5.31)

So we take the number of animals, subtract 1 (for the overall mean) and then subtract the number of degrees of freedom required to estimate the between-animal terms. In Example 5.13 we have 104 animals in total and two treatments, hence

$df_{between}$ = 104 – 1 – 8 = 95.

5.4.4.4 The mixed-model approach vs. the ANOVA-based approach

In this section we shall describe some of the advantages of using a mixed-model approach to analysing repeated measures data, compared to the ANOVA-based alternative. A discussion of this subject is given by Smith (2012).

The variance–covariance structure

We have already discussed the variance of a response: it is a measure of how spread out the results are. In an analysis of repeated measures data, however, we also need to consider the covariances. These are a measure of the degree to which pairs of responses change or vary together (co-vary).

Note that the covariance between pairs of responses is related to their correlation. To obtain the correlation between two responses we divide the covariance by

Observation	1	2	3	...	n
1	variance$_{(1)}$	covariance$_{(2,1)}$	covariance$_{(3,1)}$	...	covariance$_{(n,1)}$
2	covariance$_{(1,2)}$	variance$_{(2)}$	covariance$_{(3,2)}$	...	covariance$_{(n,2)}$
3	covariance$_{(1,3)}$	covariance$_{(2,3)}$	variance$_{(3)}$	...	covariance$_{(n,3)}$
...	...	...	...	...	...
n	covariance$_{(1,n)}$	covariance$_{(2,n)}$	covariance$_{(3,n)}$	...	variance$_{(n)}$

a measure of the variability (Snedecor and Cochran, 1989, p. 182). For responses X and Y

$$\text{correlation}_{(X,Y)} = \frac{\text{covariance}_{(X,Y)}}{\sigma_X \sigma_Y} \qquad (5.32)$$

where σ_X and σ_Y are the standard deviations of X and Y, respectively. So correlation is a (dimensionless) ratio of the covariance compared to the variance, on a scale –1 to +1.

The variances and covariances can be summarised in a single grid-like structure or (matrix) called the *variance–covariance matrix*. Assume there are n observations in the dataset. We construct an n by n grid such that:

- The main diagonal elements correspond to the n variance estimates for each of the n observations.
- The off-diagonal elements correspond to the covariances. So the $(i,j) = (j,i)$ entry is the covariance between the ith and jth observations, i.e.

In the previous section when performing the ANOVA-based analysis we assumed that:

- The variance was the same for all groups (and therefore all observations); hence the entries on the main diagonal of the variance–covariance structure are all the same (we usually denote this value by s^2, the sample variance).
- The observations were independent; hence the covariance between pairs of individual observations is equal to zero.

Observation	1	2	3	...	n
1	s^2	0	0	...	0
2	0	s^2	0	...	0
3	0	0	s^2	...	0
...	...	...	...	...	...
n	0	0	0	...	s^2

This leads to a simplified variance–covariance matrix of the form:

However, we cannot assume this simplified variance–covariance structure is true when analysing repeated measures data. As discussed above, the levels of the repeated factor cannot be randomised: day 1 must come before day 2. With almost all other factors of interest considered in this text some degree of randomisation can be performed when allocating the experimental units to the levels of these factors. We can then assume that this randomisation has, in some sense, removed any interrelationships (or covariances) between the observations. In the analysis of repeated measures data the lack of randomisation should be taken into account if the results of the analysis are to be meaningful. This can be achieved using a repeated measures mixed-model analysis approach. When using this analysis approach we can account for the relationships between responses measured on the same animal by estimating the variance–covariance structure. In particular we can decide which general structure to use when we model the variance–covariance matrix. This involves considering:

1. Variance structure: Some of these structures allow the variability of the responses to be different at each level of the repeated factor, thus relaxing the homogeneity of variance assumption.

2. Between-animal covariance structure: If the animals are selected at random, we assume that pairs of observations from different animals are independent. Hence many of the off-diagonal entries in the variance–covariance matrix are assumed to equal zero.

3. Within-animal covariance structure: Pairs of observations within-animal will be related, and so the covariances between the within-animal observations will be non-zero.

There are many general variance–covariance structures available to model the within-animal spatial relationships, these include:

Autoregressive When using this structure we assume the variability is the same at all time points. We also assume the strength of the covariance between responses measured across time is dependent on the distance between them. The size of the covariance between two observations at time points i and j is calculated using the formula:

$$s^2 \rho^{|i-j|}, \tag{5.33}$$

where ρ is the autoregressive parameter (which lies between 0 and 1) and s^2 is the sample variance. When using this structure the time points should be equally spaced for the results of the analysis to be meaningful, although this condition can be relaxed in certain statistical software packages.

Compound symmetric With the compound symmetric covariance structure we assume that the variability of the responses is the same at all time points and also that the relationship (or covariance) between the results is the same for all pairs of time points regardless of how far apart they are. With compound symmetry we only have to estimate the common variance (common across all time points) and the common covariance. This is a real benefit in experiments with small sample sizes, where not much information is collected and hence it is difficult to estimate the variance–covariance matrix with any degree of precision. However, certain assumptions are made, notably the assumption of sphericity discussed below.

Unstructured An alternative structure, where the researcher does not have to make the assumption of sphericity, is the unstructured covariance structure. With this structure the strengths of the covariances are allowed to vary for any pair of repeated measures. Additionally the variability of the responses is allowed to vary across the levels of the repeated factor. This can be useful if the responses are cell counts that are measured in several brain regions and the data are analysed using a repeated measures mixed-model analysis approach, with repeated factor Brain region. It is conceivable that the cell counts will be more variable in the larger brain regions, and this should be taken into account in the analysis.

There are, however, problems with this approach, mainly because there are many variance and covariance parameters to estimate. If there are r repeated measures per animal, then there are $(r-1) \times (r-2)$ covariance parameters and r variance parameters to estimate. This is a lot of parameters to estimate, especially if the number of animals is small and the number of time points relatively large. Unfortunately in many animal experiments this approach may produce unreliable results; see Skene and Kenward (2010) for a discussion and alternative approaches.

One of the benefits of using a mixed-model approach to analyse repeated measures data is that it allows the researcher to choose the way the variances and the spatial interrelationships are (statistically) modelled. Many variance–covariance structures, other than those described here, are available. However, it should be remembered that the more complex the variance–covariance structure, the more parameters will need to be estimated. If the study consists of only a small number of animals per group, then the parameters that define the variance–covariance structure may not be estimated with any reasonable degree of precision.

Missing data

One of the other main benefits of using the repeated measures mixed-model approach, as opposed to the ANOVA-based approach, is that the mixed-model deals with missing data (in most situations) more satisfactorily. With the alternative ANOVA-based methods it is often the case that if an animal is missing a response at one time point, then that animal is excluded from the analysis. This can be a major problem if the sample sizes are small. This is not the case in the mixed-model approach.

Sphericity

It was mentioned above that certain additional assumptions are made when conducting a repeated measures analysis as well as the usual parametric assumptions. When we perform a repeated measures ANOVA-based analysis one of the additional assumptions that we make is sphericity. Sphericity is the assumption that the variances of the estimates of the differences between the experimental groups are the same regardless of which pair of groups is being compared (Field, 1998).

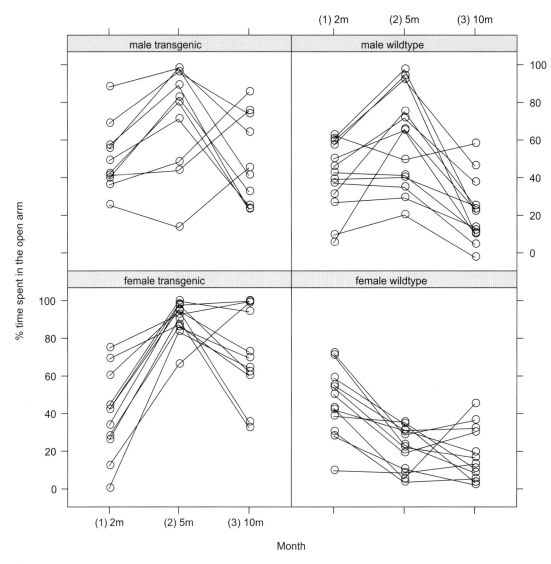

Figure 5.55. Categorised case profiles plot of the percentage time spent in the open arm of an elevated maze, from Example 5.14. Animals were assessed at 2, 5 and 10 months.

There is a test of sphericity, see Mauchly (1940), although this test is not generally recommended. For example, this test fails to detect departures from sphericity if the sample sizes are small, as is often the case in animal experiments. So using this test in animal experiments is not advised as you may never identify that the sphericity assumption does not hold. Several methods have been proposed to correct the results of the repeated measures ANOVA-based analysis if the sphericity assumption has been violated. These include the Greenhouse–Geisser, Huydt–Feldt and Wilks–Lambda adjustments. In practice most approaches generate similar conclusions, although the Greenhouse–Geisser adjustment is perhaps the most popular.

Using a mixed-model approach to analyse repeated measures data allows the researcher to avoid making

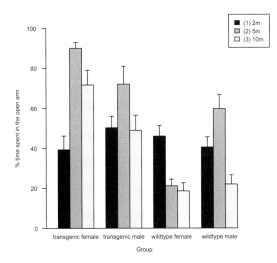

Figure 5.56. Column plot of the observed means with SEMs for the percentage time spent in the open arms of the elevated maze, from Example 5.14. Animals were assessed at 2, 5 and 10 months.

the sphericity assumption by using, for example, the autoregressive or unstructured covariance structures described above. These covariance structures allow the covariances to be different and hence do not assume sphericity.

Example 5.14: Investigating non-cognitive behaviours

It is well known that Alzheimer's disease is characterised by progressive impairment, with neuropsychiatric symptoms such as anomalous motor behaviour and anxiety. The APP/PS1 transgenic strain of mice has been shown to display increased beta-amyloid deposition and hence provides a model for Alzheimer's disease. A study was conducted to investigate the non-cognitive behaviours of these mice using the elevated maze (Pugh *et al.*, 2007). Male and female transgenic and wildtype mice were tested when 2, 5 and 10 months old. In the experimental design the two factors Genotype and Gender were fully crossed with each other and hence the design used was a repeated measures factorial design. We shall consider the percentage time spent in the open arm of the elevated maze (a measure of anxiety).

The categorised case profiles plot (generated using simulated data) reveals that the profiles of the percentage time spent in the open arm of the maze vary depending on the gender and genotype of the animal (see Figure 5.55).

There was no obvious summary measure available, and the researcher was interested in comparing the strains at each time point, hence a repeated measures analysis was required. A plot of the observed means (Figure 5.56) revealed some evidence of strain and gender differences over time. Note that in the observed means with SEMs plot, the error bars correspond to the between-animal variability (which was calculated separately for each observed

mean). If the researcher wished to investigate the effects over time, then these trends could be assessed against the within-animal variability. The within-animal variability is likely to be smaller than the between-animal variability shown on the observed means with SEMs plot.

A repeated measures mixed-model analysis was performed on the simulated data (see Table 5.22). The tests of the overall effects were calculated using the Repeated Measures Parametric Analysis module within InVivoStat.

Table 5.22 shares many similarities with the ANOVA tables described above. The terms Genotype, Gender and the Genotype:Gender interaction are tested against the between-animal variability (with 42 degrees of freedom). There is evidence that the effect of genotype varies with gender ($F_{(1,42)}$ = 6.99, p = 0.011). Overall the transgenic animals appear to spend more time in the open arm of the maze than their wildtype littermates ($F_{(1,42)}$ = 43.34, p < 0.001), although the researcher should be careful when drawing conclusions from the test of a main effect in the presence of a significant interaction.

Terms involving the repeated factor (Month) are tested against the within-animal variability (with 84 degrees of freedom). All the tests are significant, for example the Gender:Genotype:Month three-way interaction ($F_{(2,84)}$ = 12.76, p < 0.001) indicates that the profiles of the four groups in the study change over time. By considering Figure 5.56, or a plot of the predicted means generated as part of the statistical analysis (not shown), it can be seen that the percentage time spent in the open arm seems to increase at 5 months and then decrease at 10 months, with the exception of the female wildtype group.

5.4.4.5 Advantages and disadvantages of the repeated measures analysis

The advantages of the repeated measures analysis include:

- It provides the researcher with powerful and informative tests.
- It allows the researcher to answer specific questions such as: 'Does the treatment effect vary over time?'
- It allows for an overall test of the significance of the between-animal factor(s), where appropriate.
- It allows for an overall test of the significance of the repeated factor.

There are, however, some disadvantages which should be considered:

- Too many time points (we believe greater than around 15) can lead to oversensitive statistical tests. When many measurements are taken within each animal, the chances are they will be highly related. This is analogous to the issue of pseudo-replication discussed in Section 3.7.3.6. For example, in

Table 5.22. Table of tests of overall model effects from the repeated measures analysis, Example 5.14

	Num. df	Den. df	F-value	p-value
Gender	1	42	0.04	0.834
Genotype	1	42	43.34	< 0.001
Month	2	84	17.93	< 0.001
Gender:Genotype	1	42	6.99	0.011
Gender:Month	2	84	4.38	0.015
Genotype:Month	2	84	19.29	< 0.001
Gender:Genotype:Month	2	84	12.76	< 0.001

Example 3.40 (Section 3.8.1.1) it is not recommended to include the data from the 40 days in the repeated measures analysis. We suggest averaging neighbouring responses to obtain 10 averages per animal prior to carrying out any statistical tests.

- Small sample sizes and many repeated measurements can lead to an unreliable analysis. If the sample sizes are small then we cannot estimate the spatial inter-relationships of the within-animal responses (the covariance structure) with any degree of reliability.
- It leads to more complicated analyses.
- As more *p*-values are generated, the risk of finding false positives increases (see Section 5.4.8.1).
- We may have to assume sphericity, although this disadvantage can be avoided by using the repeated measures mixed-model approach.

5.4.5 Predicted means from the parametric analysis

Let us assume the researcher has carried out the statistical analysis using either a *t*-test, ANOVA or repeated measures mixed-model analysis. So far in this section we have only considered the overall tests of the experimental factors that are produced when running these analyses. However, in the analysis of animal experiments it is common practice to compare individual group means in order to investigate the experimental factors further. While there are several ways to do this, a good starting point is to consider the predicted means

generated as part of the statistical analysis, the so-called *least square (predicted) means*.

5.4.5.1 Least square (predicted) means

The method for calculating the least square (predicted) means is different from that of computing the observed means. It shares similarities with the method for generating the sums of squares described in Section 5.4.3.1. We shall describe the principle of the method with an example.

Example 5.9 (continued): A study involving three treatment groups and a control

Consider Example 5.9 as discussed in the ANOVA derivation (see Section 5.4.3.1). To calculate the predicted means consider the residuals from the statistical analysis. Consider an observation *i*, where:

$$\text{residual}_i = \text{observed}_i - \text{predicted}_i.$$

Each predicted mean is computed in such a way that the residuals (or the distances of the individual observations from their predicted means) are minimised (see Figure 5.57).

For each treatment group we therefore need a single summary measure of the residuals that can be minimised to obtain the predicted mean. Summing the residuals may appear to be a sensible summary measure, but some of the residuals will be positive and some will be negative, so a simple average of the residuals is not suitable. We use the method described above for constructing the ANOVA table and first square the residuals before summing them. This is why we use the terminology 'least square (predicted) means' as we are minimising the sum of the squares of the residuals. This approach is analogous to how we calculated the residual sums of squares in the ANOVA table.

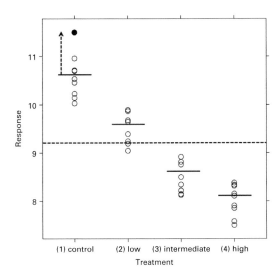

Figure 5.57. Scatterplot of the data from Example 5.9. The plot includes the grand mean of the data as a dotted line, the individual group means as solid lines and the distance of the highlighted observation from the least square (predicted) mean as an arrow.

5.4.5.2 Variability of the least square (predicted) means

As mentioned above it is usually the case that scientists report observed means alongside measures of the within-group variability. For example, the means plotted in the means with SEMs plot are the observed means and the standard errors are calculated using the within-group variability estimates. Predicted means are usually presented with the estimate of variability generated within the statistical analysis. As discussed in Section 5.2.2.1 this is, in some sense, a weighted average variability estimate, averaged over all experimental groups. In particular, we usually generate confidence intervals around the predicted means using this single variability estimate.

In practice the most commonly reported confidence interval is the 95% confidence interval. It should be noted that the 95% confidence interval is (assuming the within-group variability is roughly the same for all groups) approximately twice as large as the corresponding standard error. So if you generate a graphical plot of the predicted means with 95% confidence

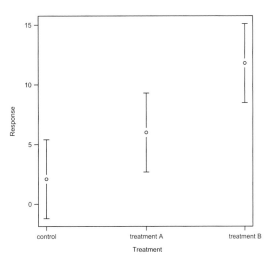

Figure 5.58. Plot of the least square (predicted) means with 95% confidence intervals, for Example 5.15.

intervals, then make sure that your audience is aware that the error bars are confidence intervals and not the more familiar standard errors... it will make your data look more variable than it really is!

Example 5.15: A single factor experiment

The following example highlights how the size of the confidence intervals of the predicted means (from a one-way ANOVA analysis) compares to the standard errors in the observed means with SEMs plot. The predicted means with 95% confidence intervals are given in Figure 5.58 and the observed means with SEMs plot is given in Figure 5.59. It can be seen that, as the sample sizes are the same across the three groups, the three 95% confidence intervals will be the same size. All three intervals use the same overall estimate of variability to generate them. The means with SEMs plot, however, employs the individual within-group variability estimates to generate the standard errors and in this case the within-group variability changes across groups. Note that most of the parametric tests described previously rely on the assumption that the variability is the same across groups and hence the means with SEMs plot does not represent the variability estimate used in the statistical analysis.

5.4.5.3 Geometric means and confidence intervals

One other benefit of using confidence intervals rather than standard errors is that they need not be symmetrical around the mean. This flexibility is useful if the

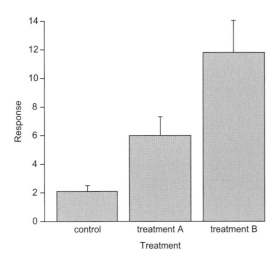

Figure 5.59. Plot of the observed means with standard errors, for Example 5.15.

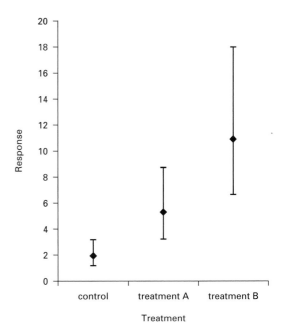

Figure 5.60. Plot of the back-transformed geometric means with 95% confidence intervals, for an experiment involving a treatment factor at three levels (control, treatment A and treatment B).

data has been log-transformed prior to the analysis to stabilise the variance. If you want to produce a means with SEMs plot in this scenario, then you may want to consider plotting the geometric means (see Section 5.2.1.4) with corresponding geometric standard errors (see Section 6.11.3).

Assume that the statistical analysis (including the calculation of the predicted means and the confidence intervals) has been carried out on the log-transformed scale. Once the predicted means and confidence intervals have been calculated (on the log scale), then they can be back-transformed onto the original scale. These means are sometimes called the back-transformed geometric means, although they are still examples of predicted means.

Example 5.15 (continued): A single factor experiment

Returning to Example 5.15, it was decided that the data required a log transformation to stabilise the variance. The researcher decided to back-transform the predicted means onto the original scale before plotting them. The plot of back-transformed geometric means, with 95% confidence intervals, is presented in Figure 5.60.

From the plot we can see that:

· The variability increases with the size of response.
· There is more variability (or uncertainly) above the predicted mean than there is below it. The response was log-normally distributed and so the variability increases as the response increases. To reflect this, the confidence intervals are larger above the mean than below.

While the first point is also addressed by the observed means with SEMs plot, the second is not. The standard error of the observed mean is, by definition, symmetrical about the mean. To avoid this, the observed means with SEMs plot would need to be produced on a log scale.

5.4.5.4 Reliability of the predicted means

When there are other factors present in the experimental design, the predicted means are more reliable than the observed means as they adjust for the effect of these additional factors. We end this section with an example of the use of predicted means to highlight this.

Example 5.16: A fertility study

An investigation was conducted to assess the effect of an intra-uterine injection of prostaglandin antagonists on mouse fertility. A series of experiments, see Biggers *et al.* (1981), was conducted to assess the effect of four prostaglandin antagonists, 7-oxa-13-prostynoic acid, 18,18,20-trimethylprostaglandin E-2, indomethacin and meclofenamic acid. The compounds were tested by injecting them into the uterine horn. Post-injection the number of embryo implantation sites was recorded. We shall focus on the experiment involving 18,18,20-trimethylprostaglandin E-2.

As each animal has two independent uterine horns it was possible to administer two different treatments (either different doses of 18,18,20-trimethylprostaglandin E-2, a saline control or the vehicle control) to each animal, one per uterine horn. Two treatments were given to each animal, where the allocation was made using a balanced incomplete block design with Animal as the blocking factor. This allowed efficient within-animal treatment comparisons to be made.

The 18,18,20- trimethylprostaglandin E-2 treatment (at four doses, Groups 3, 4, 5 and 6) and two controls (Groups 1 and 2) were administered to 30 mice over two experiments. The randomisation performed was as follows:

· Treatment pairs were randomly assigned to animals using two replicates of a balanced incomplete block design.
· The treatments within each pair were randomly assigned to the left or right uterine horns within each animal.

In this discussion we shall analyse some simulated data, using a one-way ANOVA with Animal as a blocking factor. This is different to the approach described by Biggers *et al.* (1981).

From an initial look at the data, it appeared to be the case that some animals had, on average, more implantation sites than others. This could, in part, have been due to treatment effects (as each animal did not receive all treatments) or it could have been caused by background biological variation. Following the ANOVA analysis a plot of the predicted means of the Animal factor, which took into account treatment effects, was generated. This plot revealed that there was some evidence of differences between the 30 mice (Figure 5.61).

Two plots of the treatment group means highlighted the difference between the observed and predicted means (Figures 5.62 and 5.63). The observed means with SEMs plot revealed the treatment effect, but it also hinted at a difference between the two control groups (treatments 1 and 2).

The plot of the predicted means following the ANOVA analysis takes into account that some animals appeared to have fewer implantation sites regardless of the treatments they received. This plot revealed that there was actually a much smoother dose-response relationship and also that there was no difference between the two control groups.

As the confidence intervals were the same for all groups, this plot also highlighted that the same variability estimate was used to calculate each confidence interval. Assuming that the variability estimate was the same for all groups, this overall estimate of variability was perhaps more reliable than the individual within-group variance estimates. Of course the assumption that the variance was the same across all groups may be suspect and perhaps needed further investigation.

5.4.6 Analysis of covariance (ANCOVA)

There is one other type of parametric analysis technique that the researcher may find useful and that is the

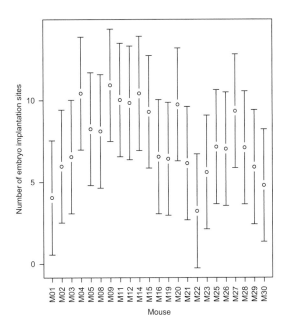

Figure 5.61. Plot of the predicted means for the individual animals with 95% confidence intervals for Example 5.16.

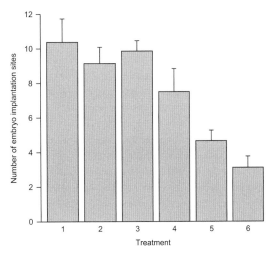

Figure 5.62. Plot of the observed means with standard errors of the treatment groups for Example 5.16.

analysis of covariance or ANCOVA. We believe this type of analysis can be used to analyse many experiments. A description of how to perform the analysis of covariance using InVivoStat is given in Section 6.3.

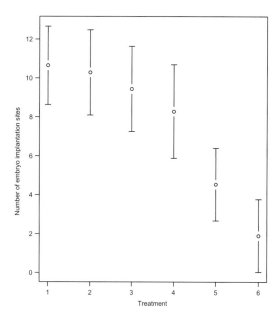

Figure 5.63. Plot of the predicted means with 95% confidence intervals of the treatment groups for Example 5.16.

Throughout this book we have tried, using both experimental design and statistical analysis, to reduce the variability (or noise) that we test the experimental hypotheses against. We achieve this by using all the available information to construct the experimental design and direct the statistical analysis. Covariates provide a further way to reduce the variability by allowing the researcher to make use of any additional information that has been recorded during the experiment. In particular, background information on the animals can be used to reduce the between-animal variability and hence improve the sensitivity of the statistical tests and/or reduce sample sizes.

In practice the researcher will have plenty of information about the animals in the study (such as body weight, age and perhaps baseline measures of the response) and it is important that this information is used in the statistical analysis. Some information, such as animal body weight, is routinely measured for husbandry purposes. Therefore it could be argued that we are always in a position to make use of covariates in the statistical analysis of animal experiments.

5.4.6.1 What is a covariate?

A covariate is a continuous numerical variable corresponding to a characteristic of the animal. It should not be confused with the covariance between pairs of responses, as described in Section 5.4.4.4.

These variables are preferably measured before the animal undergoes any experimental procedures, although this is not always the case. The purpose of the covariate is to capture some background properties of the animal that may influence the post-manipulation responses.

Possible candidates for covariates include:
- animal age;
- initial body weight;
- baseline measure of the response;
- litter size;
- time between sample collection and analysis;
- order of experimental procedures (to quantify any learning or procedural effects).

Assume that there is a strong relationship between the response (to a treatment say) and some measured baseline characteristic of the animal. Due to this relationship, animals with a high baseline level tend to have a high posttreatment response. Therefore some of the variability observed in each experimental group posttreatment can be explained by the differences already present at baseline. For example, in an experiment to measure the effect of a novel compound on locomotor activity, it was hypothesised that animals within a group that were more active at the start of the study would be likely to be the more active animals (within that group) at the end of the study, regardless of the treatment they received. Some of the variability observed within each group at the end of the study can therefore be explained by considering the baseline level of activity. The within-group variability is not entirely experimentally induced; some of it was present before the experiment started. We include the baseline locomotor activity as a covariate in the analysis to account for the variability in the response, which can be explained by considering the background behaviour of the animals.

Covariates vs. linear predictors
When performing an ANCOVA analysis certain assumptions are made, alongside the usual parametric ones.

These assumptions are considered in detail in Section 5.4.6.6. For example, we assume that the covariate is independent of, or not influenced by, the experimental factors. The covariate is a statistical device to reduce the underlying variability of the responses; it should not influence the predictions obtained when fitting the statistical model. There are other analyses, mathematically related to ANCOVA, where the researcher will want to adjust the model predictions for continuous variables that are influenced by the experimental factors. Such variables are known as *linear predictors* and the analysis is often defined as *regression analysis*. We shall discuss this analysis briefly in Section 5.4.7.

5.4.6.2 Best-fit lines and predicted lines

When performing an analysis of covariance we consider the relationship between the response of interest and the covariate. We assume this relationship is linear and hence fit straight lines to the data, one per experimental group. There are two types of lines that are described in this section and they are generated by different procedures. We define them as best-fit lines and predicted lines.

Best-fit lines
The *best-fit lines* are analogous to the observed means described in Section 5.2.1.2 and are calculated separately, and independently, for each experimental group. Best-fit lines are constructed using the least squares principle described in Section 5.4.5.1. Each line is generated such that the distances between the observations and the best-fit line are minimised. This is performed separately for each experimental group and hence the lines are independent of each other. Best-fit lines provide an insight into the underlying relationships within the dataset and are not dependent on the statistical model fitted to the data as part of the ANCOVA analysis. These lines are produced on the categorised scatterplots, as described in the next section.

Predicted lines
We also consider a second type of line, the *predicted line* (see Section 5.4.6.4). These lines are analogous to the predicted means in an ANOVA analysis. They are generated by fitting a statistical model to the data as part of the ANCOVA analysis. The predicted lines, one per experimental group, are usually parallel to each other, as discussed in Section 5.4.6.6.

5.4.6.3 Categorised scatterplot

Perhaps the easiest way to investigate candidate covariates is to plot them using a categorised scatterplot. The Y-axis on the plot corresponds to the response being analysed and the X-axis corresponds to the covariate. The pair of results per animal is then plotted on a scatterplot. It is also recommended that the scatterplot be categorised by the experimental groups (using different colours or symbols). The best-fit line for each experimental group is also included on the plot to highlight the linear relationship between the response and the covariate

Example 5.17: Effect of PFOS on cynomolgus monkey body weight

An experiment was conducted to investigate the toxicological risks associated with repeated exposure of perfluorooctanesulfonate potassium salt (PFOS) in monkeys (Seacat *et al.*, 2002). Such compounds are poorly eliminated and hence pose a possible risk to human health. The experiment consisted of both male and female monkeys receiving either the control or one of three doses of PFOS. Either four or six monkeys per sex were randomly assigned to each of the four treatment groups at the start of the study. We shall concentrate on the male monkeys in this discussion.

Many parameters were measured but we shall focus on the body weight measurement taken at the end of the dosing period (day 184 after commencement of the treatment phase). There were several candidates for use as a covariate in the analysis; we shall focus on a baseline measure of body weight and the age of the monkey at the start of the study.

A scatterplot of some simulated body weights at day 184 vs. treatment group is given in Figure 5.64. This plot revealed some evidence of an effect of treatment; however, given the between-animal variability of the response the effect was not deemed to be biologically significant.

A one-way ANOVA analysis revealed the difference between the four groups was not statistically significant ($F_{(3,20)}$ = 1.71, p = 0.198). However, we have not made use of all the information collected during the experiment. The researchers also recorded baseline body weights and the monkeys' ages. As juvenile animals usually all grow at approximately the same rate, baseline body weight is an obvious candidate for inclusion as a covariate in the statistical analysis. Animals that were lighter pre-treatment remain so posttreatment. Therefore some of the spread of body weights (within each group) can be accounted for by the baseline levels. Alternatively perhaps

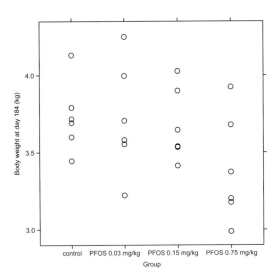

Figure 5.64. Scatterplot of monkey body weight at day 184 from Example 5.17.

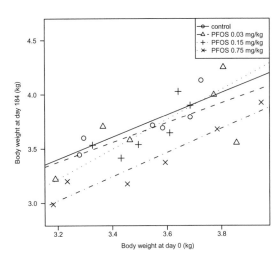

Figure 5.66. Categorised scatterplot of monkey body weight (following 184 days of treatment with PFOS or the control) vs. body weight at day 0 from Example 5.17.

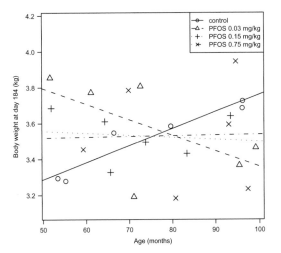

Figure 5.65. Categorised scatterplot of monkey body weight (following 184 days of treatment with PFOS or the control) vs. monkey age from Example 5.17.

the age of the monkeys could be used as a covariate. However, given the narrow age range of animals employed in the study, age is perhaps less likely to be related to the body weight at day 184.

Categorised scatterplots of the body weight at day 184 vs. the two candidate covariates are given in Figures 5.65 and 5.66.

There appears to be a strong positive relationship between body weight at day 184 and the baseline body weight. The relationship between body weight at day 184 and the age of the animal at the start of the study is less strong. This implies that the baseline body

weight will be a more influential covariate and hence will account for more of the between-animal variability.

Returning to the original scatterplot of the data, consider the observations marked a and b in the control group (Figure 5.67). Without any further information all we can say is that the difference between animal a and b's body weight at day 184 is due to the between-animal variation. However, let us consider using the baseline body weight information. It turns out that animal a was heavy at the start of the study (compared to the other animals in the control group) whereas animal b was lighter than the other animals (see Table 5.23). In other words we can explain the difference between these two animals' body weights at day 184: it is not just due to the posttreatment between-animal variability. We know why animal a had a much higher body weight at day 184 than animal b: it was because animal a was a larger animal before the study started.

Including baseline body weight in the analysis as a covariate will reduce posttreatment between-animal variability because most of the variability was present at the baseline (it was not due to the experimental procedure) and hence can be accounted for by fitting baseline body weight as a covariate in the analysis. Once the covariate is included in the statistical model, the overall test of the treatment effect is significant ($F_{(3,19)} = 4.80$, $p < 0.001$).

5.4.6.4 Predictions from ANCOVA

When conducting an ANCOVA analysis, it should be noted that the predictions from the analysis are not group means (as they would be for t-tests, ANOVA or mixed-model analyses). The predictions from the statistical model are now lines, defined as the predicted

Table 5.23. Table of body weights for animals a and b at days 0 and 184 from Example 5.17

Animal	Body weight at day 0 (kg)	Body weight at day 184 (kg)
a	3.72	4.13
b	3.27	3.45
control group mean	3.53	3.73

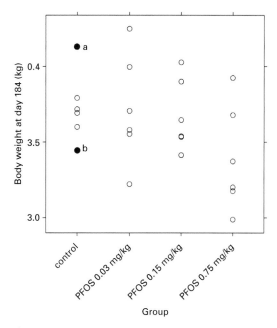

Figure 5.67. Scatterplot of the monkey body weight (following 184 days of treatment with PFOS or the control) from Example 5.17, with two animals in the control group highlighted.

lines, which model the linear relationship between the response and the covariate. There is one predicted line per group and, as commented above, the predicted lines are usually parallel.

Example 5.17 (continued): Effect of PFOS on cynomolgus monkey body weight

To begin with, consider the analysis of body weight at day 184 without including the covariate (using a one-way ANOVA analysis). It is straightforward to identify the predictions from the statistical analysis; they are simply the group means. Concentrating on the control group, the day 184 control group mean was 3.73 and this is the predicted value for all control group animals. The residual (the part of the response unaccounted for after fitting the statistical model) for animal *a* is therefore given by:

$$\text{observation}_a - \text{predicted}_a = \text{residual}_a \qquad (5.34)$$
$$4.13 - 3.73 = 0.40 \text{ (kg)}$$

and for animal *b* is:

$$3.45 - 3.73 = -0.28 \text{ (kg)}.$$

When we fit a covariate in the analysis it is not the group means that are the predictions from the statistical analysis but the predicted lines. In Example 5.17, with predose body weight fitted as a covariate in the statistical analysis, it can be shown that the predicted line for the control group is given by:

Prediction = 0.020 + 1.054 × body weight at day 0.

For each observation in the dataset the residual will be the distance (vertically) between the observation and the predicted line. For animal *a* this can be calculated using the above equation and the entries in Table 5.23:

$$\text{observation}_a - \text{predicted}_a = \text{residual}_a \qquad (5.35)$$
$$4.13 - [0.020 + 1.054 \times 3.72] = 0.19 \text{ (kg)}$$

and for animal *b* it is

$$3.45 - [0.020 + 1.054 \times 3.27] = -0.02 \text{ (kg)}.$$

These calculations are illustrated in Figure 5.68.

It can be seen that the arrows on Figure 5.68 (which highlight the residuals for animals *a* and *b*) are much smaller when baseline

body weight is included in the statistical analysis as a covariate. This improves the sensitivity of the analysis and as a result will allow the researcher to reduce the sample size in future. The property will usually hold as long as there is a strong relationship between the response and the covariate.

5.4.6.5 Predicted group means

As stated above when a covariate is included in the analysis, predictions from the analysis are predicted lines rather than predicted group means. Of course in practice most scientists do not want to report predicted lines and then make comparisons between the predicted lines. It is therefore standard practice to report the value of the predicted lines *at the overall average of the covariate*. It is these means that are presented by statistical packages as the predicted means from the ANCOVA analysis. When we make comparisons between the experimental groups in an ANCOVA analysis, it is these means (i.e. the value of the predicted lines at the average covariate) that are compared.

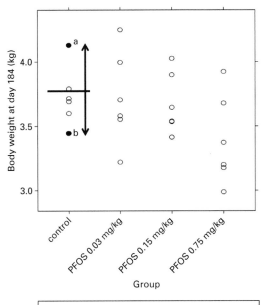

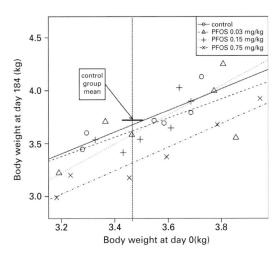

Figure 5.69. Categorised scatterplot of day 184 vs. day 0 body weight, from Example 5.17 (following 184 days of treatment with PFOS or control), with average day 0 body weight highlighted by a vertical line.

be 3.54 kg. The predicted means from the ANCOVA analysis can now be identified as the values of the predicted lines at the average body weight (see Figure 5.69). So for the control group the predicted mean is 3.75 kg and for the high dose is 3.40 kg. If we then perform a pairwise comparison to see if these two experimental groups are different, we are effectively comparing the means at the average of the covariate.

5.4.6.6 Assumptions for ANCOVA

While there are undoubted benefits from including a suitable covariate in the statistical analysis, the researcher must be careful. There are three assumptions, as well as the usual parametric assumptions, that we make when fitting a covariate. These assumptions are partly due to features of the ANCOVA approach described above. If they do not hold then the conclusions drawn from the analysis of covariance may be invalid or at least compromised.

Is it worth fitting the covariate?
When the researcher identifies a possible covariate, a decision must be made whether to include the covariate in the statistical analysis. While not strictly an ANCOVA assumption, when fitting a covariate the researcher is tacitly assuming there is an underlying relationship

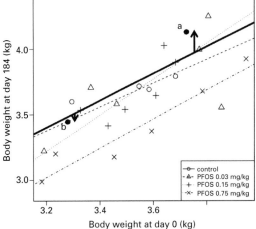

Figure 5.68. Scatterplot of monkey body weight, from Example 5.17 (following 184 days of treatment with PFOS or the control) and categorised scatterplot of day 184 vs. day 0 body weight, with two animals in the control group highlighted on both plots. On the lower figure, the dotted lines correspond to the best-fit lines and the solid line corresponds to the predicted line for the control group.

Example 5.17 (continued): Effect of PFOS on cynomolgus monkey body weight

Returning to Example 5.17, first we calculate the average baseline body weight of all the animals in the study. This value turns out to

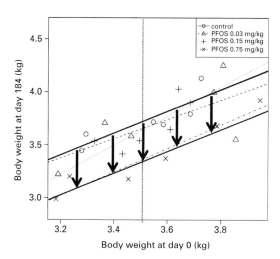

Figure 5.70. Categorised scatterplot of day 184 vs. day 0 bodyweight, from Example 5.17 (following 184 days of treatment with PFOS or control), with comparison between the PFOS 0.75 mg/kg treated group and the control group highlighted.

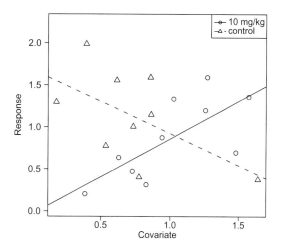

Figure 5.71. Categorised scatterplot of a response vs. covariate from Example 5.18, where there is a significant interaction between the covariate and the Treatment factor (the best-fit lines are not parallel).

(or correlation) between the response and the covariate. As mentioned above, the relationship between the response and the covariate should be approximately linear and the slope of the predicted lines should not be close to zero.

Experimental group by covariate interaction
When performing the analysis of covariance, one of the assumptions made is that the underlying linear relationship between the response and the covariate is the same for each group, i.e. there is not group by covariate interaction and hence the best-fit lines are approximately parallel.

As discussed above, the predicted means, and any comparisons between the predicted means, are calculated at the average value of the covariate. In theory if the relationships between the response and the covariate are approximately the same for all experimental groups, i.e. the best-fit lines on the categorised scatterplot are all roughly parallel, then the level of the covariate at which we make these comparisons is irrelevant in the sense that the differences between the experimental groups are maintained at all values of the covariate (Figure 5.70). So in the analysis we force the predicted

lines to be parallel. This is only sensible if the best-fit lines are also roughly parallel.

Example 5.17 (continued): Effect of PFOS on cynomolgus monkey body weight

In Figure 5.70 the predicted lines for the control and 0.75 mg/kg PFOS group are included. As the best-fit lines are approximately parallel it can be seen that the parallel predicted lines are similar to the best-fit lines and hence the size of the difference between the two groups is independent of the level of the covariate at which the comparison is made.

In the statistical analysis we assume there is no interaction between the experimental groups and the covariate, and hence the predicted lines are parallel. This is not the case for the best-fit lines on the categorised scatterplot, which are allowed to vary depending on the within-group relationships. The categorised scatterplot therefore provides a useful way to assess the assumption that there is no interaction between the experimental groups and the covariate. If the best-fit lines on the plot are not parallel (which occurs when there is an interaction between the experimental factor(s) and the covariate) then the assumption that the predicted lines are parallel may not be valid.

Example 5.18: Significant interaction between the treatment factor and covariate

In this example, see Figure 5.71, there is an interaction between the covariate and the Treatment factor. Clearly the lines are not parallel and the relationship between the response and covariate varies

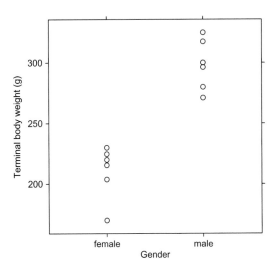

Figure 5.72. Scatterplot of terminal animal body weights from Example 5.19, categorised by the gender of the animals.

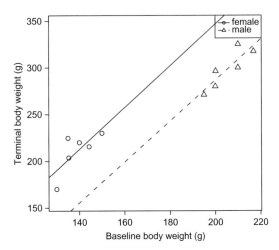

Figure 5.73. Scatterplot of terminal vs. baseline animal body weights from Example 5.19, categorised by the gender of the animals and including the predicted lines from ANCOVA.

depending on the treatment. This in itself may be an interesting finding. The treatment is having an effect on the response/covariate relationship and the size of the treatment effect appears to vary depending on the level of the covariate.

If we include the covariate in the analysis, then we force the two predicted lines to be parallel (and hence they will be almost horizontal). The predicted means will be similar (the average covariate is 0.88 kg). Hence we would conclude that there is no significant difference between the two treatments ($F_{(1,16)}$ = 1.14, p = 0.301). Clearly this is slightly misleading in this case.

Covariate is not influenced by the experimental factors

The third assumption, as mentioned above, we make when fitting a covariate is that it is not influenced by the experimental factor(s). If this assumption does not hold then the predicted means (and the difference between the predicted means) will be influenced by the covariate. Remember the predicted means are calculated at the average value of the covariate. If there are no experimental effects on the covariate, then this is a reasonable approach to take. However, as we shall see in Example 5.19, if there is an experimental effect on the covariate, then the predictions from the analysis may not reflect the observed data.

Remember, we fit the covariate purely as a tool to reduce the variability. Including it in the statistical analysis should not influence the estimates of the

experimental group means. As long as there are no significant experimental effects on the covariate then this will be the case. In general the assumption of no experimental effect on the covariate will usually hold, or can be assumed to hold, if the covariate is measured before and experimental manipulation occurs.

Example 5.19: Gender effect on the baseline body weight covariate

Consider an experiment involving both male and female Wistar rats. Figure 5.72 is a scatterplot of the terminal body weight data recorded when the rats were 12 weeks old. This revealed (as expected) that the males were significantly heavier than the females. The males weighed on average 298 g whereas the females weighed 211 g.

Assume body weight was also recorded at the beginning of the experiment (when the rats were 8 weeks old) revealing that the males were heavier than the females at the start of the study. Consider the categorised scatterplot of the terminal vs. baseline body weights, see Figure 5.73, which includes the parallel predicted lines from the ANCOVA.

While the males were significantly bigger than the females at the end of the study, they were also larger at the start. As discussed above, in the analysis of covariance the predicted means are made at the average level of the covariate, averaged over males and females. This overall average body weight at the start of the study was 172 g. If we now look at the categorised scatterplot we see an interesting finding. The females' predicted terminal body weight is higher than the males'! Males have a predicted mean of 225 g and females have a predicted mean of 284 g (see Figure 5.74).

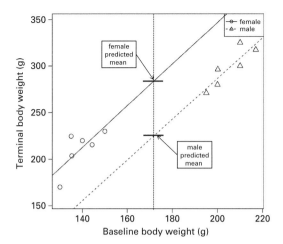

Figure 5.74. Scatterplot of terminal vs. baseline animal body weights from Example 5.19, categorised by the gender of the animals, with the predicted means from ANCOVA illustrated.

Clearly the conclusion from the analysis of covariance is misleading, but the problem is not the analysis of covariance itself. Unfortunately the assumption of no experimental effects on the covariate (sex effects in this case) does not hold. Effectively the analysis is predicting what the terminal body weight of a male or female Wistar rat would be given that the animals had an initial body weight equal to the overall average baseline body weight, even though it is unlikely that such an animal of either sex exists.

It is also apparent from Figure 5.74 that we have predicted means that are outside the ranges of the original data. This will increase the variability of these predicted means. The further away from the data that we make a prediction, the less certain we are of the accuracy of that prediction.

5.4.6.7 Strategy for when the independence assumption does not hold

In the previous section we described the assumptions that are made when performing an ANCOVA analysis, in particular that the covariate is independent or not influenced by the experimental factors. When this assumption does not hold then the covariate, which in theory should only be a device to reduce the variability, will influence the predictions from the statistical model.

While the assumption of independence will usually hold if the covariate is measured pretreatment, there are examples where this is not the case. For example, consider the case where baseline activity is used as a

covariate in the statistical analysis of a locomotor activity response. If the experiment consists of wildtype and knockout mice, where the gene knockout is known to influence activity, then there may be a difference at baseline between the strains. Although this difference is expected, it does imply the independence assumption underpinning the ANCOVA does not hold.

We can avoid breaking this assumption by first performing an adjustment to the covariate that removes any treatment-related effects on the covariate (Milliken and Johnson, 2002, pp. 543–52). Effectively we remove any experimental group related effects from the covariate before performing the ANCOVA analysis.

Example 5.19 (continued): Gender effect on the baseline body weight covariate

Returning to Example 5.19, it was observed that the covariate was not independent of the experimental groups. In particular there was, as expected, a gender effect on the baseline body weight. It was shown above that this affected the reliability of the results of the statistical analysis.

This problem could have been avoided by first subtracting the covariate group means from the individual covariate responses. We first subtract the average male baseline body weight from all the individual male baseline body weights. We repeat the process for the females. These new adjusted baseline body weights, which are centred on zero for both sexes, are plotted in Figure 5.75.

The predicted means from ANCOVA using this adjusted baseline body weight covariate are now much more sensible (298 g for males and 211 g for females). The standard errors of the predicted mean for the males in these three analyses are:
- 8.7, in the ANOVA analysis ignoring baseline information;
- 18.9, in the analysis using the baseline body weight as a covariate;
- 5.5, in the analysis using the adjusted baseline body weight as a covariate.

This reduction in variability, between the two ANCOVA analyses, is because in the latter analysis the predicted mean was calculated at zero, the midpoint within the range of the (adjusted) baseline body weight data, whereas in the unadjusted baseline body weight ANCOVA analysis the predicted mean was calculated at a point outside the range of the male baseline body weight data. This could help reduce the sample sizes in future studies.

Some authors recommend always doing this adjustment to a covariate before fitting it in the statistical model as it removes all the (however subtle) experimental related effects from the covariate. This also implies that the covariate will not influence the difference between predicted means and the predicted means themselves will be within the spread of the data

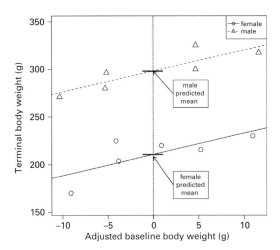

Figure 5.75. Scatterplot of terminal animal body weight vs. adjusted baseline body weight from Example 5.19, categorised by the gender of the animals, with the least square (predicted) means from ANCOVA illustrated.

and hence be estimated more efficiently. This strategy is certainly recommended in Example 5.19, as there does appear to be a big reduction in the between-animal variability that can be achieved by fitting baseline body weight as a covariate.

We end this discussion of the analysis of covariance with two special cases that could involve the use of covariates.

5.4.6.8 ANCOVA and stratified randomisation

As discussed above in Section 4.2.1, a stratified randomisation will *increase* the between-animal variability of the data. Assume animals are assigned to treatment groups using the baseline responses to stratify the randomisation. Let us also assume that as researcher is using baseline information to stratify the randomisation there is a strong relationship between the pre- and posttreatment responses. Now, as described in Section 4.2.1, this randomisation will effectively force the spread of baselines (within each group) to be as large as possible. If there is a strong relationship between pre- and posttreatment responses, then forcing the range at baseline to be artificially high will have a similar effect on the posttreatment responses. In other words, it will increase the variability of the posttreatment responses,

compared to the variability resulting from a completely random allocation.

If animals were randomised to the experimental groups using a baseline stratified randomisation (which we would recommend) then the researcher should also include the baseline in the analysis as a covariate (or alternatively as a blocking factor) to remove the additional variability introduced when using the stratification process.

5.4.6.9 Change from baseline responses

When baseline measures of a response are recorded, it seems to be common practice in the analysis of animal experiments to first calculate a change from baseline response. This can either be the percentage change from baseline or the actual change from baseline. The analysis of the change from baseline then proceeds using the techniques described in Sections 5.4.3 and 5.4.4.

This analysis technique is popular because there are several perceived benefits:

- It is assumed that by calculating the change from baseline we will, in some sense, reduce the animal-to-animal variability by normalising the response.
- If there is an overall difference between the groups at baseline then that difference may bias the experimental group comparisons. By calculating the change from baseline response, then this bias will be reduced or eliminated.

Unfortunately this approach is only valid in certain special cases. In many cases the adjustment can be misleading and can actually increase the between-animal variability of the analysed response. An alternative approach, which as we shall see is more widely applicable and avoids these problems, is to analyse the original response and include the baseline measure in the analysis as a covariate.

Between-animal variability

As mentioned above, it is often assumed that normalising the response using baseline measures will reduce the between-animal variability. However, this is not always the case. The baseline measure will also have an associated variability just as the response does. If you calculate the ratio:

$$\text{Ratio} = \text{Response} / \text{Baseline} \times 100\% \qquad (5.36)$$

or the actual difference between them:

Actual difference = Response – Baseline   (5.37)

then the variability of the change from baseline response will involve both the variability of the response and the variability of the baseline measure.

This increase in the variability of the change from baseline response, caused by including the baseline variability, must be balanced against the reduction in the between-animal variability achieved by the normalisation process itself. However, if the response variability is small, compared to the baseline variability, then the derived change from baseline response may be more variable than the original response. In the authors' experience it tends to be the case that statistical significance is less pronounced when analysing a change from baseline response, compared to a suitable analysis of the original response.

Instead of analysing the change from baseline response, the baseline information should be used as a covariate in the analysis. Using this approach we can reduce the between-animal variability, as described above, without introducing the baseline variability into the analysis. In other words, the variability in the analysis of covariance is still just the variability of the response. The covariate does not directly increase the variability of the response analysed.

Example 5.3 (continued): MRI quantification of the thymus

In Example 5.3 we discussed an experiment to assess the ability of magnetic resonance imaging (MRI) to measure the volume of the thymus accurately in mice compared to a more established histological technique (Brooks *et al.*, 2005). In the study mice received either the vehicle or one of three doses of dexamethasone, a compound known to reduce the size of the thymus. Mice were imaged one week prior to dosing and two days after dosing. The categorised case profiles plot (Figure 5.76) gives an indication of the responses observed.

Both the posttreatment thymus volume and the percentage change in thymus volume were analysed. Interestingly the effect of the treatment on the percentage change response was less significant than it was when analysing the posttreatment volume. The reason for this can be seen by considering Figure 5.76. While the posttreatment measures were tight, in particular in the animals that received dexamethasone, the baseline measures were much more variable. Dexamethasone has a strong effect on the thymus, but there is a physical limit to the reduction in size that can be achieved. So while the spread of the baselines represents the natural between-animal variability, the spread of the post-dose responses highlights the physical limitation of the model, i.e. all thymus volumes in the dexamethasone-treated groups were reduced to approximately the same size.

When we analysed the percentage change from baseline response all the variability of the baseline measurements was introduced into the variability of the percentage change response. This was not the case when the posttreatment responses were analysed without any baseline adjustment.

In our opinion the reader should heed this warning. Never carry out a change from baseline analysis without first plotting the data to see if it is appropriate. In this example if we had not plotted the data first then we may have analysed the more variable percentage change response, thus missing a potentially significant posttreatment effect.

Biasing the results when there is no real relationship

There is a second pitfall if the researcher fails to plot the data when analysing a change from baseline response. Consider the situation where there is no underlying relationship between the baseline and the response. Perhaps the baseline measurements were taken too far in advance of the treatment phase, or maybe the variability in the assay is such that the relationship is not apparent.

Now, assuming that there is no relationship, if we had carried out an analysis of the change from the baseline response, we would artificially reduce the size of the response for those animals that happened to have a large baseline relative to the others. Conversely we would artificially increase (relatively) the response for those animals with small baselines. This can lead to misleading results and conclusions.

When fitting a covariate the researcher should first consider a categorised scatterplot of the response vs. the covariate. This will immediately reveal if there is a relationship between them. More importantly, the adjustment made by the covariate depends on the strength of the response vs. covariate relationship. So in situations where the relationship between baseline and the response is weak, then the adjustment made by fitting the covariate will be negligible.

Varying the relationship between post-manipulation and baseline responses

Let us assume that we want to remove any baseline differences that may bias the treatment comparisons using a change from baseline response. For the change from baseline to be free of baseline effects, then the

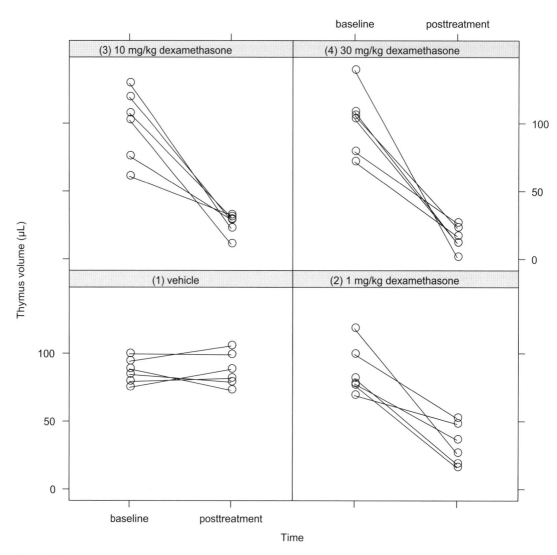

Figure 5.76. Categorised case profiles plot of the MRI measured thymus volume in mice, categorised by four treatment groups for Example 5.3.

relationship between the baselines and the treatment responses must satisfy certain properties. If these properties are not satisfied, then unfortunately we may not completely remove the bias caused by baseline differences.

Example 5.17 (continued): Effect of PFOS on cynomolgus monkey body weight

Consider Example 5.17 described above, where there was a significant positive relationship between day 184 and baseline body weight responses. A plot illustrating the overall relationship between the two body weight responses is given in Figure 5.77.

Due to this underlying relationship between baseline and day 184 body weights, it appears that normalising the body weight using either the actual change from baseline or the percentage change from baseline will reduce the between-animal variability and remove the influence of (however subtle) baseline differences from the analysis.

Let us assume there is a linear relationship between the posttreatment and the baseline responses, i.e.

$$\text{Response} = a \times \text{Baseline} + b, \tag{5.38}$$

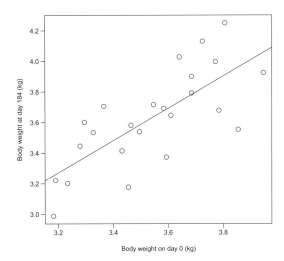

Figure 5.77. Scatterplot of the overall relationship between monkey body weight (following 184 days of treatment with PFOS or the control) and baseline body weight from Example 5.17.

for some constants a and b. This is the standard equation for a line:

$$y = ax + b. \tag{5.39}$$

Now the percentage change from the baseline can be written as:

$$(\text{Response} / \text{Baseline}) = ([a \times \text{Baseline} + b] / \text{Baseline})$$
$$= (a + b / \text{Baseline}). \tag{5.40}$$

So the percentage change from baseline is only free of baseline effects if $b = 0$, i.e. the predicted line passes through the origin.

For the actual change from baseline we have:

$$\text{Response} - \text{Baseline} = [a \times \text{Baseline} + b] - \text{Baseline}$$
$$= (a - 1) \times \text{Baseline} + b. \tag{5.41}$$

The actual change from baseline response is only free of the influence of the baseline if $a = 1$, i.e. there is a one-to-one relationship between the post-dose responses and baseline responses.

Unless these conditions hold, then the actual (or percentage) change from baseline will still be influenced by differences at the baseline. Fitting the baseline as a covariate overcomes this limitation. The covariate simply estimates the actual relationship between the baseline and posttreatment responses and makes an adjustment based on the strength of the relationship. It does not require $b = 0$ or $a = 1$.

Example 5.20: Dog telemetry studies

In dog telemetry studies, see Aylott *et al.* (2011), dogs are fitted with a telemetric device in a surgical procedure. Following a suitable period of time to allow the dogs to recover, test compounds can be assessed. Heart rate, blood pressure and parameters derived

from an electrocardiogram (ECG) trace are measured at baseline and then continuously for up to 48 hours post-dose of the compound. During this period the animal may be active, resting or sleeping. Hence the relationship between baseline and post-dose responses will vary over time due to the animals' level of activity. An analysis of the actual change from baseline, which requires a one-to-one relationship at all time points if it is to be free of baseline effects, will clearly be misleading at certain time points, for example when the dogs are asleep.

In practice we believe the safest option is to always use the covariate approach rather than a change from baseline approach:

- It is more general, coping with any relationship between the response and baseline regardless of the strength of the relationship.
- It does not adversely increase the variability of the response being analysed.
- It does not require the relationship to be one-to-one, or alternatively that the predicted relationship must go through the origin.

5.4.7 Regression analysis

In the previous section a continuous numerical variable was included in the statistical analysis as a device to reduce the underlying variability. These numerical variables, defined as covariates, were not influenced by the experimental factors. As long as this condition held, then their inclusion in the statistical analysis did not influence the predicted means from the analysis.

In Example 5.19 the covariate was influenced by the experimental groups and therefore the predicted means from the analysis were also affected. This led to erroneous conclusions. Sometimes, however, we require this adjustment, for example in the analysis of organ weight data in safety assessment studies (Shirley, 1977).

When we know the numerical variable is not independent of the treatment, but we want to adjust for the effect it has on the response, then we say that the numerical variable is a linear predictor rather than a covariate. The purpose of including it in the statistical analysis is not only to reduce the variability but also to provide an adjustment to the predicted means. This analysis approach is commonly known as regression analysis, rather than analysis of covariance, although the mathematical derivation is the same.

Example 5.21: Organ weight assessment in toxicology studies

When assessing the effect of a test compound on, say liver weight, we would want to first remove any apparent treatment effect on liver weight that was actually caused by an effect on the overall body weight of the animal (Shirley, 1977). For example, if the test compound has a side effect that makes the test animals lose their appetite, then they may consume smaller quantities of food compared to the control animals. This will reduce their overall body weight (and hence also the liver weight) of the animals treated with the compound compared to the control animals. So the reduction in liver weight may be simply due to a reduction in body weight and not related to any specific toxicological effect on the liver. When we look at the effect of the test compound on the liver we would want to first remove any effect caused by overall changes in body weight. This can be achieved by fitting terminal body weight as a linear predictor. The predicted means will then be adjusted for any differences in terminal body weight, as described in Example 5.19.

We argue that we are not fitting terminal body weight as a covariate in this analysis. The role of terminal body weight is not merely to reduce the between-animal variability. It is also fitted as a linear predictor and is included in the analysis to adjust the predicted liver weight means for any (treatment-related) terminal body weight differences.

5.4.8 Multiple comparison procedures

While ANOVA and ANCOVA tables contain the overall tests of significance, and the predicted means with confidence intervals provide an illustration of the results of the statistical analysis, the researcher will probably want to compare the individual experimental group means. The approaches that can be employed include *post hoc* tests, planned comparisons and multiple comparison procedures. As this part of the statistical analysis can be of primary importance when analysing data generated in animal experiments, these tests attract more attention in this field than in many other scientific disciplines. Unfortunately for the researcher, this area of statistics is a controversial one. Statisticians are not in general agreement about which approaches are the most appropriate to use.

In this section we shall discuss some of the issues surrounding multiple comparison procedures. When making our recommendations we assume the researcher has carried out a well-designed experiment and has decided in advance which comparisons are of interest.

The analysis will therefore not involve a data-trawling exercise, where many tests are performed and only the significant ones reported.

5.4.8.1 The risk of finding false positives and false negatives

Let us assume an experiment has been conducted involving a treatment group and a control group. If the two group means are compared using a *t*-test, and the test is performed at the significance level α (usually fixed at 5%), then effectively the researcher is accepting a 5% risk that a rejection of the null hypothesis is a false positive (the Type I error rate, see Section 2.3.5). In other words, if the conclusion is that the treatment appears to have had an effect, then there is a 5% chance that this conclusion is incorrect.

Family-wise error rate (FWE)

In most experiments the researcher will make more than one comparison between the experimental groups. This set of tests is defined by many authors as the *family of tests* (for example, Ludbrook, 1998). Unfortunately as the number of comparisons made increases, and hence the size of the family of tests increases, the risk of finding a false positive result also increases. This is known as the *family-wise error rate* (FWE). It is the chance, or probability, of making at least one false positive conclusion within the family of tests.

To control the family-wise error rate (i.e. maintain the significance level at the nominal level α regardless of the number of comparisons made) we can employ a multiple comparison procedure, which should help reduce the risk of finding false positive results. There are many such procedures available, some are stricter (and hence offer more protection against making false positives) than others. The general principle is that for a result to be statistically significant, the result should, in some sense, be more pronounced. This way the researcher is, in theory, less likely to declare results significant that are, in reality, just due to chance.

Alongside the risk of finding a false positive result (the Type I error), we also need to consider the risk of finding a false negative result, the Type II error (see

Section 2.3.5). Now if β denotes the statistical power of the test, then

$$\text{Type II error} = 1 - \beta. \tag{5.42}$$

In Section 2.3.5 it was noted that as the chance of finding a false positive conclusion decreases, so the chance of finding a false negative increases (and the statistical power decreases). Hence some of the multiple comparison procedures may be considered more powerful than others, in that you are more likely to declare a true positive result, but these tests do not provide such strong protection against the false positive risk. The researcher should bear this in mind when considering other scientists' results and the procedures they used to generate them.

False discovery rate (FDR)

From the above description it should be apparent that if you wish to control the risk of getting an individual false positive result (and control the FWE), then as the number of comparisons increases so does the size of effect required to achieve statistical significance. While in many situations the comparisons (which are planned in advance) are relatively small in number, in some animal experiments many comparisons are performed. Examples include neuroimaging, where thousands of voxels are compared (see Bennett *et al.*, 2009) or the analysis of microarray data. If you are making a large number of comparisons then any multiple comparison adjustment can become so large that there is little chance of finding any statistically significant results.

An alternative, and seemingly sensible approach, is to try to control the *proportion* of false positives at a set level (α) rather than to try to make sure there are no individual false positive results. This is known as controlling the *false discovery rate* (FDR). It should be noted that approaches aimed at controlling the FDR are less strict than those that control the FWE. Some false positives are allowed: it is only the proportion that is controlled. They are therefore more powerful as a result. When using such tools the researcher is more likely to achieve statistical significance, although some of the results may be false positives.

It should be noted that *p*-values generated using procedures that control the FDR have a subtly different meaning to those calculated as part of the FWE procedures. As discussed above in Section 2.3.2, the latter represents the probability of observing a result as or more extreme than the one found by running the experiment if the null hypothesis were true (and hence we compare them against α). When performing a procedure that controls the FDR we accept there will be false positive results, hence these *p*-values do not represent the same risk.

In situations where many comparisons are made, procedures that control the FDR may be preferable to those that control the FWE as otherwise true positive results can be missed (Bennett *et al.*, 2009).

Guarding against risks

Many procedures are available; however, the choice of a multiple comparison procedure will depend on the level of risk (of getting a false positive or false negative result) that the scientist is prepared to take. Some procedures guard against the risk more than others and are therefore less powerful. The scientist needs to be aware of the risk level when carrying out an analysis so that false positive results can be identified when conducting future confirmatory experiments. The choice of procedure should be made in advance (based on an acceptable level of risk) and *not* by a *post hoc* data-trawling exercise that involves looking at many different procedures to find the one that gives the desired results!

The choice of multiple comparison procedure will also depend on the context in which the results are to be employed (see Section 2.4), that is whether the analysis is being performed as:

- an exploratory analysis, where the scientist is exploring ideas or generating hypotheses;
- a confirmatory analysis, where the scientist is trying to prove a hypothesis or arrive at a definitive conclusion.

In many cases the analysis will be between these extremes. It may be the case that there are several read-outs that lead to decisions based on the balance of evidence. In an exploratory analysis, unprotected tests (least significant difference tests or planned comparisons, as discussed below) may be employed. These tests should be used alongside estimates of the size of the effects with confidence intervals. In a confirmatory analysis, the scientist may require a fully-fledged multiple comparison procedure to reduce the risk of finding false positives.

In this section we shall also consider statistical tools for dealing with the risk of finding false positives: multiple comparison procedures are only one of a number of techniques available. In practice there are many non-statistical safeguards that help the scientist avoid making false positive conclusions. These include:

- Experiments may be repeated to confirm a significant result.
- The novel compound may be assessed in several different animal models (note this is the biological model as opposed to the statistical model).
- Knowledge about the size of the biologically relevant effect and the background variability of the response may be used when assessing the effectiveness of a novel compound.

These practical safeguards are as important as the multiple comparison procedures described in this section and hence should always be considered alongside any statistical techniques.

5.4.8.2 Choosing the family of tests

The first problem that should already be apparent to the reader is the somewhat arbitrary choice of the family of tests (Miller, 1981, pp. 31–5). As stated above the larger the number of tests being made, the larger the family of tests, hence the risk of finding a false positive result is higher and therefore the greater the adjustment for multiplicity needs to be. So the size of the family of tests influences the impact of the multiple comparison procedure, but what defines the family of tests? It could be:

- An individual comparison. The family of tests is of size one and hence no multiple comparison adjustment is necessary.
- The set of comparisons made on an end point in an experiment. If an experiment consists of four treatments, each compared to the control, then the family of tests is of size four per end point analysed.
- All comparisons made in an experiment. Assume that there are three end points measured in an experiment. If there are four comparisons made at

each end point, then the total number of comparisons made is $4 \times 3 = 12$. This is the size of the family of tests.

- All the comparisons made on a treatment. Assuming a treatment is tested in several different experiments before a decision is made on its efficacy, should we adjust for all the comparisons made during the development of the treatment?
- All the comparisons you have ever generated.

Clearly the last two are not sensible choices, but this does highlight the problem when defining the family of tests, as Miller (1981, p. 35) comments: 'There are no hard-and-fast rules for where the family lines should be drawn.' Ludbrook (1998) suggests that: 'A family of hypotheses is all those actually tested on the results of a single experiment.' This should be a sensible choice in many scenarios.

In practice we suspect most researchers would be more comfortable with using the second of our options above, but this is a somewhat arbitrary decision and could impact on the conclusions drawn from the statistical analysis. Even if the researcher decides to follow this strategy to define the family of tests, there may still be practical pitfalls when employing a multiple comparison procedure in the statistical analysis. We highlight this with two different examples.

Example 2.4 (continued): MRI assessment of a transgenic phenotype

Consider the experiment described in Section 2.4 to compare the volumetric changes observed in the brain regions of wildtype and TasTPM transgenic mice (Maheswaran *et al.*, 2009). The size of several brain regions was measured at four time points using MRI. The differences between the volume of the brain regions in the wildtype and transgenic mice were assessed. We assume that the family of tests defined by the researcher was the total number of comparisons made in the statistical analysis of the experiment.

Now in reality only a couple of brain regions were of direct interest. However, using an MRI technique allowed the researcher to measure the volume of many more brain regions. This led to a paradox. If volume measurements from many brain regions were taken, and an assessment made of the effect of strain in each of these brain regions, then the family of tests (and hence the false positive risk) would be larger than would have been the case if only a few brain regions had been assessed in the same experiment. Hence the influence of the multiple comparison procedure needs to be greater to control the increased false positive risk when more brain regions are assessed. In other words the researcher will be penalised for assessing more of the (available) information.

It is conceivable that the strain effects in the regions of interest will be statistically significant if we make a multiple comparison adjustment for the family of tests only involving comparisons in the brain regions of interest. However, if we make comparisons across all available brain regions, and then perform a multiple comparison procedure adjustment for this much larger family of tests, then we may find that none of the results are statistically significant.

So should we only make the comparisons of interest, even though we have the ability to collect and assess additional information? Clearly it seems absurd to avoid assessing possibly useful information from the experimental animals (which is readily available) simply because it may compromise the statistical analysis. One solution to this dilemma is to make one adjustment for the comparisons that are of interest, i.e. the comparisons deemed important before running the study. This would be a confirmatory analysis (see Section 2.4). A second less stringent multiple comparison procedure can then be applied to the wider exploratory analysis where false positives are perhaps more likely to occur because the hypotheses being tested were not planned in advance and the analysis is effectively a data-trawling exercise. If there are significant results in the exploratory analysis, then the scientist should perhaps try to verify these results in future independent experiments as they could be false positives.

Example 5.10 (continued): Anti-diabetic effects of epigallocatechin gallate

In Example 2.4 the researcher has to decide whether the family of tests involves multiple end points (where each brain region is classed as an end point). However, it may be the case that there are choices to be made within a single end point.

Consider the experiment described above to assess the effect of epigallocatechin gallate (EGCG), a catechin found in green tea, on type 2 diabetes in rodents (Wolfram *et al.*, 2006). The experiment consisted of five groups, including 2.5, 5.0 or 10.0 g/kg of EGCG in the diet (*n* = 9), a placebo control (*n* = 9) and a positive control of thiazolidinedione rosiglitazone at 72 mg/kg of diet (*n* = 5). The positive control was included to show the experimental procedure worked. As a comparison it could be argued that it has a different status in the analysis to the treatment comparisons back to the control. Fewer animals may have been allocated to the positive control as it was not of direct interest. In particular though, should we include this comparison in the family of tests? When applying a multiple comparison procedure adjustment (to the treatment comparisons as they are of primary interest) should we also adjust for an additional comparison involving the positive control, hence reducing the power of the treatment comparisons? We would suggest that as this comparison has a different purpose to the treatment comparisons there is no need to include it in the family of tests.

5.4.8.3 Unadjusted tests

Before we consider a selection of the many multiple comparison procedures available to the researcher we shall describe the tests that do not make any adjustment for

multiplicity; these include multiple *t*-tests, least significant difference (LSD) tests and planned comparisons. Of the three tests discussed in this section the LSD tests and planned comparisons will in many cases give the same individual *p*-values; however, the process involved in generating them is philosophically different.

Multiple t-tests

The simplest method that could be used to perform pairwise comparisons between experimental groups is to carry out many individual *t*-tests. By this we imply the researcher separates the data from the two groups to be compared. The data from these two groups is then analysed using a *t*-test. While this approach is commonly applied in practice there are a number of reasons why it is not recommended; see Elashoff (1981) for example. This approach can increase the false positive risk.

When using the multiple *t*-tests approach the estimate of the between-animal variability, which the difference between the group means is assessed against, may be unreliable. Remember the *t*-test uses a signal-to-noise ratio. To produce a reliable test result we need an accurate estimate of both the group means and the underlying variability of those means. If we want a more reliable estimate of the group means, then most researchers appreciate that this can be achieved by increasing the sample size. The same is true of the variance estimate. In the multiple *t*-test approach the between-animal variance estimate is calculated using the animals from only two of the experimental groups. Why use only two groups of animals to estimate the between-animal variability when more groups, and hence more animals, are available? By isolating two groups from the full dataset, and calculating the variability based on those two groups only, we get a less reliable estimate of the variability. The variance estimate obtained could be artificially small (and lead to an increase risk of finding a false positive) or artificially high (and lead to an increased risk of finding a false negative).

As the variability estimate is different for each *t*-test, then the results of the multiple *t*-tests will not be directly comparable. It is possible that the largest observed difference between two group means is not as statistically significant as the smallest difference. This is clearly an odd result that would be hard to justify in practice (and may indicate the homogeneity of variance assumption does not hold). If we can make the assumption that the variability is the same across all experimental groups, perhaps using a transformation of the data, then we should use this single estimate of variability for all comparisons between the group means. This single estimate is calculated using more information and hence will be more reliable. This can be observed by considering the degrees of freedom. The residual degrees of freedom, for example generated in the ANOVA table (see Section 5.4.3.1), are usually greater than the residual degrees of freedom for the individual *t*-tests.

Example 5.22: A drug comparison trial

Consider the following example consisting of two treatment groups and a control group. There were four animals per treatment group and it was planned in advance to compare each treatment group back to the control. A plot of the observed means with SEMs is given in Figure 5.78.

Let us assume that the two treatments were compared back to the control using two separate *t*-tests. It turns out that treatment A was significantly different from the control (*p* = 0.047) whereas treatment B was not (*p* = 0.060), even though the difference between treatment B and the control was greater than the corresponding difference between treatment A and control.

There are several reasons why the conclusions of this analysis are unsound. It appears, perhaps just by chance, that the treatment A responses are less variable than either the control or treatment B responses. So when we computed the individual *t*-tests, the variability estimate used in the treatment A vs. control comparison was smaller than the variance estimate used in the treatment B vs. control comparison. Given that there were only four animals per group, a more reliable estimate of the underlying variability of the response could have been obtained by considering all animals, for example using a one-way ANOVA approach to provide a single more reliable estimate of the between-animal variability.

Of course it may be the case that the responses from one of the treatment groups are genuinely less variable than the others. This can happen, for example, when the responses from the control group are less variable than those in the treated groups. Perhaps different animals respond differently to the treatment, whereas they react to the control in the same way. In such cases an ANOVA-based analysis may not be appropriate (the single variance estimate is not reliable) and in such cases the responses should be transformed to homogenise the variances across groups. If it is not possible to find a suitable transformation then the researcher should consider using the non-parametric tests rather than resort to individual *t*-tests (see Section 5.5.1.2).

The remaining approaches described in this section use all of the data to estimate the variability of the response.

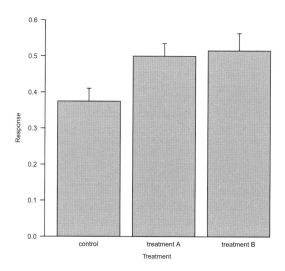

Figure 5.78. Plot of the observed treatment means with standard errors, for Example 5.22.

This implies that the statistical tests are using a more reliable and reproducible estimate of the variability and hence the test results are more reliable than those generated using the multiple *t*-tests approach.

Least significant difference test

The least significant difference (LSD) test is similar to performing multiple *t*-tests. All possible pairwise comparisons between the group means are made in (we would argue) a data-trawling exercise. The crucial difference between this approach and using multiple *t*-tests is that the LSD test uses the same variability estimate for all individual tests. It is (in some sense) the variability estimate averaged over all groups and can be found, for example, in the ANOVA table (the MS_{Residual} term). For each pair of means, calculate:

$$t = \frac{(\bar{y}_i - \bar{y}_j)}{\sqrt{\dfrac{s^2}{(1/n_i + 1/n_j)}}} \quad \text{for } 1 \le i \ne j \le x, \tag{5.43}$$

where $\bar{y}_i$ is the *i*th group mean with sample size n_i, $\bar{y}_j$ is the *j*th group mean with sample size n_j, s^2 is the estimated variance (the MS_{Residual}) term and x is the number of experimental groups. The value t is compared to a *t*-distribution with the residual term's degrees of freedom, as for a *t*-test.

In theory the results from the LSD test will be more reliable than doing multiple *t*-tests as they use the same overall estimate of variability. However, it should be stressed that if you do need to compare everything to everything in a data-trawling exercise, then there is still a risk of finding false positive results. The LSD test offers no direct protection against this risk.

Example 5.22 (continued): A drug comparison trial

Returning to Example 5.22, let us assume that the LSD test had been used to compare the treatment groups. Using this analysis approach, treatment B was (statistically) significantly different from the control ($p = 0.037$) whereas treatment A was not ($p = 0.057$). This, we argue, is a more reliable result. Both these LSD tests used the same estimate of variability, but because the effect observed for treatment B was larger than that observed for treatment A, it is sensible that the treatment B vs. control p-value was smaller. A plot of the predicted means with 95% confidence intervals, which also uses the single estimate of the variability, is given in Figure 5.79. The final comparison, treatment A vs. treatment B, was not significant ($p = 0.799$).

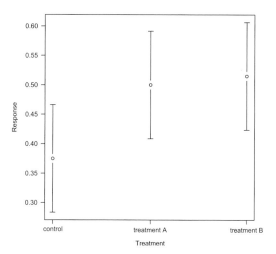

Figure 5.79. Plot of the predicted treatment means with 95% confidence intervals, for Example 5.22.

Planned comparisons

When a researcher reports that an LSD test was performed, we believe this should imply all pairwise comparisons have been made in a data-trawling exercise. In animal experiments we believe this procedure is rarely applied. Usually the hypotheses of interest have been decided in advance and the experimental groups chosen accordingly. In Example 5.22 it is likely that the comparisons of interest are treatment A vs. control and treatment B vs. control. The third comparison (treatment A vs. treatment B) is of less interest. We feel this analysis strategy is much more closely aligned to general practice in animal research. The decision about which comparisons to make is usually taken well in advance of performing the analysis and the experimental design will reflect this.

If the researcher only considers those comparisons that were planned in advance, then these tests are known as planned comparisons (Snedecor and Cochran, 1989, pp. 226–8). Planned comparisons are a strategy for only carrying out the comparisons that are of interest. The tests are not data driven. They are a much more controlled way of conducting a statistical analysis and as a result, we argue, will guard against making false positives conclusions. As stated by Armitage *et al.* (2002, p. 227): 'When comparisons are made which

flow naturally from the plan of the experiment or survey, the usual *t* test [unadjusted test] is appropriate.' If the researcher states that planned comparisons (as opposed to LSD tests) have been used then this implies the analysis was not a data-trawling exercise but a controlled process. We believe that many analyses defined as being LSD tests in the literature are actually planned comparisons because only the comparisons of interest are ever considered.

Implementation of LSD tests and planned comparisons

We stated above that the *p*-values generated from LSD tests and planned comparisons are the same in most cases: it is the underlying philosophy behind the tests that is different. However, in some statistical packages the two tests are calculated using different approaches and this can result in different *p*-values being generated.

In some statistical packages if the LSD test (or any other *post hoc* test) is selected, then the means that are compared are the observed means and not the least square (predicted) means from the analysis. In other words any blocking factors and/or covariates will be ignored when calculating the means. Curiously the variance estimate used in the LSD test is usually the residual mean square entry in the ANOVA or ANCOVA table and hence the variance estimate is adjusted for these effects.

The planned comparisons are always performed on the least square (predicted) means and take into account any covariate and/or blocking factor. If you are in any doubt about this, then it is always safest to use the planned comparisons option in the statistical software package, rather than risk using the LSD test.

Within InVivoStat's Single Measure Parametric Analysis module, planned comparisons can be produced by selecting the unadjusted (LSD) test. This will generate all possible pairwise comparisons on the least square (predicted) means rather than on the observed means. Generating all pairwise tests in this fashion is similar to the LSD approach except we perform the tests on the least square (predicted) means. In practice it is assumed that users of InVivoStat are not interested in all of the p-values generated but will select only those planned *a priori*. Other statistical software packages may require the user to enter the planned comparisons manually. This allows much more complicated and versatile comparisons to be made (other than pairwise tests involving one group versus another).

5.4.8.4 Stepwise multiple comparison procedures that control the FDR

The methods described so far do not offer direct control over the risk of finding false positive results. In this section a procedure is described that controls the false discovery rate. While not commonly applied in practice, controlling the FDR is perhaps more aligned with the process that researchers follow.

The Benjamini–Hochberg procedure

Benjamini and Hochberg (1995) developed a procedure that controls the proportion of false positive results rather than trying to ensure there are no individual false positive results. It can be applied when many comparisons are made and involves applying an adjustment to the unadjusted p-values. The following shows how to compute the adjustment to the p-values by hand:

1. Calculate the unadjusted p-values, either using the LSD or planned comparison approaches. Assume c p-values have been generated.

Table 5.24. Table of the adjustments to the p-values that are made when using the Benjamini–Hochberg procedure

Unadjusted p-value	Adjusted p-value†
p_1	$p'_1 = [c / 1] \times p_1$
p_2	$p'_2 = [c / 2] \times p_2$
...	...
$p_{(c-1)}$	$p'_{(c-1)} = [c / (c-1)] \times p_{(c-1)}$
p_c	$p'_c = [c / c] \times p_c$

†To preserve the monotonicity of the p-values, if $p'_{(i+1)} < p'_i$ then replace $p'_{(i+1)}$ with p'_i ($1 \leq i \leq c - 1$).

2. Rank the p-values in order of significance, smallest first. Label them $p_1, ..., p_c$.
3. Multiply the ith p-value by c / i as highlighted in Table 5.24, where

$$p'_i = [c / i] \times p_i. \qquad (5.44)$$

4. Working *up* the table, starting with the largest p-value, as soon as an adjusted p-value is less than α then:
   a) The corresponding comparison (and all comparisons with smaller adjusted p-values) is declared significant.
   b) All comparisons corresponding to larger p-values are declared non-significant.

Example 5.23: Multiple comparison adjustment

Assume an analysis has been carried out on experimental data and the p-values for the planned comparisons are 0.001, 0.009, 0.019, 0.020 and 0.250. Using the Benjamini–Hochberg procedure (testing at the significance level $\alpha = 0.05$ or 5%):

The largest p-value p_5 is non-significant:
(5 / 5) × 0.250 = 0.250 > 0.05
The second largest p-value p_4 is significant:
(5 / 4) × 0.020 = 0.025 < 0.05

Therefore the comparisons corresponding to the p-values p_1, p_2 and p_3 are also declared significant.

5.4.8.5 Simultaneous multiple comparison procedures that control the FWE

Following on from Section 5.4.8.4, two sets of approaches are now described that can be used to control the family-wise error rate. The first set involves simultaneously adjusting all the comparisons. The second set involves making the adjustments in a step-wise fashion, working through the set of comparisons and only stopping when significance (or non-significance, depending on the procedure) is reached. To begin with we shall consider the simultaneous comparison procedures as they are commonly applied in practice.

The Bonferroni procedure

The Bonferroni multiple comparison procedure (Bonferroni, 1936) is a well-known procedure that is straightforward to perform. It is often applied, we argue, in many cases unnecessarily. The procedure can be considered to be strict, especially when many comparisons are made, and hence the chance of finding a true positive result (the statistical power) of this procedure is lower than for other multiple comparison procedures. For a discussion of some of the misuses of the Bonferroni procedure, see Nakagawa (2004).

Assume that the researcher wishes to make c comparisons and this is the size of the family of tests that needs adjusting for. The hypotheses of interest are then assessed using a modified significance criterion. If the test is to be performed at the significance level α then rather than declaring a comparison significant if the p-value is less than or equal to α, the result is declared significant if:

$$p\text{-value} \le \alpha / c. \tag{5.45}$$

Alternatively (and equivalently) the unadjusted p-value can be multiplied by c and then compared against α directly, i.e.

$$[p\text{-value}] \times c \le [\alpha / c] \times c = \alpha. \tag{5.46}$$

It is common practice, when using computer programs to carry out multiple comparison procedures, to perform adjustments to the p-values (and compare these against α) rather than assess the unadjusted p-values against a reduced significance level. Although the latter approach is used to describe some of the procedures in this chapter, when comparing the results of the different procedures we shall employ the former approach.

For example, if ten comparisons are assessed at the 5% significance level, then the p-values have to be smaller than:

$$\alpha / 10 = 0.05 / 10 = 0.005$$

to be declared statistically significant. This is quite a strict criterion for animal experiments, where (ethically acceptable) small sample sizes will inevitably reduce the statistical power. Making ten comparisons in an experiment may seem to be an unusually large number; however, this can easily be achieved if the responses are measured at multiple time points in a study.

Although by definition the Bonferroni procedure may be quite strict, in practice the situation is often worse. Many statistical software packages, when calculating the Bonferroni adjusted p-values, also assume that the researcher wants to compare everything to everything. This is usually more comparisons than are of interest. So not only is the Bonferroni adjustment unduly strict, but many software packages adjust for more comparisons (or a larger family of tests) than is really necessary. For this reason we would urge the reader to be careful if a statistical software package is used to perform the Bonferroni procedure.

The Dunn–Šidák procedure

The Dunn–Šidák procedure (Šidák, 1967) is similar to the Bonferroni procedure; however, the significance level we test against is not α / c but

$$1 - (1 - \alpha)^{1/c}. \tag{5.47}$$

The Dunn–Šidák procedure is an improvement on the Bonferroni procedure as the value we test against is slightly larger than the equivalent Bonferroni value. However, it still has the same drawbacks as the Bonferroni procedure described above. More importantly it also requires the individual tests to be independent of each other. By independent we imply that the tests, and hence the p-values, are not related to each other. There could be a lack of independence if the researcher makes comparisons (on data generated from the same animals) at several time points in a repeated measures analysis. As observations measured on each animal are related, the comparisons based on

Table 5.25. Table of the values that p-values are tested against for the LSD, Bonferroni and Dunn–Šidák procedures, with a significance level of 0.05, for various sizes of families of tests

Size of family of tests	LSD	Bonferroni	Dunn–Šidák
1	0.0500	0.0500	0.0500
2	0.0500	0.0250	0.0253
3	0.0500	0.0167	0.0170
4	0.0500	0.0125	0.0127
5	0.0500	0.0100	0.0102
6	0.0500	0.0083	0.0085
7	0.0500	0.0071	0.0073
8	0.0500	0.0063	0.0064
9	0.0500	0.0056	0.0057
10	0.0500	0.0050	0.0051
15	0.0500	0.0033	0.0034
20	0.0500	0.0025	0.0026

these observations, and hence the corresponding p-values, will also be related. For example, let us assume the researcher had recorded the heart rate of resting animals (in treatment and control groups) every second for 60 seconds. Within the repeated measures analysis the two groups are compared at each time point, i.e. 60 comparisons are made. It should be obvious that these tests will probably be highly related. If each animal's heart rate was constant across the minute, then effectively the researcher has measured the same heart rate 60 times per animal and has not recorded 60 independent pieces of information. The analysis should reflect this. If one p-value is significant, chances are all the others will be too.

Table 5.25 contains the critical values that the p-values are assessed against when using the LSD, Bonferroni and the Dunn–Šidák procedures with a significance level of 0.05.

The Tukey HSD procedure
Tukey (1953) proposed a multiple comparison procedure that aims to keep the risk of finding a false positive, at a user-defined significance level, when all possible pairwise comparisons are made. It is therefore an appropriate procedure to use if you are going on a data-trawling exercise and want to compare everything to everything, i.e. the family of tests is of size $c = x \times (x - 1)$, where x is the number of experimental groups.

If, however, you only wish to make a few selected comparisons, then this procedure will be overly strict and hence there is a risk of making false negative conclusions in the statistical analysis.

The researcher should also be aware, when making all pairwise comparisons, that the corresponding p-values will not be independent of each other. For example, consider an experiment that consists of three treatment groups, A, B and C, and the researcher wants to compare A vs. B, A vs. C and B vs. C. The last comparison is a linear combination of the first two, and hence the three comparisons are not independent of each other.

The Tukey HSD procedure is based on the Studentised range statistic, which is used to identify the critical value beyond which all pairwise comparisons are declared significant (Toothaker, 1993, p. 60). For each pair of means we begin by calculating the t-values, as described for the LSD test. These t-values are compared to the α level critical value of the Studentised range distribution for x means (as opposed to the critical values of a t-distribution with the residual degrees of freedom, as was the case in the LSD test). Tables of these critical values are available in many statistical textbooks, although in practice statistical software will perform all the necessary calculations.

This test is an exact test, which turns out to be somewhat conservative if the sample sizes are unequal or when there are covariates present. By conservative we imply that if the user decides to accept a 5% risk of finding a false positive, then the actual risk of finding a false positive (using this procedure) will be less than 5%. While this may appear beneficial it does imply that the statistical power of the analysis is compromised.

The Tukey–Kramer procedure

The Tukey–Kramer procedure (Kramer, 1956) is similar to the Tukey HSD procedure described above, but includes an adjustment to account for unequal sample sizes.

The Scheffé procedure

The Scheffé multiple comparison procedure (Scheffé, 1953) adjusts for not only all pairwise comparisons, but also more complicated comparisons involving linear combinations of the group means. With this method the risk of finding a false positive for any possible comparison is held at the significance level α. Because the Scheffé procedure deals with a more general situation than just pairwise comparisons between group means, it is stricter than the other techniques. In our experience an animal researcher usually wants to make pairwise comparisons between the group means, so this procedure is not recommended.

The Dunnett procedure

Comparing all the treatment groups back to a control group is perhaps the most common set of comparisons that are made when analysing data from animal experiments. Dunnett (1955, 1964) considered this situation and the procedure he proposed is a popular choice amongst researchers.

The Dunnett procedure is a modification of the t-test. The null hypothesis (that there is no difference between the treatment group and the control group) is rejected if the difference between the treatment group mean and the control group mean is greater than a number that is a function of a critical value (calculated using the multivariate normal distribution) and the variability of the data. To begin with the t-values are calculated (for the comparisons involving the control group), as described for the LSD test. These t-values are compared to $d\alpha(x - 1, f)$, the critical value based on $x - 1$ (the number of treatment groups) and f (the

residual degrees of freedom) for the Dunnett procedure. The $d\alpha(x - 1, f)$ values are tabulated in many statistical textbooks, although in practice statistical software will perform all the necessary calculations.

While the Dunnett procedure is undoubtedly a useful procedure there are some issues that should be considered before using this procedure. The procedure was designed for comparing $x - 1$ unrelated independent groups back to a single (control) group (Miller, 1981, p. 76). So if you have $x - 1$ different treatments, then you can use the Dunnett procedure to compare all treatment groups back to the control group. Increasing doses of a single compound are related to each other and so care must be taken when using the Dunnett procedure in this situation.

The researcher should also be aware that the Dunnett procedure should only be used if the experimental design consists of a single factor, Treatment say, and all treatments are compared to the control. Hence the family of tests is of size $x - 1$. The procedure is not applicable if a factorial design is employed. If there are two crossed factors (for example Treatment at x levels and Strain at two levels) in the experimental design, then there will be more than one control group to compare to (in this case a wildtype control group and a transgenic control group). One approach you should not take is to carry out the Dunnett procedure twice, once per strain. In this case the two multiple comparison adjustments assume the family of tests is of size $x - 1$. We feel this family is half the true size as you are comparing all groups back to the control for both the transgenics and the wildtypes. If you do want to adjust for multiplicity, then you should adjust for all the $2 \times (x - 1)$ comparisons.

Example 5.22 (continued) – A drug comparison trial

We return to the drug trial considered above, which consisted of two treatment groups and a control. We now consider the adjusted p-values obtained using some of the simultaneous multiple comparison procedures discussed in this section (see Table 5.26).

It is interesting to note that the only statistically significant result at the 5% level (treatment B vs. control) was obtained using the unadjusted LSD test, although the Dunnett procedure revealed some evidence of an effect. The researcher would need to decide if this was a true effect or really a false positive result by considering, for example, the size of the observed effect. It also highlights how the p-values contain more information and should not simply be used as a tool to decide on significance/non-significance.

Table 5.26. Table of the *p*-values (unadjusted and adjusted) for the LSD, Bonferroni, Tukey and Dunnett procedures

Comparison	LSD	Bonferroni	Tukey HSD	Dunnett
treatment A vs. control	0.057	0.170	0.127	0.099
treatment B vs. control	0.037	0.110	0.085	0.065
treatment B vs. treatment A	0.799	1.000	0.963	–

5.4.8.6 Stepwise multiple comparison procedures based on group differences that control the FWE

As an alternative to the simultaneous adjustment procedures described so far, there are several methods available that make adjustments in a stepwise fashion. It can be argued that there is an improvement in statistical power if a stepwise approach is applied (Shaffer, 1995), although these methods are not universally accepted within the statistical community. We begin by describing two popular methods, the Newman–Keuls and Duncan procedures. These approaches are based on comparing the size of the difference between the group means to test dependent critical values.

The Newman–Keuls procedure

To begin this section two methods are considered, the Newman-Keuls procedure and Duncan's multiple comparison procedure. We discuss them because there are theoretical concerns with these methods that the reader should be aware of. In particular it is well known that neither approach controls the risk of finding a false positive (Ludbrook, 1998).

The Newman–Keuls procedure was first devised by Newman (1939) and then popularised by Keuls (1952). The procedure involves comparing the size of the difference between two means against a set of least significant ranges. Essentially the treatments are grouped together into sets of means such that the treatment means within each set are not statistically significantly different from each other.

Assume there are *x* experimental groups to be compared. The groups are numbered $T_1, T_2, ..., T_x$ such that

$$T_1 \le T_2 \le ... \le T_x.$$

The process begins by calculating the $x - 1$ least significant ranges $R_2, R_3, ..., R_x$ where

$$R_p = r_\alpha(p,f)\sqrt{s^2/n}, \ (2 \le p \le x), \tag{5.48}$$

where *n* is the sample size, $r_\alpha(p,f)$ is the upper α percentage point of the Studentised range for groups of *p* means with *f* error degrees of freedom and s^2 is the estimated variance (the $MS_{Residual}$). For unequal sample sizes we replace *n* with the harmonic mean n_h where:

$$n_h = \frac{x}{\sum_{i=1}^{a}(1/n_i)}, \tag{5.49}$$

where n_i is the *i*th group sample size.

The procedure is performed in a sequential manner:
- The difference between T_x and T_1 is compared against R_x.
- The difference between T_x and T_2 is compared against R_{x-1}.

The procedure continues until:
- The difference between T_x and T_{x-1} is compared against R_2.

The process is then repeated but starting with:
- The difference between T_{x-1} and T_1, which is compared against R_{x-1}.

The process continues until all $x(x-1)/2$ pairwise comparisons have been made, i.e. when
- The difference between T_2 and T_1 is compared against R_2.

If the observed difference between the means is larger than the corresponding least significant range then we conclude that the two means are significantly different from each other. To avoid contradictions, no difference between a pair of means is considered significant if the two means involved lie between two other means that were not declared significantly different.

The Newman–Keuls procedure is popular amongst researchers, as it is a powerful technique. The process also appears to be a sensible approach as it is aligned with the purpose of running many statistical analyses. The researcher may want to know which sets of treatments are different rather than identifying which pairs of treatments are statistically significantly different from each other. Many statisticians, however, do not recommend this procedure because it does not control the risk of finding a false positive conclusion (Holland and Copenhaver, 1988). If you want to reduce the risk of finding false positive results (and hence decide to use a multiple comparison procedure) then you should at least employ a method that controls the risk of finding a false positive conclusion.

Duncan's multiple range procedure

Duncan's multiple range procedure (Duncan, 1955) is a modification of the Newman–Keuls procedure. The procedure is almost identical to the above method, except that the least significant ranges (the $R_i's$ defined above) are calculated using increasing levels of the false positive risk. The risk of finding a false positive result is given by

$$1 - (1 - \alpha)^{c-1}. \tag{5.50}$$

This procedure will produce a larger set of significant results (including true and false positives) than the Newman–Keuls procedure but there is an increased risk of finding a false positive (Curran-Everett, 2000). Duncan's multiple range procedure may give the most significant results of all the multiple comparison procedures, but it is dangerous to use this procedure as it does not offer the protection that most of the other multiple comparison procedures provide.

5.4.8.7 Stepwise-based multiple comparison procedures based on *p*-values that control the FWE

The methods described in the previous section control the family-wise error rate by making a simultaneous adjustment across all comparisons. However, stepwise approaches provide powerful alternatives that control the family-wise error rate and hence are procedures that the researcher should consider using.

The Holm procedure

The Holm procedure (Holm, 1979) is a simple procedure to apply as it involves making adjustments to the unadjusted LSD/planned comparison *p*-values. This procedure focuses attention on those comparisons that are of interest to the researcher and not all possible pairwise tests. The following description shows how to compute the adjusted *p*-values by hand in a series of stages:

1. Calculate the unadjusted *p*-values, either using the LSD or planned comparison approaches. Assume c *p*-values have been generated.
2. Rank the *p*-values in order of significance, smallest first. Label them $p_1, ..., p_c$.
3. Multiply the ith *p*-value by $(c - i + 1)$ as highlighted in Table 5.27, where

$$p'_i = (c - i + 1) \times p_i. \tag{5.51}$$

4. Working *down* the table, starting with the smallest unadjusted *p*-value, as soon as an adjusted *p*-value is greater than α then:
   a) The corresponding comparison (and any comparisons with larger adjusted *p*-values) is declared non-significant.
   b) Any comparisons corresponding to smaller adjusted *p*-values are declared significant.

It can be seen that this approach is similar to the Bonferroni approach, but whereas in the Bonferroni approach the adjustment to the *p*-values involves multiplying them all by c, in this procedure the *p*-values are multiplied by a sliding scale of levels between 1 and c.

Example 5.23 (continued): Multiple comparison adjustment

Assume an analysis has been carried out on experimental data and the *p*-values for the planned comparisons are 0.001, 0.009, 0.019, 0.020 and 0.250.

Using the Holm procedure (testing at the significance level $\alpha = 0.05$ or 5%):

The smallest *p*-value p_1 is significant: $0.001 \times 5 = 0.005 < 0.05$

The second smallest *p*-value p_2 is significant:

$0.009 \times 4 = 0.036 < 0.05$

Table 5.27. Table of the adjustments to the p-values that are made when applying the Holm and Hochberg procedures

Unadjusted p-value	Adjusted p-value†
p_1	$p'_1 = (c) \times p_1$
p_2	$p'_2 = (c-1) \times p_2$
...	...
$p_{(c-1)}$	$p'_{(c-1)} = (2) \times p_{(c-1)}$
p_c	$p'_c = (1) \times p_c$

†To preserve the monotonicity of the p-values, if $p'_{(i+1)} < p'_i$ then replace $p'_{(i+1)}$ with p'_i $(1 \leq i \leq c-1)$.

The third smallest p-value p_3 is non-significant:

$0.019 \times 3 = 0.057 > 0.05$

Therefore the comparison corresponding to the larger p-values, p_4 and p_5, is also declared non-significant.

The Hochberg procedure

The Hochberg procedure (Hochberg, 1988) is more powerful than the Holm procedure when the comparisons tested can be assumed to be independent of each other (see Section 5.4.1.4). This procedure, which involves making a similar adjustment to the unadjusted p-values as is applied in the Holm procedure, can also be easily carried out by hand:

1. Perform stages 1–3 as above for the Holm procedure.
2. Working *up* the table, starting with the largest p-value, as soon as an adjusted p-value is less than α then:
   a. Declare the corresponding comparison (and all comparisons with smaller adjusted p-values) significant.
   b. Any comparisons corresponding to larger adjusted p-values are declared non-significant.

Example 5.23 (continued): Multiple comparison adjustment

Assume an analysis has been carried out on experimental data and the p-values for the planned comparisons are 0.001, 0.009, 0.019, 0.020 and 0.250.

Using the Hochberg procedure (testing at the significance level $\alpha = 0.05$ or 5%):

The largest p-value p_5 is non-significant: $1 \times 0.250 = 0.250 > 0.05$
The second largest p-value p_4 is significant: $2 \times 0.020 = 0.040 < 0.05$

Therefore the comparisons corresponding to the p-values, p_1, p_2 and p_3, are also declared significant.

Note that when using the Holm procedure only p_1 and p_2 were declared statistically significant. This highlights the additional power of the Hochberg procedure.

The Hommel procedure

The Hommel procedure is a stepwise procedure that is more powerful than either Holm or Hochberg (Blakesley *et al.*, 2009). The disadvantage of this procedure is that it is not as easy to perform the calculations as it is for the other two. Using the Hommel procedure, we reject all hypotheses whose p-values are less than or equal to α / j, where:

$$j = \max\{i \in \{1,\ldots,c\} : p_{(c-i+k)} > k\alpha / i, \text{ for } k = 1,\ldots,i\}. \quad (5.52)$$

We shall omit any further details as in practice such calculations can easily by performed by a computer package. A more detailed description is given in Hommel (1988).

The Benjamini–Hochberg procedure

Before we end this section we shall briefly return to the Benjamini–Hochberg procedure discussed in Section 5.4.8.4. While this procedure controls the FDR, rather than the FWE, in principle it is similar to the Holm and Hochberg procedures. All three involve applying adjustments to the p-values, as defined in Tables 5.24 and 5.27. These adjusted p-values are then compared to the significance level α.

Conclusion

Table 5.28 summarises the properties of the Holm, Hochberg and Hommel stepwise multiple comparison procedures.

Example 5.22 (continued): A drug comparison trial

Returning to the drug trial considered above consisting of two treatment groups and a control group. We now consider the results obtained using the some of the stepwise multiple comparison procedures discussed in this section (see Table 5.29). In this simple case, all three multiple comparison procedures gave similar results.

5.4.8.8 The gateway ANOVA approach

A related procedure that deserves special attention is the so-called gateway ANOVA approach (Holson *et al.*, 2008). This procedure, which results in protected tests, has a long history and is popular amongst researchers.

Table 5.28. Table of the properties of the Holm, Hochberg and Hommel procedures

Multiple comparison procedure	Property	When to use†
Holm	More powerful than Bonferroni when controlling the FWE	When comparisons are not independent and calculations to be performed by hand
Hochberg	More powerful than Holm but assumes independence of comparisons	When comparisons are independent and calculations to be performed by hand
Hommel	Most powerful technique considered in this section to control the Type I error rate	When the researcher has access to packages able to perform the required calculations

†To control the false discovery rate, rather than the family-wise error rate, use the Benjamini–Hochberg procedure.

Table 5.29. Table of p-values (unadjusted and adjusted) for the LSD, Holm, Hochberg and Hommel procedures

Comparison	LSD	Holm	Hochberg	Hommel
treatment A vs. control	0.057	0.113	0.113	0.113
treatment B vs. control	0.037	0.110	0.110	0.085
treatment B vs. treatment A	0.799	0.799	0.799	0.799

However, it should only ever be seen as a rule of thumb.

The general principle of the gateway ANOVA approach is that to make any comparisons between the experimental group means, the overall test in the ANOVA table has to be significant. The argument is that if the overall test in the ANOVA table is non-significant, then it is more likely that any statistically significant pairwise comparisons are false positives. The approach was suggested by the eminent statistician R. A. Fisher and hence any test that is only carried out conditional on the overall ANOVA test is called a Fisher's protected test.

This strategy has been shown (through simulation) to be a useful tool in reducing the false positive risk in certain special cases. In general, however, there are many situations where this approach is not valid. We argue that most if not all animal experiments fall into one of these situations! As Hsu (1996, p. 177) comments:

Not only does performing a test of homogeneity [gateway test] *first not guarantee the probability of an incorrect assertion to be less than α … it might guarantee this probability to be (conditionally) greater than α if multiple comparison results are only reported when the test of homogeneity rejects* [i.e. the gateway test is significant].

The following scenarios imply the gateway ANOVA approach should not be relied upon.

Type of test used

The gateway ANOVA approach was developed under the assumption that the researcher wants to make all pairwise comparisons between the groups using multiple t-tests or the LSD test. However, unless the experimental design involves only two or three independent groups, it can be shown that the gateway ANOVA approach is not strong enough to guard against finding false positives.

There is also no need to apply Fisher's protection to any of the multiple comparison procedures listed above (Holson *et al.*, 2008). These procedures, such as Dunnett, Hommel and Hochberg, are designed to reduce the risk of finding false positives. In other words there is no need to apply more than one safeguard against false positives in a single analysis. This can seriously reduce the power of the experiment.

Treatment structure

The overall tests in the ANOVA table are global tests. They should not be confused with local inferences involving specific group mean comparisons. When the gateway ANOVA approach is used it is tacitly assumed that the experimental groups have no structure. By that we imply all groups have equal status in the experiment. The researcher can then make any number of comparisons (perhaps all pairwise comparisons) between the group means. In this scenario using a gateway ANOVA approach is meaningful as the overall test in the ANOVA table also treats all groups equally. However, even in this scenario, as mentioned above, once there are more than three groups the approach is no longer reliable.

In many experiments the treatments do have a structure. You may have a control group that has a different status in the experiment to the treated groups because you plan to compare all treatments back to the control (and you do not plan to compare the treatments to each other). If you have more than one factor in the experimental design, then there will be a structure to the group means. You probably would not want to compare the wildtype treated group to the transgenic control group, for example. The ANOVA table tests do not take this complex experimental structure into account. ANOVA is purely a test to see if the individual means are different from each other.

In certain circumstances a positive control may have been included in the experiment, which again has a different status in the experimental design to the treatment groups. Such control groups allow the researcher to check whether the experimental procedure has worked. In theory, if the experimental procedures were successful there should be a significant difference between the control and the positive control. In such cases it is the significance of the comparison between the positive control and the control that should be used to decide if the treatment comparisons can be made rather than the overall ANOVA table test. Perhaps the test of the positive control effect should be performed regardless of the significance of the overall ANOVA test.

Example 5.24: Assessing the effect of pyroglutamylated RFamide peptide 43

A study was conducted to assess the effect of pyroglutamylated RFamide peptide 43 (QRFP43) on the stimulation of the hypothalamic-pituitary-gonadal axis (Patel *et al.*, 2008). ICV-cannulated rats (*n* = 9 to 14) were injected with QRFP43 at doses of 0.3, 1 or 3 nmol, saline or neuropeptide Y (NPY) at 3 nmol (the positive control). Several parameters were measured; we shall focus on the food intake measured over the first hour post-injection.

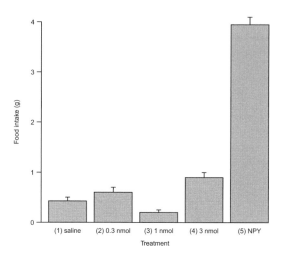

Figure 5.80. Plot of the observed treatment means with standard errors, from Example 5.24.

While the data analysed here has been simulated, the pattern observed in the means, as given in Figure 5.80, is similar to that presented in the original paper. From this plot it is clear that there is a significant difference between the saline and NPY groups.

If the positive control (NPY) group is included in the statistical analysis, then it is almost certain that the overall test of the treatment effects in the one-way ANOVA table will be significant. If the positive control is excluded from the one-way ANOVA analysis, then the overall treatment effect may not be significant. So if the overall treatment test in the ANOVA table is used as a gateway test, then the researcher could be in a position where comparisons of the doses of QRFP43 to saline can only be made if the positive control is included in the experimental design and statistical analysis. Clearly this is a strange position to be in.

The real problem here is that the overall treatment test in the ANOVA table does not take into account the structure of the treatments. In this example we have a positive and saline control, which have a different status in the experiment to the QRFP43-treated groups. The overall test in the ANOVA table does not take this into account whereas the pairwise tests do.

All pairwise tests

As discussed above, in most animal experiments there is a distinct structure to the treatments and the researcher knows in advance exactly which comparisons to make. This is rarely all possible comparisons. Remember using the gateway ANOVA approach tacitly implies that you want to compare everything to everything.

The overall test within the ANOVA table can be seen as an average treatment effect assessment. So if you have many treatments, most of which have the same effect, then the overall ANOVA test may not be significant even though there are significant differences between some of the treatments. These significant effects have effectively been lost because most of the treatments are not different from each other. This begins to be a problem when the number of groups is greater than three and gets worse as the number increases.

Example 5.25: Dose-response assessment

An experiment was conducted to assess the effect of increasing the doses of a test compound on animals. The experiment consisted of four increasing doses of a compound and a vehicle. Now there is a distinct structure to these treatments, not only can they be separated into two types, the control group and the treated groups, but they are also ordered on the dose scale. The researcher knows in advance exactly which pairwise comparisons need to be made, i.e. comparisons of each treatment group back to the control group. Perhaps the overall dose related trend will also be assessed.

To begin with the data was plotted (see Figure 5.81). We can see from the plot that there is some evidence of a decrease in the response as the dose of the compound increases. It may not be large but the trend appears consistent across the doses. We can deduce this because we know there is an ordering to the treatment groups.

Now let us assume we decided (unwisely) to use the gateway ANOVA approach to guard against false positives. It turns out that the overall test of the treatment effect in the ANOVA table is not significant at the 5% level ($F_{(4,35)}$ = 2.31, p = 0.068). In this case we would not make any pairwise comparisons between the treated groups and the control group.

Is this a sensible approach? Perhaps. However, remember the overall test in the ANOVA table was a global test and did not use all the available information. We know that:

a) There is a structure to the treatments (i.e. they were on an increasing dose scale).

b) We only planned to make certain pairwise tests (treatment groups vs. control group).

If we ignored the gateway ANOVA result, as we argue we should have done in this case, then we would have found significant differences between treatments and the control. Using planned comparisons we achieved significance at the highest two doses (p = 0.021 and p = 0.010, respectively). Even using the Hommel procedure, which is designed to reduce the false positive risk, we still achieved significance at the top dose (p = 0.040). Was it a real effect or a false positive? Obviously this would have depended on the biological relevance of the decrease, but given that there was a decreasing trend across all doses we may have concluded that the effect observed was real. Hopefully this conclusion would have been verified in a follow-up experiment, perhaps involving higher doses.

In conclusion then, the gateway ANOVA approach has certain limitations and should be used carefully.

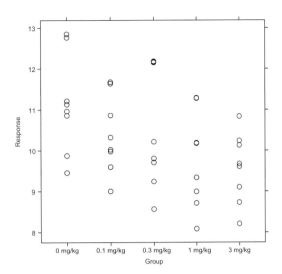

Figure 5.81. Scatterplot of the data from Example 5.25.

While it is certainly worthwhile looking at the ANOVA table, to make overall assessments of the experimental effects, it should not stop you making the individual (and presumably planned) comparisons on the individual experimental group means. We recommend you should report the results of the overall ANOVA table tests, perhaps as a footnote.

5.4.8.9 Multiple comparison procedures in statistical software packages

As mentioned above, when carrying out most of the multiple comparison procedures, many packages assume you want to make all pairwise comparisons between the group means. The packages then adjust for a family of tests of this size. So if you have x treatments, the multiple comparison procedures in most packages will adjust for all $x \geq (x - 1)$ pairwise comparisons. We believe that in many animal experiments the researcher does not want to make all possible pairwise comparisons, hence the default multiple comparison adjustment made by the computer package will be unduly strict. Such automated multiple comparison procedures should be avoided, unless all pairwise comparisons are required.

The researcher should also confirm whether the software package is making comparisons on the observed means or the least square (predicted) means. In many packages the multiple comparison procedures are performed on the observed means and do not take into account any covariates or blocking factors present in the experimental design.

Multiple comparison procedures available within the InVivoStat analysis modules include:

- Single Measure Parametric Analysis module: Unadjusted (LSD/planned comparisons), Benjamini–Hochberg, Bonferroni, Dunnett, Hochberg, Holm, Hommel and Tukey (see Section 6.3)
- Repeated Measures Parametric Analysis module: Unadjusted (LSD/planned comparisons) (see Section 6.4)
- Non-Parametric Analysis module: Unadjusted (Wilcoxon), Behrens–Fisher's and Steel's (see Section 6.6)

With the exception of the unadjusted procedures, InVivoStat adjusts for all possible pairwise comparisons in these modules. To allow more control over the family of tests to adjust for, i.e. if you only want to adjust for a few comparisons, the user also has the option of using the p-value adjustment module, see Section 6.5, where only the p-values of interest are adjusted for. The procedures available in this module include Benjamini–Hochberg, Bonferroni, Hochberg, Holm and Hommel.

5.4.8.10 Recommendations

Given all the procedures described in this section (and this list is by no means exhaustive), which procedure should be used? To some extent this depends on the level of risk of finding a false positive that the researcher is prepared to take and also whether the analysis performed is exploratory or confirmatory. There are, however, a few general rules that can be followed. We stress these are only our opinions and are not universally accepted by all statisticians.

False discovery rate

We believe if you are concerned about finding false positive results, then you should consider using a procedure that controls the false discovery rate. Such procedures, such as Benjamini–Hochberg, are statistically powerful, if less stringent, than those that control the family-wise error rate.

Family-wise error rate

All pairwise comparisons If you do plan to compare everything to everything in a data-trawling exercise, then you should use a procedure such as the Tukey HSD procedure (if the sample size is the same across all groups) or Tukey–Kramer procedure (if the sample sizes are different).

All-to-one comparisons If your experimental design has only one (Treatment) factor and you plan to compare all treatments back to one (the control) then the Dunnett procedure can be used.

Planned comparisons If you are only carrying out certain pre-planned comparisons in a controlled fashion then you can use the unprotected planned comparisons. If you do want to be certain that you do not have false positive results then we recommend manually adjusting these p-values using either:

- Hochberg: If you do not have access to a computer to carry out the computations and the comparisons are independent.
- Holm: If you do not have access to a computer to carry out the computations and the comparisons are not independent.
- Hommel: If you do have access to a computer to carry out the computations, but only if you can define the set of comparisons to include in the family of tests.

5.5 Other useful analyses

To end this chapter on statistical analysis we shall consider some additional statistical tests that may be of use to the animal researcher. These tests are applicable in specific situations and should be employed when the assumptions of the parametric tests described in Section 5.4.1 do not hold. These tests include the non-parametric tests, the tests of proportions and survival analysis.

5.5.1 Non-parametric analyses

All of the analyses considered so far in this text can be described as parametric. The parametric tests provide the researcher with a flexible, powerful and easy-to-use family of statistical tests. We also argue that crucially (in the analysis of animal experiments) the parametric tests allow the experimental design employed (i.e. block designs) and also any additional information collected (i.e. covariates) to be accounted for in the statistical analysis.

As discussed above we make certain assumptions when carrying out a parametric analysis. Occasionally these assumptions do not hold and alternatives are required. In this section we shall consider some of the non-parametric tests. These tests require fewer assumptions to be made than the parametric equivalents, and hence they provide an alternative analysis strategy in certain situations. If the assumptions of the parametric analysis do not hold then these tests can be more powerful than the parametric equivalents. It can also be shown that for certain tests, for example the Mann–Whitney test discussed below, they have similar levels of statistical power as the parametric equivalents, even when the parametric assumptions hold.

5.5.1.1 When to use a non-parametric test

There are several situations where the researcher should consider using a non-parametric test. We discuss some of the more common cases.

The homogeneity of variance assumption does not hold

One of the assumptions of the parametric analysis is that the variability is approximately the same across all groups. If this assumption does not hold then the researcher should first try to transform the response variable, perhaps using a log or square root transformation. Hopefully this will stabilise the variance across the groups. However, in certain situations none of the transformations resolve this problem. For example, it may be the case that the variability of the response is not related to the size of the response. A scatterplot of such a response is given in Figure 5.82.

In this example the treatment groups with the largest within-group variability (B and D) do not have the largest mean response. So neither a log nor square root transformation will homogenise the variability across the four treatment groups. In this situation the researcher should consider using a non-parametric test.

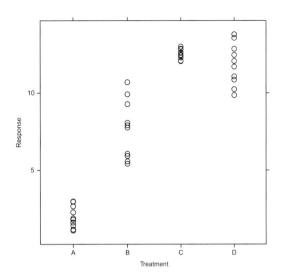

Figure 5.82. Scatterplot of the responses from an experiment involving four treatments, A, B, C and D, where the variability in treatment groups B and D is greater than in treatment groups A and C.

The responses are not continuous and/or the residuals are not normally distributed

When we carry out a parametric analysis we assume that the data are continuous and therefore the residuals can be normally distributed. There are, however, occasions where it is not possible to measure a continuous response. For example, the researcher may have to measure a discrete response (see Section 3.2.1.1) and hence the data generated are not continuous. If a parametric approach is applied to this non-continuous response then the residuals may not be normally distributed.

If a count response is measured, and the set of counts observed consists of many distinct values, then for the purposes of the analysis it could be assumed to be continuous. The response can then be analysed using a parametric analysis approach. If the counts recorded consist of only three or four distinct values, then clearly this is not continuous.

Whether the distribution of the residuals breaks the normality assumption depends on the number of different responses observed and the range of these responses. If the response has an observable range of 0 to 100 counts, but only the values 0, 1, 99 and 100 were recorded, then clearly it should not be assumed to be continuous with normally distributed residuals. However, if there were many different counts observed between 0 and 100, then the researcher may feel the response can be assumed to be continuous and hence proceed with a parametric analysis (assuming the other parametric assumptions hold).

There are no fixed rules on whether a response can be assumed to be continuous or not. Given that there will always be a calibration limit on the measuring device used in the experiment, it could be argued that no response is truly continuous! As a rule of thumb (and this really is only a rule of thumb) we believe that if the response variable contains at least eight different values, with a reasonable spread of responses (within each group) across these eight values, then it can be assumed to be continuous. If in doubt the researcher should contact a statistician for advice as alternative techniques may be available.

Clearly responses that are binary can never be assumed to be continuous and in fact should be analysed using more specialised tests, such as those discussed in Section 5.5.2.

The responses are constrained

The assumption that the residuals are normally distributed implies that the responses can be measured at any numerical value: in theory the range should be unbounded above and below. In practice there will be practical, physical and ethical constraints on the response that may compromise this assumption. For example, many responses are bounded below by zero.

If the researcher feels that practical constraints are influencing the behaviour of the response, i.e. if many responses lie on a boundary and hence have near-zero variability, then a non-parametric test may be more appropriate.

Example 5.26: Hotplate pain model

An experiment was conducted to assess the effect of an analgesic in the hotplate pain model. Following treatment an animal's paw was placed on a hotplate (at 55ºC) and the time to withdraw the paw was recorded. For ethical reasons the maximum amount of time that an animal's paw can be left on the hotplate is 30 seconds – this prevents any tissue damage. If an animal does not withdraw its paw after 30 seconds have elapsed, then the animal is removed from the hotplate and a censored observation of 30 seconds recorded.

If the dataset contains many responses that are censored, then it may be better for the researcher to use non-parametric tests to analyse the data. There are limits though, even with non-parametric tests, as certain assumptions are still made in such analyses. If all the results are censored for one of the experimental groups, then this group should be removed from the dataset prior to statistical analysis. This situation can occur, for example, if a positive control or high dose of a compound is included in the experiment and the treatment effect is so strong that all animals achieve the ethical limit. Alternatively, the survival analysis technique, described in Section 5.5.3, could be applied.

5.5.1.2 Non-parametric tests

In general non-parametric tests are performed on the ranked data. The responses are ranked in order of size, where the largest observation is given rank 1. This ranking is carried out ignoring the experimental design. An example of ranking is given in Table 5.30.

The majority of the non-parametric tests are carried out on the ranks rather than the original responses. As the response data are ignored, and the ranking used in the analysis instead, it can be seen that information will be lost when performing non-parametric tests.

Apart from relaxing some of the parametric assumptions, the ranking technique also implies that the results of the statistical analysis are less likely to be influenced by any outliers. For example, the largest observation in the dataset may appear to be an outlier on the original scale, but it is given rank 1 regardless of the actual numerical value. In other words the observation will be given the same rank regardless of how extreme it is.

Table 5.31 lists some parametric tests and the equivalent non-parametric tests.

For more details of the calculations involved in performing these tests, see Armitage *et al.* (2002, pp. 272–89). A description of how to carry out some of these tests within InVivoStat's non-parametric analysis module is given in Section 6.6.

The Mann–Whitney test

As an example of the calculations involved when performing one of the statistical analyses given in Table 5.31, we shall consider the Mann–Whitney test.

Table 5.30. Ranking applied when performing a non-parametric test

Treatment	Response	Rank
drug	0.963	1
drug	0.948	2
drug	0.862	3
drug	0.852	6
drug	0.776	8
drug	0.616	12
drug	0.554	13
drug	0.546	14
drug	0.539	15
drug	0.35	22
drug	0.297	23
drug	0.249	24
drug	0.112	27
vehicle	0.859	4
vehicle	0.853	5
vehicle	0.845	7
vehicle	0.712	9
vehicle	0.675	10
vehicle	0.655	11
vehicle	0.488	16
vehicle	0.449	17
vehicle	0.444	18
vehicle	0.429	19
vehicle	0.405	20
vehicle	0.395	21
vehicle	0.207	25
vehicle	0.158	26
vehicle	0.083	28

To perform this test we first add together the ranks of the observations in each of the two groups (the R_i's) and then calculate

$$U_i = R_i - \frac{n_i(n_i+1)}{2}(i = 1, 2),$$ (5.53)

where R_i is the sum of the ranks of the ith group and n_i is the sample size of the ith group. To perform the Mann–Whitney test, the minimum of U_1 and U_2 (defined as U) is compared to significance tables that can be found in many statistical textbooks. Alternatively, for large sample sizes (greater than about 20), we can compute

Table 5.31. Table of parametric and equivalent non-parametric tests

Parametric test	Non-parametric test
Unpaired t-test	Wilcoxon rank sum test (also known as) Mann–Whitney test
Paired t-test	Wilcoxon matched pairs test
One-way ANOVA	Kruskal–Wallis test
One-way ANOVA with blocks	Friedman's test
Dunnett	Steel's
LSD test	Behrens–Fisher-type tests

$$z = \frac{U - \dfrac{n_1 n_2}{2}}{\sqrt{\dfrac{n_1 n_2 (n_1 + n_2 + 1)}{12}}},$$ (5.54)

which is approximately normally distributed and can hence be assessed against the critical values of the normal distribution.

The principle of the Mann–Whitney test is that the smaller U is, the greater the difference between the sum of the ranks of the two groups. This implies that it is more likely that there is an overall shift in the distribution of the observations between the two groups and hence there is a significant treatment effect.

The Mann–Whitney test is the non-parametric equivalent of the unpaired t-test. It can be shown (Lehmann, 1999, p. 176) that if the normality assumption holds then the statistical power of the Mann–Whitney test is about 95% of that of the t-test. If the normality assumption does not hold then this non-parametric test is considerably more powerful than the t-test.

5.5.2 Testing the difference between proportions

In certain situations the researcher may not be able to measure a continuous response. Perhaps the only response that can be measured, given the animal model, is nominal, ordinal or binary. With these responses, the animals within each experimental group can be divided into a number of categories, each category corresponding to one of the finite levels of the response.

Example 5.27: Assessment of laparoscopic techniques in the treatment of malignant abdominal disease

In the late 1990s it was postulated that wound metastases were created when laparoscopic techniques were used to resect tumours. A study, involving the injection of a tumour cell line in rats, was conducted to assess this (Mathew *et al.*, 1996). As part of the experiment rats (*n* = 12 per group) were given an injection in the left flank abdominal musculature with a suspension of mammary adenocarcinoma tumour cells, causing a tumour to develop in the lateral abdominal wall. After 7 days, the animals underwent either a laparoscopy or laparotomy followed by tumour resection. Following a further 7 days, the animals were killed and their wound metastases assessed. Table 5.32 summarises the results of this experiment, where the response was either presence or absence of microscopic metastases.

It can be seen from the table that the type of surgery had a significant effect on wound metastases. In such cases, where the response is a binary measure, the parametric and non-parametric approaches so far considered cannot be applied. The researcher may want to investigate whether the proportion of animals with microscopic metastases varied between the two surgical groups.

5.5.2.1 Analysis procedure

In this section we shall describe two tests that can be used to analyse binary, nominal or ordinal responses, the chi-squared test and Fisher's exact test. The analysis procedure involves testing to see if the proportion of animals in each of the response categories varies depending on the experimental group. With these tests, we are investigating the proportion of animals within each category and not the total number. So, for example, if there were twice as many animals allocated to the control group compared with the treated groups, then (assuming there were no treatment-related effects) we would expect to see twice as many animals in the control group with a specific response compared to the treated group.

The process begins, as described in Section 2.3.1, by formulating the null and alternative hypotheses:

H_0: The chance (or probability) of an animal being associated with any given response category is the same regardless of which experimental group they are allocated to.

Table 5.32. Table of the responses from Example 5.27. Animals were categorised depending on whether wound metastases were observed or not

Response type	Surgery type	
	laparoscopy	laparotomy
microscopic metastases present	10	2
microscopic metastases absent	2	10

H_1: The chance (or probability) of an animal being associated with any given response category varies depending on which experimental group they are allocated to.

Both the chi-squared test and Fisher's exact test effectively ask the question: 'Given the observed pattern of responses across the experimental groups, what is the chance of seeing this pattern of results, or a pattern even more extreme, when in reality the response is not influenced by the experimental group?'

If, for each group, the number of animals observed within each response category is greater than five, then the researcher should consider using the chi-squared test. If in one of the response categories the number of animals is less than five, as is often the case in animal experiments, then Fisher's exact test is usually the preferred test. This latter test makes fewer assumptions, but is more computationally intensive to perform. We shall describe both tests in the following sections. Descriptions of how to perform the chi-squared test and Fisher's exact tests using InVivoStat are given in Section 6.12.

5.5.2.2 Chi-squared test

For each combination of response category and experimental group we work out the number of animals we would expect to see in each combination (assuming the null hypothesis is true) given the total number of animals:

a) in each experimental group;

b) within each response category, summed across all experimental groups.

We then compare these calculated values to the values actually observed in the experiment. If the expected results (under the null hypothesis) and the observed results are approximately the same, then we can conclude the null hypothesis is true. If the expected and observed results are sufficiently different, then we conclude the null hypothesis is not true, and hence the alternative hypothesis is accepted.

Example 5.28: Congenital Cytomegalovirus

Congenital *Cytomegalovirus* (CMV) infection during pregnancy is known to cause long-term new-born morbidity, mental retardation and sensorineural hearing loss. A study was conducted to assess whether the antiviral agent cyclic cidofovir could prevent transmission of CMV infection from mother to offspring (Schleiss *et al.*, 2006).

Guinea pigs ($n = 5$ in the saline control group and $n = 4$ in the cyclic cidofovir treatment group) were challenged with the guinea pig CMV prior to mating and then given either the placebo or the treatment during pregnancy. The numbers of dam and premature pup deaths were assessed (from a total of $n = 20$ pups in the saline control group and $n = 21$ in the cyclic cidofovir treatment group). In the placebo group, one dam and four pup deaths were observed whereas in the treatment group there were none (see Table 5.33).

As death was a binary response (guinea pigs were either alive or dead) it was felt that a chi-squared test could be used to assess the treatment effect. Given the small number of animals ($n = 0$) in one of the response/treatment group combinations this test is perhaps not ideal (and Fisher's exact test is more reliable) but for the purposes of this discussion we shall continue.

The test begins by calculating the row totals (25 placebo animals and 25 treated animals) and the column totals (45 alive and 5 dead). Given these row and column totals we then calculate the expected number of animals in each category under the assumption that there is no treatment-related effect. The (i,j)th entry in this table is given by:

$$\text{Expected total}_{i,j} = \frac{\text{Row}_i \text{ total} \times \text{Column}_j \text{ total}}{\text{Total number of animals}}. \tag{5.55}$$

For example, the expected number of living placebo animals was $25 \times 45/50 = 22.5$. The expected totals, along with the row and column totals, are presented in Table 5.34.

We then work out how far the observed responses are from the expected responses. We do this using the following approach:
(a) Calculate the differences between the observed and expected results.
(b) Square the individual differences calculated in (a) (squaring makes all differences positive).
(c) For each squared difference, divide through by the expected value.
(d) Add up the ratios calculated in (c).

Table 5.33. Mortality results from Example 5.28. Guinea pigs (numbers of dams and pups are added together) were categorised into one of two categories

	alive	dead
placebo	20	5
treatment	25	0

In this case we calculate:

$$\frac{(20-22.5)^2}{22.5} + \frac{(5-2.5)^2}{2.5} + \frac{(25-22.5)^2}{22.5} + \frac{(0-2.5)^2}{2.5} = 5.56.$$

This number is the test statistic and from this we can work out the probability of getting a result as extreme (or more extreme) than the one observed if the null hypothesis of no treatment effect is true. To do this we assume that the test statistic is approximately chi-squared distributed. We can then predict how likely it is that we can observe such a large test statistic, or one larger, if there was in reality no treatment-related effect.

The assumption that the test statistic is approximately chi-squared distributed has been shown to be reliable when there is a large number in both the row and column totals and also for each combination of response and group. When there are fewer than five animals in one of the contingency table combinations then this assumption may not hold.

For the case where there are only two experimental groups and the response is binary, it can be shown that the test statistic is not quite chi-squared distributed. A commonly applied technique to adjust the test statistic in this situation is Yates' continuity correction. To apply this correction we reduce the difference between the observed and expected responses by ½ prior to squaring. So we add ½ onto the negative differences and subtract ½ from the positive differences:

$$\frac{(20-22.5+\frac{1}{2})^2}{22.5} + \frac{(5-2.5-\frac{1}{2})^2}{2.5} + \frac{(25-22.5-\frac{1}{2})^2}{22.5} + \frac{(0-2.5+\frac{1}{2})^2}{2.5} = 3.56.$$

In this case $p = 0.059$, i.e. there is a 5.9% chance of observing these results, or something more extreme, if there was, in reality, no real difference between the groups. In this case we would therefore conclude the null hypothesis was true and that there was no difference between the groups. However, given that the sample size in one of the groups was less than five, perhaps Fisher's exact test would give a more reliable result.

5.5.2.3 Fisher's exact test

With Fisher's exact test we calculate all possible outcomes of the experiment that would have resulted in

Table 5.34. Expected responses from Example 5.28. Guinea pigs were categorised into one of two categories

	alive	dead	column totals
placebo	22.5	2.5	25
treatment	22.5	2.5	25
row totals	45	5	50

the row/column totals given in the contingency table. We can do this because each animal's response can only be one of a distinct set of values and so there is a finite number of experimental outcomes. For each of these experimental outcomes we calculate the probability of it occurring, assuming the null hypothesis is true. By using this technique we can determine exactly what is the probability of observing the set of experimental results we obtained *or something more extreme* under the assumption that the null hypothesis is true and there is no experimental group related effect.

In practice the number of possible experimental outcomes that will need to be assessed becomes large as the total number of animals increases. So in larger experiments this approach may not be computationally feasible. However, given the power of modern computers, it should be possible to use Fisher's exact test in many animal experiments.

Example 5.28 (continued): Congenital Cytomegalovirus

As the number of deaths in the treated group was less than five, it can be argued that the Fisher's exact test is a more appropriate test to use than the chi-squared test. To perform this test we begin by calculating, given the row and column totals, the probability (under the null hypothesis) of achieving the observed 20/5/25/0 split. This is given by the hypergeometric probability function:

$$\text{Probability} = \frac{(R_1! \times R_2! \times C_1! \times C_2!)}{(N! \times a_{11}! \times a_{12}! \times a_{21}! \times a_{22}!)} \tag{5.56}$$

where R_i is the *i*th row total, C_j is the *j*th column total, N is the total number of animals in the experiment and a_{ij} is the number of animals in the *i*th row and *j*th column. The ! symbol is the factorial symbol, where $x! = x \times (x-1) \times (x-2) \times ... \times 2 \times 1$ and $0! = 1$. So $3! = 3 \times 2 \times 1 = 6$.

For the observed result we calculate:

Probability of observing the 20/5/25/0

$$\text{split} = \frac{(25! \times 25! \times 45! \times 5!)}{(50! \times 20! \times 5! \times 25! \times 0!)} = 0.025 \text{ or } 2.5\%.$$

This is only one of the possible experimental outcomes though. As each animal must be present in one of the four categories (as a result of the random allocation process and the response to the treatment) we can work out the probability of every possible split of the 50 animals that would result in the observed row/column totals under the null hypothesis. So we can start with the 21/4/24/1 split, then the 22/3/23/2 split and so on. For each unique combination (and there are obviously many of them) we work out the probability of achieving such a result using the above formula.

Now Fisher's exact test result is the chance of observing (under the null hypothesis of no experimental group effect) a split in the 50 animals that is as extreme or more extreme than the one that was actually observed. A more extreme split will have a probability that is smaller than the one we calculated for the observed split (2.5% in this case). So we add up all the individual probabilities that are as small (or smaller) than the one we calculated for the observed split. This sum corresponds to the Fisher's exact test *p*-value result. It is exact because we have considered all possible experimental outcomes to arrive at this conclusion.

The *p*-value is the chance (or probability) of achieving the observed result (or one more extreme) if the null hypothesis of no experimental group effect is true. As long as the resulting *p*-value is less than or equal to 0.05 (or 5%) we can claim that the null hypothesis is not true. In other words if the *p*-value is less than 0.05, and the null hypothesis is true, then there is only a 5% chance of getting such an extreme result. We can conclude this chance is too small and hence the alternative hypothesis is accepted.

In this case the *p*-value was 0.050, to three decimal places, so there was evidence of a difference at the 5% level.

5.5.3 Survival analysis

In this final section we shall describe another type of analysis that the researcher may require when assessing data generated from animal experiments, namely survival analysis. We shall give a brief introduction of this analysis technique and some of its applications. A fuller account is available in Kleinbaum and Klein (2005, Chapters 1 and 2). A description of how to perform a survival analysis using InVivoStat is given in Section 6.15.

Consider an experimental situation where the response of interest is the time to an event. The event can be an animal responding to a stimulus, for example the tail flick test in pain research or the time to paw withdrawal in the hotplate pain model. Alternatively it could be the time of death, for example in a carcinogenicity study (Semela *et al.*, 2007). There are two complications when analysing time-to-event data that imply we should not use the parametric tests to analyse the data.

Responses may be censored

For certain animals we may not be able to measure the actual response time or the time of death. For example, in the tail flick test there will be an ethical limit on the length of time that the animal can be tested. Some animals will not respond within the time limit and hence it is impossible to know the animals' true response times. In carcinogenicity studies the experiment is conducted for a fixed period of time (usually up to 2 years) and hence we do not know when animals that were alive at the end of the study would have died if the study had continued. In such long-term studies animals may die of non-treatment-related causes (the so-called accidental deaths). We do not know exactly when the animal would have died (due to the treatment regime) only that it would have been greater than the time of its accidental death. We need to take this into account when assessing treatment-related survival time. In these cases we say that the observation is censored as we do not know the actual response time. All we do know is that it is greater than a certain value.

In animal studies the time limit is usually a value imposed by the study protocol, and hence will be the same value for all animals in the experiment. In general this need not be the case. In clinical trials, for example, the limit may vary as patients can drop out of an experiment (and become a censored observation) at any time during the trial.

Responses may be skewed

In certain situations the responses may be skewed and hence the residuals will not be normally distributed. For example, if there is an ethical limit on the response, and many animals achieve the limit, then the data will be right-skewed. In the extreme case all the responses in an experimental group are censored. This can occur if an experiment includes a positive control, and all animals achieve the boundary due to the treatment having a large effect.

Both of these issues, the censored responses and the skewed distribution of the observed responses, imply that we should not use the standard methods already described above to analyse the data. An alternative approach is to use survival analysis techniques.

Example 5.29: Cecal ligation model of sepsis

A well-established model of sepsis is the cecal ligation and puncture model in rodents. The model involves ligating the cecum and puncturing the exposed cecal pouch in two places. The punctured cecal pouch is then squeezed to allow faecal material to enter the peritoneal cavity. Unfortunately there can be significant variability in the mortality associated with this model and so a study was conducted to evaluate the influence of length of the cecum ligation as a determinant of mortality (Singleton and Wischmeyer, 2003). The study consisted of six groups, with the level of ligation ranging between 5% and 35% of the cecum. The animals were monitored for 4 days after surgery. In the study the mortality ranged from all animals in the group with a 35% ligated cecum compared to none in the group with a 5% ligated cecum. The experimental results revealed a clear effect related to percentage ligation on mortality. However, as the data were censored and the residuals were not normally distributed a parametric analysis approach could not be used to analyse the data.

5.5.3.1 The survival function

Rather than estimate the experimental group means and test to see if one mean is different from another, we calculate the survival function. One definition of the survival function $S(t)$ is that it is the probability, or chance, that an animal will survive beyond time t. We can assume the decrease over time in the probability of surviving can be modelled using either:

- A curve (in a similar way to the dose-response methodology discussed in Section 3.6.1). Examples include the exponential or Weibull curves.
- The Kaplan–Meier non-parametric approach.

The latter seems to be a more reliable approach when the group sizes are small.

To calculate this survival function we begin by dividing the time course into a series of time bins, in this case days posttreatment. Let us assume we want to calculate the probability of an animal in group 1 surviving the first day. This is simply:

$$S(1) = \frac{(n_1 - j_1)}{n_1}, \tag{5.57}$$

where n_1 is the number of animals in that group alive at the start of the study and j_1 is the number that died during day 1.

Now, assuming there are no censored (or accidental) deaths on day 1, the probability of an animal not dying during day 2 will be:

$$\frac{([n_1 - j_1] - j_2)}{[n_1 - j_1]} = \frac{(n_2 - j_2)}{n_2}, \tag{5.58}$$

where $n_1 - j_1 = n_2$ is the number of animals alive at the beginning of the second day and j_2 the number of animals that died during the second day. However, this is not the probability of an animal in group 1 surviving the first two days. An animal must first survive day 1 before it can survive day 2. The chance of an animal surviving day 2 (given that it has also survived day 1) can be calculated by multiplying together the probability of it surviving day 1 and the probability of it surviving day 2, i.e.

$$S(2) = \frac{(n_1 - j_1)}{n_1} \times \frac{(n_2 - j_2)}{n_2}. \tag{5.59}$$

In general then, to calculate the probability of an animal in a given group surviving time interval t, we need to calculate

$$S(t) = \prod_{i=1}^{t} \left[\frac{(n_i - j_i)}{n_i} \right]^{\delta_i} \tag{5.60}$$

where n_i is the number of animals alive in that group at the start of time interval i, j_i is the number in that group that died during interval i and $\delta_i = 0$ if there were no deaths in that group in interval i and 1 otherwise. $\prod$ is used to denote that we calculate a separate value of the term in square brackets for each time period from 1 up to t and then multiply them together, i.e.

$$S(t) = \left[\frac{(n_1 - j_1)}{n_1} \right]^{\delta_1} \times \left[\frac{(n_2 - j_2)}{n_2} \right]^{\delta_2} \times \ldots \times \left[\frac{(n_t - j_t)}{n_t} \right]^{\delta_t}. \tag{5.61}$$

The purpose of δ_i is that if there are no deaths in that group in interval i, then the ith term does not contribute to the survival function (as $x^0 = 1$, for any value of x). Note also that the n_i's will need to be reduced by any accidental deaths that occurred in that group during the previous interval.

Once we have calculated the Kaplan–Meier survival function separately for each group at each time point we can plot the results on a Kaplan–Meier survival plot. This gives a visual indication of the results of the experiment.

Example 5.29 (continued): Cecal ligation model of sepsis

The Kaplan–Meier survival plot for Example 5.29 is given in Figure 5.83.

5.5.3.2 Comparing groups

While it is useful to generate the survival function, we also may want to know whether the rates of survival vary between the experimental groups. This assessment of group differences can be performed using a log-rank test. We shall describe the log-rank test for the simpler case where there are only two groups. The derivation, in particular of the variance estimate, is more complex when there are more than two groups and requires estimating the covariances between the groups (see Kleinbaum and Klein, 2005, p. 94). In general, however, the approach described here can be generalised to more than two groups and software packages will routinely perform the calculations.

The null hypothesis for the log-rank test is that there are no differences in the survival function for each of the groups. In other words the animals have the same chance of dying or responding in a given time interval regardless of which group they are allocated to.

For each time interval, as defined above, we calculate the observed and estimated number of responders in a similar fashion to that described in Section 5.5.2.2 for the test of proportions. Table 5.35 summarises the interval i results from an experiment involving two groups. For interval i we calculate the expected number of responders E_{ij} in group j, where:

$$E_{i1} = \frac{R_{i1} \times C_{i1}}{n_i} \text{ and } E_{i2} = \frac{R_{i2} \times C_{i2}}{n_i}. \tag{5.62}$$

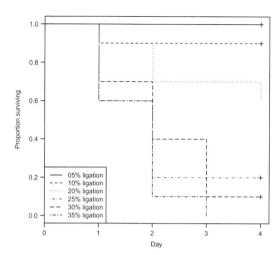

Figure 5.83. Kaplan–Meier survival plot for Example 5.29, the cecal ligation model of sepsis.

We also require an estimate of the variance V_i at interval i. This can be estimated using the formula:

$$V_i = \frac{(R_{i1} \times R_{i2} \times C_{i1} \times C_{i2})}{n_i^2 (n_i - 1)}.$$ (5.63)

If we add up the E_{i1}'s, E_{i2}'s and V_i's across all time intervals then we obtain an estimate for the expected total number of responders in each group (assuming the null hypothesis is true) and an estimate for the total variance (E_1, E_2 and V, respectively). For the test we

Table 5.35. Expected responses for an example involving two factors categorised in one of two categories at interval i

	Observed results at interval i		
	responder	non-responder	Total
group 1	a_i	b_i	R_{i1}
group 2	c_i	d_i	R_{i2}
Total	C_{i1}	C_{i2}	n_i

also require the total number of observed responders in each group (O_1 and O_2, respectively).

We now calculate the log-rank statistic:

$$\chi^2 = \frac{(O_1 - E_1)^2}{V}.$$ (5.64)

which is chi-squared distributed with one degree of freedom. Note if there are G groups in the experiment, then this test will involve a chi-squared test with $G - 1$ degrees of freedom.

Example 5.29 (continued): Cecal ligation model of sepsis

The data was analysed using the log-rank test described above and it was discovered that there was a significant difference between the six group ($\chi^2 = 37.34$, with five degrees of freedom, $p < 0.001$). This is perhaps as expected, given the observed decrease in survival rates as the percentage ligation increases.

Analysis using InVivoStat

InVivoStat is a free-to-use statistical software package developed specifically for animal researchers. It consists of a series of modules, which produce graphical plots, summary statistics and statistical analyses. In this chapter we shall discuss how to use InVivoStat, describe the individual modules and consider some of the technical details of the analyses.

6.1 Getting started

InVivoStat can be downloaded from the website: www.invivostat.co.uk. Once installed it can be accessed via the Windows start menu.

6.1.1 Data import

Data can be imported into InVivoStat from Excel (using the xls or xlsx file formats) or from a text editor using the csv (comma delimited) format. It is recommended that the final dataset is first created in Excel, including all data manipulations, before importing into InVivoStat. If the Excel file contains multiple worksheets, then the user is prompted to select one of the worksheets to import into InVivoStat. Multiple datasets can be opened within InVivoStat but they must be imported individually.

Datasets cannot contain commas in either the variable names or within the body of the data. Variable names cannot also contain the symbols: ~ (tilde), + (plus) or * (asterisk), as these characters are used internally within InVivoStat. Users will not be able to import datasets that include these characters.

The majority of analyses can be performed using the two data formats described in this section. There are also a couple of specialised data formats required for certain modules within InVivoStat, but these are described in the appropriate section. Regardless of the format required a few general principles apply to all datasets:

- The results of each response measured during the experiment should be arranged in a single column of the dataset.
- Variable names should be entered in the first row of the dataset (in Excel).
- Missing data should be left as empty cells (in Excel).
- No text should be placed in numerical response columns (other than the title in the first row). If any text is included then InVivoStat will assume the column contains only non-numeric data.

6.1.1.1 Single measure format

If each animal is assessed once only for each of the responses, then the dataset should be arranged in the single measures format. Several different responses can be measured but each one is placed in a separate column. Each row of the dataset corresponds to the observations from one animal. Other variables are included in the dataset to define, for example, the treatment factor(s), blocking factors and any covariates. Table 6.1 contains the first 14 rows of such a dataset. The dataset involves two responses (touch and body weight, measured pre- and posttreatment), strain and gender of the animal and the treatment that it receives. There is also a blocking factor at two levels.

Table 6.1. Table of the first 14 rows of a dataset in single measure format

Animal	Strain	Treatment	Gender	Block	Body weight pretreatment	Body weight posttreatment	Touch response
1	transgenic	0 mg/kg	male	I	0.85	0.81	2
2	transgenic	0 mg/kg	male	I	0.69	0.98	2.5
3	transgenic	0 mg/kg	male	I	0.38	0.10	3
4	transgenic	0 mg/kg	male	I	0.19	0.97	3.5
5	transgenic	1 mg/kg	male	I	0.84	0.84	6
6	transgenic	1 mg/kg	male	I	0.78	0.71	5.5
7	transgenic	1 mg/kg	male	I	0.41	0.99	8
8	transgenic	1 mg/kg	male	I	0.50	0.44	8.5
9	transgenic	5 mg/kg	male	II	0.72	0.30	7.5
10	transgenic	5 mg/kg	male	II	0.16	0.52	6
11	transgenic	5 mg/kg	male	II	0.26	0.17	9
12	transgenic	5 mg/kg	male	II	0.69	0.99	8.5
13	transgenic	0 mg/kg	female	I	1.02	0.42	9
14	transgenic	0 mg/kg	female	I	1.71	0.73	6.5
...	...	...	...	...	...	...	...

Table 6.2. Table of the first 14 rows of a dataset in repeated measures format

Animal	Treatment	Day	Response
1	A	1	1.53
1	A	2	1.09
1	A	3	1.07
1	A	4	1.81
2	A	1	1.04
2	A	2	1.51
2	A	3	1.25
2	A	4	1.44
3	A	1	1.08
3	A	2	1.68
3	A	3	1.58
3	A	4	1.27
4	B	1	2.48
4	B	2	2.61
...	...	...	...

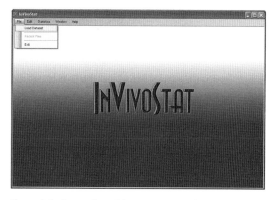

Figure 6.1. Screenshot of the input screen of InVivoStat.

6.1.1.2 Repeated measures format

If a response is measured repeatedly for each animal, for example observations are taken over time, then the dataset must be arranged in a slightly different format to that described above. In this format the measurements recorded for each response are still placed in a single column and so each animal is represented in multiple rows of the dataset. Two additional variables must be included in the dataset to identify the levels of the repeated factor and also the levels of the Animal factor that each observation corresponds to. Other variables, corresponding to the treatment factor(s), blocking factors and covariates can also be included as extra columns in the dataset. These datasets are described as long and thin. Table 6.2 contains the first 14 rows of a dataset where each row corresponds to an individual animal at a time point. The

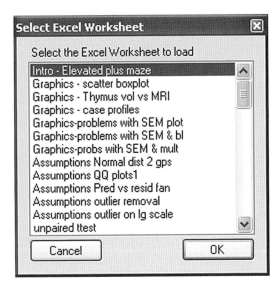

Figure 6.2. Screenshot of the Microsoft Excel™ input screen of InVivoStat when there are multiple sheets in the Excel file.

dataset involves one response (measured on each of the 4 days), the treatment that the animal receives along with the Animal and Day variables.

6.1.2 Importing a dataset into InVivoStat: Excel import

The dataset can be loaded from the File menu (see Figure 6.1):

File → Load Dataset

The Excel file is selected, using standard Windows methodology. If the file has multiple worksheets, then the user is prompted to select one of the worksheets to import (see Figure 6.2).

6.1.3 Importing a dataset into InVivoStat: text file import

A csv version of the dataset can be opened directly in InVivoStat from the File menu:

File → Load Dataset

The user should then navigate to the csv file using standard Windows methodology.

6.1.4 Data management

It is recommended that any data manipulations are performed in Excel prior to importing the data into InVivoStat. However, there are a few operations that can be carried out within InVivoStat itself. Clicking on a column header (variable name) will sort the dataset by that variable.

The dataset can be edited within InVivoStat if the 'Allow Editing of Data' option has been selected prior to opening the dataset. This option is available within the Options window:

Statistics → Options → Allow Editing of Data

Individual observations can be deleted from the dataset by highlighting the cell and pressing delete on the keyboard. Individual observations can also be edited if required. Note that any edits to the data must be completed and finalised (by clicking off the active cell in the dataset) before running the analysis.

The user can also include a copy of the data, as analysed by InVivoStat, in the output. This can be selected within the Options window:

Statistics → Options → Output Data with Results

6.1.5 Running an analysis

Once the dataset has been imported into InVivoStat, the user begins an analysis by opening the module of choice. The modules can be accessed by selecting the appropriate option from the Statistics drop-down menu. Each module window contains two tabs.

Settings

On this tab the user selects all the options required to conduct the analysis. This includes the dataset to use in the analysis, the variable selection and the choice of analysis results.

Results

Once the options have been selected the user moves to the Results tab. The analysis process begins with module-specific data checks. If any of these checks reveal

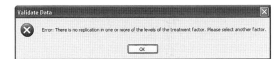

Figure 6.3. Screenshot of an InVivoStat error message.

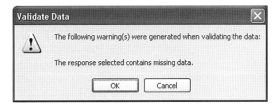

Figure 6.4. Screenshot of an example of an InVivoStat warning message.

issues with the dataset, then warning or error messages are produced. If no messages are generated then the Results tab is displayed with the results of the analysis, including a description of the analysis and any content-specific references. If selected, the output also includes a copy of the data.

6.1.6 Warning and error messages

When running an analysis, InVivoStat performs a series of checks on the dataset prior to analysis. These can be categorised as error messages or warning messages, depending on the severity of the problem. Error messages are differentiated from warning messages by a red cross. An example of an error message is given in Figure 6.3.

If an error message is displayed, the analysis will not proceed. The user must return to the dataset and make changes where necessary, as described in the error message.

Warning messages are for information only and are identified by a yellow triangle. They may highlight the need for user intervention, but in most cases they merely identify a possible issue within the dataset. The user can proceed with the analysis following a warning message. An example of a warning message is given in Figure 6.4.

6.1.7 Log file

Once the analysis has been completed, the user can view the log file, which contains additional information about the analysis. The log is available by clicking on the 'View Log' button next to the report URL on the top right-hand side of the Results window. The log should also be reviewed if the analysis results have not been generated as expected and the output is incomplete (i.e. no references are included at the end of the output).

Viewing the log may give the user valuable information to help explain why InVivoStat did not complete the requested analysis.

6.1.8 Exporting results

Once the results have been generated then they can be exported in a number of formats. All results can be cut and pasted into other packages by either right clicking on the plots (then select copy) or highlighting the text or tables and right clicking. *To paste a plot into another software program, remember to use the 'paste special' command and paste as a bitmap.* An output file is stored as a html file on the user's computer. The location of this file is shown at the top of the output window (see Figure 6.5).

Clicking on the save icon (see Figure 6.5) allows the user to save the output in a number of different formats including html, mht and text. We recommend using mht as this will save text, tables and figures together in a single file. Once created, an mht file can be opened directly in Microsoft Word. This method preserves all output formatting. Once open, individual results and figures can then be cut and pasted into other software using standard Microsoft Windows methodology.

6.2 Summary Statistics module

The Summary Statistics module in InVivoStat is available from the Statistics drop-down menu entitled 'Summary Statistics'. The interface is shown in Figure 6.6.

The Summary Statistics module allows the user to generate summary statistics of the numerical variables

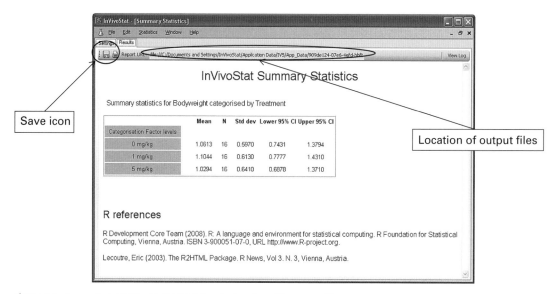

Figure 6.5. Screenshot of InVivoStat highlighting the location of the output files.

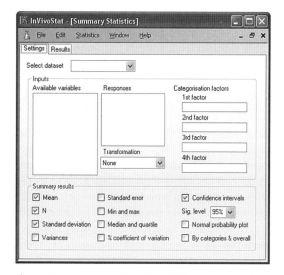

Figure 6.6. Screenshot of the InVivoStat Summary Statistics module interface.

within the dataset, as described in Section 5.2. Multiple variables can be selected and the summary statistics can be broken down by up to four different categorisation factors.

6.2.1 Analysis procedure

The analysis procedure is illustrated in Figure 6.7.

Input selection

1. Dataset selection: The analysis begins by selecting a dataset from the drop-down list of available imported datasets.
2. Response(s) selection: Multiple responses can be selected by dragging and dropping from the 'Available variables' list into the 'Responses' box.
3. Response transformation: The user can transform the response variables using the $\log_{10}$, $\log_e$, square root or arcsine transformations.
4. Categorisation factor(s) selection: Up to four factors (with either numeric or categorical factor levels) can be selected for categorising the results by. Simply drag and drop the factors from the 'Available variables' list into the 'Categorisation factor' boxes.

Output selection

5. The user should select the output options by highlighting the required summary statistics.

Table 6.3. Summary statistics for Response 1 categorised by Treatment and Strain

	Mean	N	Std dev	Std error	Lower 95% CI	Upper 95% CI
Categorisation Factor levels						
0 mg/kg transgenic	1.0454	8	0.6353	0.2246	0.5143	1.5765
0 mg/kg wildtype	1.0770	8	0.5966	0.2109	0.5783	1.5758
1 mg/kg transgenic	1.1371	8	0.6058	0.2142	0.6306	1.6436
1 mg/kg wildtype	1.0738	8	0.6597	0.2332	0.5223	1.6253
5 mg/kg transgenic	0.9811	8	0.6355	0.2247	0.4498	1.5123
5 mg/kg wildtype	1.0789	8	0.6874	0.2430	0.5042	1.6536

Table 6.4. Overall summary statistics, ignoring the categorisation factor(s), for Response 1

	Mean	N	Std dev	Std error	Lower 95% CI	Upper 95% CI
Response 1	1.0655	48	0.6044	0.0872	0.8900	1.2411

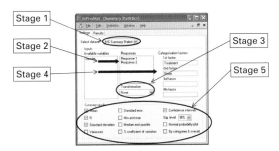

Figure 6.7. Screenshot illustrating the five-stage process for the InVivoStat Summary Statistics module.

6.2.2 Worked example

In the following example various summary statistics for Response 1 were calculated. The summary statistics were categorised by two factors, Treatment and Strain. The summary statistics were calculated separately for each combination of the two factors (see Table 6.3) and also overall, ignoring the categorisation factor (see Table 6.4).

6.3 Single Measure Parametric Analysis module

The Single Measure Parametric Analysis module in InVivoStat is available from the Statistics drop-down menu. The interface is shown in Figure 6.8. The Single Measure Parametric Analysis module performs many of the parametric tests described in Section 5.4 including the ANOVA, ANCOVA and *t*-tests. This module allows the user to fit multiple treatment factors, blocking factors and a single covariate. Interactions involving the treatment factors are included in the statistical analysis whereas interactions involving the blocking factors are not.

6.3.1 Analysis procedure

The analysis procedure is illustrated in Figure 6.9.

Input selection

1. Dataset selection: The analysis begins by selecting a dataset from the drop-down list of available imported datasets.

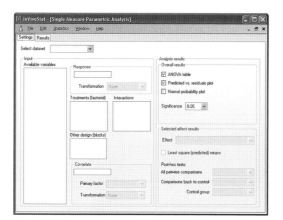

Figure 6.8. Screenshot of the InVivoStat Single Measure Parametric Analysis module interface.

2. Variable selection: Once the dataset has been selected, the user can select the variables for analysis by dragging and dropping them from the 'Available variables' list into the 'Response', 'Treatments (factorial)', 'Other design (blocks)' and 'Covariate' boxes.

3. Response transformation: Once selected, the user can apply a transformation to the response: $\log_{10}$, $\log_e$, square root, rank or arcsine. If a covariate has been selected, this will be transformed using the same transformation as the response, although this can changed manually if required.

4. Primary factor selection: If a covariate is selected, then the user can select the Primary factor. This factor is used to categorise the scatterplot produced as part of the output (see Section 6.3.2). The Primary factor should ideally be one of the factors of interest.

Output selection

5. ANOVA table: This option produces overall tests of the significance of the factors, interactions and covariates present in the statistical model (see Section 5.4.3).

6. Predicted vs. residuals plot: This plot allows the user to check the homogeneity of variance assumption of the parametric analysis (see Section 5.4.1.3).

7. Normal probability plot: This plot allows the user to check the normality assumption of the parametric analysis (see Section 5.4.1.2).

8. Significance level: The user can also choose the significance level for the tests, the default being 0.05 or 5%.

9. Selected effect: This is the effect that the user is interested in investigating further.

10. Least square (predicted) means: InVivoStat produces a plot of the predicted means of the term in the statistical analysis that corresponds to the Selected effect. These predicted means take into account terms included in the statistical analysis, such as the covariate (see Section 5.4.5).

11. All pairwise comparisons: This option produces all pairwise comparisons between the least square (predicted) means of the term corresponding to the Selected effect. The user has the option of adjusting the p-values for multiple comparisons. Options include Holm, Hochberg, Hommel, Benjamini–Hochberg, Tukey and Bonferroni (see Section 5.4.8).

12. Comparisons back to control: This option produces all-to-one comparisons between the least square (predicted) means of the term corresponding to the selected effect. The user should select the group (to compare all other groups to) from the drop-down list. This option is only available if a factor is Selected as the selected effect. The user has the option of adjusting the p-values for multiple comparisons. Options include Holm, Hochberg, Hommel, Benjamini–Hochberg, Dunnett and Bonferroni.

Output details

1. Response and covariate: InVivoStat identifies the response being analysed and also the covariate (if one is selected). This section also describes any transformations that have been applied.

2. Scatterplot of the data: InVivoStat produces a scatterplot of the data. The X-axis corresponds to the levels of either the single treatment factor or the highest-order interaction between the treatment factors and the Y-axis corresponds to the response.

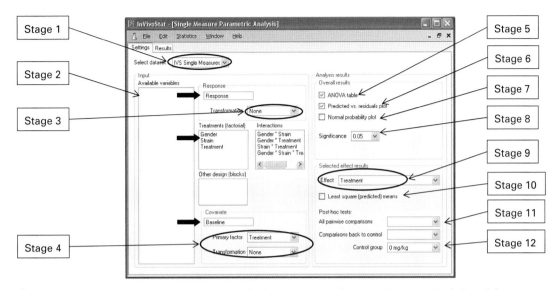

Stage 1

Stage 2

Stage 3

Stage 4

Stage 5

Stage 6

Stage 7

Stage 8

Stage 9

Stage 10

Stage 11

Stage 12

Figure 6.9. Screenshot illustrating the 12-stage process for the InVivoStat Single Measure Parametric Analysis module.

3. Categorised scatterplot of the data (ANCOVA only): When fitting a covariate in the statistical analysis, certain assumptions are made (see Section 5.4.6.6). This plot allows the user to assess these assumptions. Given below the plot is a description of the assumptions and also advice on how the plot should be used to assess them.

4. ANOVA/ANCOVA table: The ANOVA/ANCOVA table contains tests of the overall effects. InVivoStat uses the type II sums of squares in the statistical model fitting process (Armitage *et al.*, 2002, pp. 355–6). Any statistically significant results are described below the table.

5. Diagnostic plots: If requested, InVivoStat produces the predicted vs. residuals plot and the normal probability plot. The residuals presented on the predicted vs. residuals plot are the externally Studentised residuals (see Section 5.4.1.5).

6. Plot of the least square (predicted) means: InVivoStat produces a plot and table of the least square (predicted) means from the analysis with confidence intervals.

7. All pairwise comparisons: InVivoStat produces a table of all pairwise comparisons between the levels of the factor or interaction corresponding to the Selected effect. As well as the size of the difference between the means, and associated confidence intervals, InVivoStat also provides *p*-values to test the statistical significance of the differences. These *p*-values are either unadjusted for multiplicity or presented with a multiple comparison adjustment (see Section 5.4.8).

8. All-to-one comparisons: InVivoStat produces a table of all-to-one pairwise comparisons between the levels of the factor or interaction corresponding to the Selected effect. As well as the size of the difference between the means, and associated confidence intervals, InVivoStat provides *p*-values either unadjusted for multiplicity or with a multiple comparison adjustment (see Section 5.4.8).

9. References: Finally, references for the methods applied in the analysis are given.

6.3.2 Worked example

A behavioural experiment was conducted that consisted of three factors of interest: Strain, Gender and Treatment. Baseline responses were also measured and it was decided to investigate if these measurements could be used as a covariate to reduce the between-animal variability. The data was analysed using the Single Measure Parametric Analysis module.

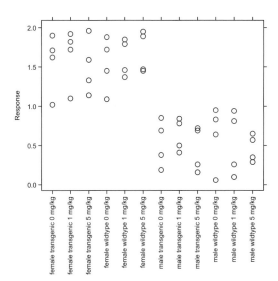

Figure 6.10. Scatterplot of the responses, categorised by the combinations of Strain, Gender and Treatment.

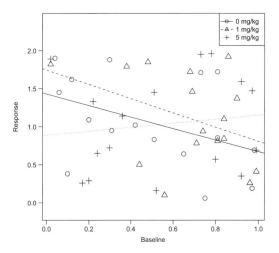

Figure 6.11. Categorised scatterplot of the Response vs. Baseline covariate, categorised by the primary factor (Treatment).

The scatterplot of the original data, see Figure 6.10, highlighted the clear difference between the responses from the male and female animals. Given the underlying variability of the responses (which appear to be similar across all experimental groups), there did not appear to

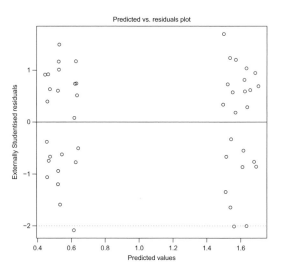

Figure 6.12. Externally Studentised residuals vs. the predicted values from the statistical model.

be any obvious outliers. If, however, the within-group standard deviations were used to identify outliers, perhaps using the rule that any observation beyond two standard deviations is deemed to be an outlier, then the two low observations in the female transgenic 0 mg/kg and 1 mg/kg groups would have been declared outliers. We argue these results are probably not outliers, given the variability observed in the other groups.

The categorised scatterplot, with best-fit lines (see Section 5.4.6.3), highlighted that there was no strong relationship between the response and baseline measurements (Figure 6.11). This indicated it may be unwise to include the baseline measurement as a covariate in the statistical analysis. For the purposes of this illustration, however, we shall proceed with the ANCOVA analysis rather than reanalyse the data without the covariate.

Table 6.5 is the three-way ANCOVA table. The baseline covariate was not significant ($F_{(1,35)} = 0.03, p = 0.873$). There was, however, a significant overall difference between males and females ($F_{(1,35)} = 120.37, p < 0.001$). None of the other terms were statistically significant.

The predicted vs. residuals plot (see Figure 6.12) highlighted that there was no need to transform the data. The sizes of the residuals for the groups with the

Table 6.5. Three-way ANCOVA table

	Sums of Squares	Degrees of Freedom	Mean Square	F-value	p-value
Baseline	0.00	1	0.00	0.03	0.873
Gender	12.62	1	12.62	120.37	< 0.001
Strain	0.01	1	0.01	0.05	0.822
Treatment	0.04	2	0.02	0.21	0.809
Gender:Strain	0.01	1	0.01	0.07	0.799
Gender:Treatment	0.06	2	0.03	0.27	0.763
Strain:Treatment	0.05	2	0.03	0.25	0.783
Gender:Strain:Treatment	0.04	2	0.02	0.21	0.812
Residuals	3.67	35	0.10		

Table 6.6. Pairwise comparisons of the levels of Strain and Dose

Comparison	Difference	Lower 95% CI	Upper 95% CI	Std error	p-value
female transgenic 1 mg/kg vs. female transgenic 0 mg/kg	0.085	-0.389	0.559	0.233	0.718
female transgenic 5 mg/kg vs. female transgenic 0 mg/kg	-0.051	-0.523	0.421	0.232	0.828
female wildtype 1 mg/kg vs. female wildtype 0 mg/kg	0.090	-0.384	0.563	0.233	0.703
female wildtype 5 mg/kg vs. female wildtype 0 mg/kg	0.161	-0.310	0.631	0.232	0.492
male transgenic 1 mg/kg vs. male transgenic 0 mg/kg	0.106	-0.359	0.571	0.229	0.647
male transgenic 5 mg/kg vs. male transgenic 0 mg/kg	-0.076	-0.547	0.395	0.232	0.745
male wildtype 1 mg/kg vs. male wildtype 0 mg/kg	-0.087	-0.557	0.384	0.232	0.710
male wildtype 5 mg/kg vs. male wildtype 0 mg/kg	-0.155	-0.620	0.309	0.229	0.502

lower predicted responses (with a mean around 0.5) were similar to those groups with the higher predicted responses (with a mean around 1.6).

As the researcher wished to compare the treatments to control separately for each Gender/Strain combination, the 'All pairwise comparisons' option was selected. Table 6.6 contains selected results of interest from the table of all pairwise comparisons of the levels of the Gender:Strain:Treatment three-way interaction.

The table of all pairwise comparisons revealed that none of the treatment group means were significantly different from control. If the user wished to adjust these p-values for multiplicity (see Section 5.4.8), then all p-values of interest should be extracted from this table and the P-Value Adjustment module employed to make an adjustment for multiplicity based on the correct number of comparisons.

6.3.3 Technical details

In this section we consider some of the technical details of the Single Measure Parametric Analysis module. In particular we describe how to use this module to analyse data generated when employing some of the experimental designs defined in Chapter 3.

6.3.3.1 Analysis of large factorial experiments

A factorial experiment is defined as an experiment conducted to assess two or more crossed factors of interest (see Section 3.5). As discussed above, such experiments allow the researcher to investigate the interactions between factors.

In Section 3.5 we differentiated between small and large factorial designs. Large factorial designs usually consist of many factors and therefore inevitably involve many combinations of the levels of the individual factors. To keep experiments manageable (and ethically justifiable) the sample size at each combination of the factor levels has to be small. The purpose of these experiments is to investigate the overall effect of the factors (and their interactions) rather than make pairwise comparisons between the predicted means. The sample size at each of the combinations of the factor levels is not sufficiently large to make meaningful pairwise comparisons between the predicted means. So the set of results from the analysis of such experiments should include an ANOVA/ANCOVA table, diagnostic plots and a plot or table of the least square (predicted) means. It is not recommended that the researcher make any pairwise comparisons when using large factorial designs.

6.3.3.2 Analysis of small factorial experiments

In practice many of the factorial experiments carried out will employ small factorial designs. These designs involve fewer factors, perhaps two or three at most, with a suitably large sample size at each combination of the levels of the factors so that pairwise comparisons between the means are sufficiently powered (see Section 3.5.3).

Care must be taken when making pairwise comparisons between the levels of the factors in the statistical analysis. You should not compare levels of a factor if a higher-order interaction involving that factor is statistically significant. For example, consider a two-way factorial experiment involving factors Gender and Treatment where the Gender by Treatment interaction is statistically significant. This implies that the effect of the treatment varies depending on the sex of the animal. So it would be misleading to compare the levels of the Treatment factor ignoring gender. The treatment comparisons should be made separately for each sex.

In general you should only compare the levels of a factor if all interactions involving that factor are not statistically significant, in which case it can be argued that the non-significant interaction(s) should be removed from the statistical model. InVivoStat uses this approach when carrying out an analysis of data generated from small factorial experiments.

- InVivoStat always produces the ANOVA table including all factors of interest and all interactions involving these factors. This allows the user to investigate the significance of all the terms in the analysis including the higher-order interactions. We define this as the *full statistical model*.

- If the user selects the highest-order interaction as the Selected effect, then InVivoStat uses the full statistical model when making the pairwise comparisons between the levels of this interaction.

- If the user selects one of the factors of interest as the Selected effect, then InVivoStat uses a *reduced statistical model* when calculating the least square (predicted) means and pairwise comparisons. This reduced statistical model will include all the factors but will not include any of the interactions involving the Selected effect.

- For analyses involving more than two treatment factors of interest, if the user selects a Selected effect that is an interaction but not the highest-order interaction, then InVivoStat uses a *reduced statistical model* when calculating the least square (predicted) means and pairwise comparisons, where any higher-order interactions involving the Selected effect are excluded.

For example, consider an experimental design with two crossed factors (Treatment and Strain). The data generated were analysed in InVivoStat using a two-way ANOVA approach where Treatment, Strain and the Treatment by Strain interaction were included in the statistical analysis. If the researcher selected the Treatment factor as the Selected effect, then the Treatment by Strain interaction would have been removed from the statistical model prior to making the pairwise comparisons of the levels of the Treatment factor.

This approach helps the researcher to avoid the situation where, for example, the levels of a factor are compared in the presence of a statistically significant two-way interaction in the statistical model. If the two-way interaction is significant, then the levels of the two-way interaction should be compared rather than the levels of a factor in the presence of the interaction. The latter comparisons may be misleading for the reasons highlighted above.

Example 6.1: Assessing the effect of maternal separation

An experiment was conducted to assess the long-term effect of maternal separation on behavioural and neuroendocrine indices (Slotten *et al.*, 2006). Male and female rat pups were assigned to either a treatment group (which underwent maternal separation for 3 hours on postnatal days 3–15) or a non-handled control group. For simplicity we shall consider only the female pups in this discussion. Various tests were performed on the animals over time, but we shall focus on the measurement of plasma corticosterone levels. Animals in each treatment arm were either restrained for 20 minutes prior to being humanely killed, or killed immediately upon removal from the home cage. There were therefore two factors in the experiment: Treatment (levels: maternal separation and non-handling) and Restraint (levels: no restraint and restraint). The full-factorial design used is illustrated in Figure 6.13.

The *full statistical model* for the analysis included:

Factors: Treatment, Restraint
Two-way interaction: Treatment:Gender

· If the user chose the two-way interaction as the Selected effect, then the *full statistical model* would be used to calculate the pairwise comparisons.
· If the user selected one of the factors as the Selected effect (for example Treatment), then the *reduced statistical model* used to make the pairwise comparisons would have included:
Factors: Treatment, Restraint

When the statistical model used in the analysis (to compute the pairwise comparisons) is not the *full statistical model*, a warning is included in the analysis log. For example, if the user decided to investigate the effect of the treatment then the Treatment factor

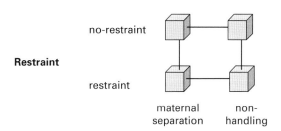

Figure 6.13. Full-factorial experimental design used in Example 6.1.

should be chosen as the Selected effect. This would have generated the following message in the log:

You have selected to plot/compare levels of a main factor in the presence of a higher-order interaction(s). This should only be carried out if the higher-order interaction(s) are not statistically significant. In the following we have removed these interaction(s) from the model prior to making the comparisons. The actual model fitted is Response ~ Restraint + Selected effect

Note that in this case the Selected effect was Treatment and hence

Response ~ Restraint + Selected effect

corresponded to

Response ~ Restraint + Treatment.

The '~' notation is used by the statistical language R when the term on the left-hand side of an equation is the variable being analysed and the term(s) on the right-hand side corresponds to the factors, interactions and any covariates in the statistical model.

6.3.3.3 Analysis of experiments involving blocking factors

The statistical analysis of data generated from experiments employing block designs, or more generally experiments where the researcher wishes to include a blocking factor in the analysis, can easily be carried out within the Single Measure Parametric Analysis module.

Recall that the purpose of including a blocking factor in an analysis is simply to reduce the underlying (unaccounted for) variability (see Section 3.4.2). We achieve this by removing the variability that can be explained by the levels of the blocking factor. So if an experiment was conducted over 2 days, and all the results on day

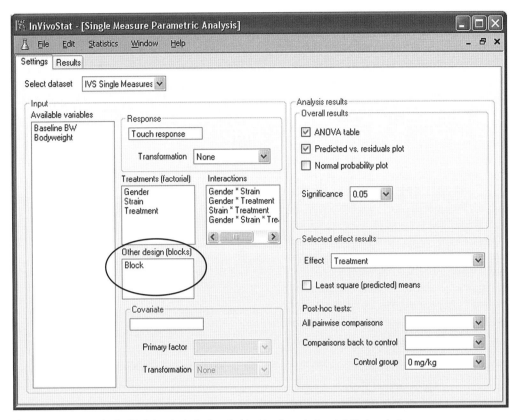

Figure 6.14. Screenshot highlighting the inclusion of a blocking factor in the statistical analysis.

2 were higher than on day 1, then this extra variability could be removed by fitting Day as a blocking factor in the analysis.

Two things should be apparent to the reader from the above statement:

- We do not want to conduct a test to see if the levels of the blocking factor are significantly different. It does not matter if there is a significant difference between day 1 and day 2: all that matters is that we account for the day-to-day variability in the analysis.
- We do not expect the treatment effect to be different within each block. So the results may all be higher on day 2, but this increase will affect all animals (regardless of the treatment they receive). In other words we assume there are no interaction(s) between the treatment factor(s) and the blocking factor(s).

Recall the randomisation recommended for a block design. We randomise treatments to the animals separately for each block. By considering this randomisation it can be shown that, referring to the two bullets above:

- There is no randomisation-based justification for testing whether the levels of the blocking factor are significantly different from each other.
- There is no randomisation-based justification for including any interactions involving the blocking factors in the statistical analysis.

InVivoStat does not provide the user with the ability to assess the pairwise differences between the means of the levels of the blocking factor(s). Nor does it include any interactions involving the blocking factor(s) in the statistical analysis.

When using the Single Measure Parametric Analysis module, selecting a blocking factor involves simply dragging and dropping the relevant variable from the 'Available variables' list into the 'Other design (blocks)'

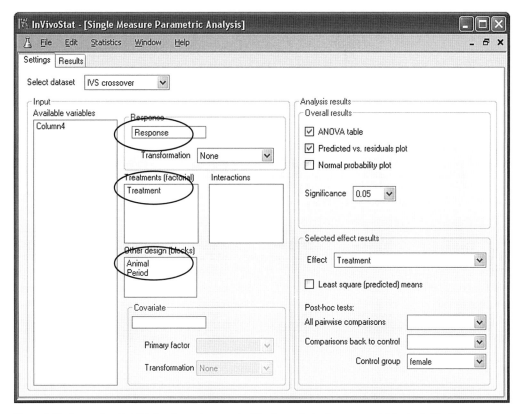

Figure 6.15. Screenshot highlighting the options required for the analysis of a crossover trial using InVivoStat.

box (see Figure 6.14). Other options are the same as above in the analysis of factorial experiments.

6.3.3.4 Analysis of crossover trials

In a crossover trial each animal receives two or more of the treatments over time and hence is measured repeatedly over time. Assuming only one observation is taken per animal per test period, then the data can be analysed using the Single Measure Parametric Analysis module. As long as the animals are randomly assigned to the treatment sequences, and the treatments themselves are randomly assigned to the treatment labels of the design, then we can assume independence between the observations measured for each animal. Effectively, as discussed in Section 3.4.9, a crossover design is a special case of a two-way block design.

In the dataset the user will need to include a variable indicating which test period the measurement was taken in and a second variable indicating the animal that the response was taken from (along with variables defining any treatment factors and so on). The dataset for a crossover trial will contain one row per animal per test period. As discussed in Section 3.4.9, this combination corresponds to the experimental units in a crossover trial. The dataset will also contain variables defining which animal the response corresponds to (Animal factor) and which test period the measurement was taken in (Test period factor). These factors should be dragged and dropped into the 'Other design (blocking)' box in the Single Measure Parametric Analysis module interface. This implies that the Animal factor will be defined as a fixed factor in the analysis of crossover trials. It is possible in other statistical packages to define

Animal as a random factor, but the benefits are minimal especially if each animal receives all treatments during the experiment.

Figure 6.15 illustrates the options required when analysing a crossover trial. The selection implies that no interactions involving either Animal or Test period will be included in the statistical analysis. This agrees with the general analysis procedure described in many textbooks, for example Jones and Kenward (2003, pp. 205–8).

6.3.3.5 Analysis of designs with missing factor combinations

The Single Measure Parametric Analysis module will not allow the user to analyse data if there are any missing combinations of the levels of the factors of interest. Instead a warning message is given highlighting the problem. This issue can occur if the experimental design is not of full-factorial type. There are two possible solutions:

- As described above, manually combine two factors together and use this new combined factor in the analysis instead of the two original factors.
- Move one of the treatment factors into the 'Other design (blocks)' box. This has the effect of omitting the interaction between the two factors from the analysis. However, you can then only compare the levels of the single treatment factor within InVivoStat. If you are interested in the levels of the interaction itself, then this approach will not allow you to make any pairwise tests between the levels of the interaction. In this case the first option is perhaps more appropriate.

6.4 Repeated Measures Parametric Analysis module

The Repeated Measures Parametric Analysis module in InVivoStat is available from the Statistics drop-down menu entitled 'Repeated Measures Parametric Analysis'. The interface is shown in Figure 6.16.

The Repeated Measures Parametric Analysis module performs a repeated measures mixed-model analysis. The module allows the user to fit multiple treatment factors, blocking factors and a single covariate. All interactions involving the treatment factors are included in the statistical analysis whereas interactions involving the blocking factors are not.

6.4.1 Analysis procedure

The analysis procedure is illustrated in Figure 6.17.

Input selection

1. Dataset selection: The analysis begins by selecting a dataset from the drop-down list of available imported datasets.
2. Variable selection: Once the dataset has been opened, the user can select the variables to include in the analysis by dragging and dropping them from the 'Available variables' list into the 'Response', 'Treatments (factorial)', 'Other design (blocks)', 'Covariate', 'Repeated factor' and 'Subject factor' boxes. The subject factor (usually Animal), a repeated factor and at least one treatment factor must be selected before the analysis can proceed.
3. Response transformation: Once selected, the user has the option of applying a transformation to the response: $\log_{10}$, $\log_e$, square root, rank or arc-sine. If a covariate has been selected, this will be transformed using the same transformation as the response, although this can be changed manually if required.
4. Primary factor selection: If a covariate is selected, then the user has the option of selecting the Primary factor. This factor is used to categorise the scatterplot produced as part of the output. The Primary factor should ideally be one of the factors of interest.
5. Covariance structure: Finally the user can select a covariance structure to quantify the spatial interrelationships between the within-animal observations (see Section 5.4.4.4). The default option is the compound symmetric structure (all observations within-animal are equally correlated). Other options include autoregressive (recommended if the repeated factor is Time and the time points are equally spaced) or unstructured (recommended if

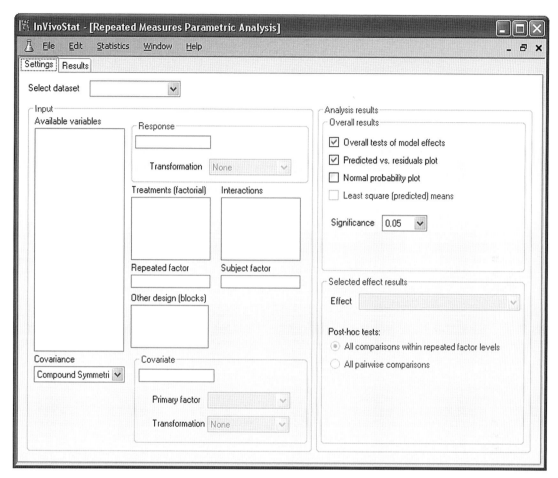

Figure 6.16. Screenshot of the InVivoStat Repeated Measures Parametric Analysis module interface.

the sample sizes are not too small). These options can be selected from the drop-down list.

Output selection

6. Overall tests of model effects: This option produces overall tests of the significance of the factors, interactions and covariates present in the statistical model.

7. Predicted vs. residuals plot: This plot allows the user to check the homogeneity of variance assumption of the parametric analysis where appropriate (see Section 5.4.1.3).

8. Normal probability plot: This plot allows the user to check the normality assumption of the parametric analysis (see Section 5.4.1.2).

9. Least square (predicted) means: The Repeated Measures Parametric Analysis module produces a plot of the least square (predicted) means (with confidence intervals) of either the treatment factor across the levels of the repeated factor (if only a single between-animal factor is included in the analysis) or the highest-order interaction across the levels of the repeated factor (if multiple between-animal factors are included in the analysis).

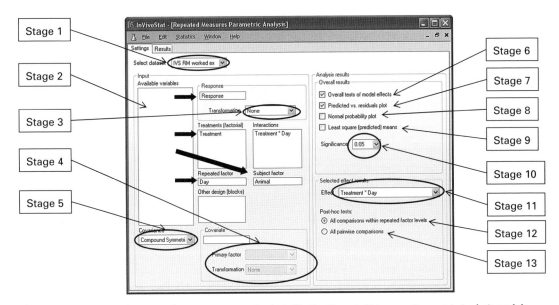

Figure 6.17. Screenshot illustrating the 13-stage process for the InVivoStat Repeated Measures Parametric Analysis module.

10. Significance level: The user can also choose the significance level for the tests, the default being 0.05 or 5%.

11. Selected effect: This is the effect the user wishes to investigate further.

12. All pairwise comparisons within repeated factor levels: This option produces all pairwise comparisons (within each level of the repeated factor) between the least square (predicted) means of the term corresponding to the Selected effect.

13. All pairwise comparisons: If the user wishes to assess how the individual factor levels change across the levels of the repeated factor, then the 'All pairwise comparisons' option should be selected. This option can potentially produce many pairwise tests, so only those comparisons planned in advance should be considered.

Output details

1. Response, covariance structure and covariate: InVivoStat identifies the response being analysed, the covariance structure used and also the covariate (if one is selected). This section also describes

any transformations that have been applied to the response and covariate.

2. Categorised case profile of the data: InVivoStat produces a categorised case profile of the data (see Section 5.3.4). The plot is categorised by either the treatment factor (if only a single between-animal factor is included in the analysis) or the levels of the highest-order treatment interaction (if multiple between-animal treatment factors are included in the statistical analysis).

3. Categorised scatterplot of the data: When fitting a covariate in a statistical analysis, certain assumptions are made (see Section 5.4.6.6). This plot allows the user to assess these assumptions. Given below the plot is a list of the assumptions and also advice on how the plot can be used to assess them. The scatterplot is categorised by the levels of the Primary factor at each level of the repeated factor.

4. Table of overall tests of model effects: The ANOVA-style table contains overall tests of the significance of the terms present in the statistical model. Any statistically significant results are described below the table.

5. Diagnostic plots: If requested InVivoStat produces the predicted vs. residuals plot and the normal probability plot. The residuals on the predicted vs. residuals plot are the standardised residuals as these provide a test for outliers (see Section 5.4.1.5). Any observation with a residual greater (or less than) three could be considered an outlier. Care should be taken though when using this plot as the within-animal variability is used in the calculation to standardise the residuals.

6. Plot of the least square (predicted) means: InVivoStat produces a plot and table of the predicted means of either the treatment factor at each level of the repeated factor (if only a single between-animal factor is included in the analysis) or the highest-order interaction at each level of the repeated factor (if multiple between-animal factors are included in the analysis). Also included on the plot are confidence intervals around the predicted means, calculated using the between-animal variability.

7. Pairwise comparisons on the least square (predicted) means: InVivoStat produces a table of all pairwise comparisons between the levels of the term corresponding to the Selected effect. This can be performed either at each level of the repeated factor or across the levels of the repeated factor. As well as the size of the difference between the means, and confidence intervals, InVivoStat also provides p-values to assess the significance of these differences. A list of statistically significant comparisons is given below the table.

8. References: Finally, references for the methods applied in the analysis are given.

6.4.2 Worked example

Consider an experiment where animals were administered one of three treatments (factor Treatment, levels: A, B and C). The response of each animal to the treatment was then measured once per day for 4 days (factor Day, levels: 1, 2, 3 and 4). The data were analysed using the Repeated Measures Parametric Analysis module. As the time points were equally spaced, it was assumed that the within-animal covariance structure was autoregressive. The options selected are highlighted in Figure 6.18.

Categorised case profiles plot

A categorised case profiles plot revealed a large treatment effect (Figure 6.19). It also revealed that each animal's response to treatment was stable over time. Perhaps a one-way ANOVA on the mean summary measure (the average of each animal's responses over the 4 days) could have been analysed instead.

Table 6.7 lists the tests of the overall model effects. There was a significant effect of Treatment ($F_{(2,6)} = 448.9$, $p < 0.001$) but no overall effect of Day ($F_{(3,18)} = 0.42$, $p = 0.742$) or any evidence that the effect of the treatment varied over time ($F_{(6,18)} = 1.35$, $p = 0.287$).

Using the approach described in Section 5.4.4.3, the Treatment factor was tested against the between-animal variability (denominator degrees of freedom is 6) whereas the Day factor and the Treatment by Day interaction were tested against the within-animal variability (denominator degrees of freedom is 18). We can see this by considering the total number of animals and days:

$$
\begin{aligned}
\text{Between-animal df} \quad &= \quad \text{No. of animals} \\
&\qquad - df_{\text{mean}} - df_{\text{Treatment}} \\
&= \quad 9 - 1 - 2 \\
&= \quad 6.
\end{aligned}
$$

$$
\begin{aligned}
\text{Within-animal df} \quad &= \quad \text{No. of animals} \times \\
&\qquad (\text{No. of time points} - 1) \\
&\qquad - df_{\text{Day}} - df_{\text{Treatment:Day}} \\
&= \quad 9 \times (4-1) - 3 - 6 \\
&= \quad 18.
\end{aligned}
$$

The predicted vs. residuals plot indicated there was no need to transform the data (see Figure 6.20). The variability appears similar across the range of the predicted values. The pairwise tests between treatments are given in Table 6.8. The tests revealed significant differences between the treatment means at all time points.

6.4.3 Technical details

Repeated measures analyses are carried out in InVivoStat using a mixed-model implementation within the nlme package in R (Pinheiro *et al.*, 2008). With this

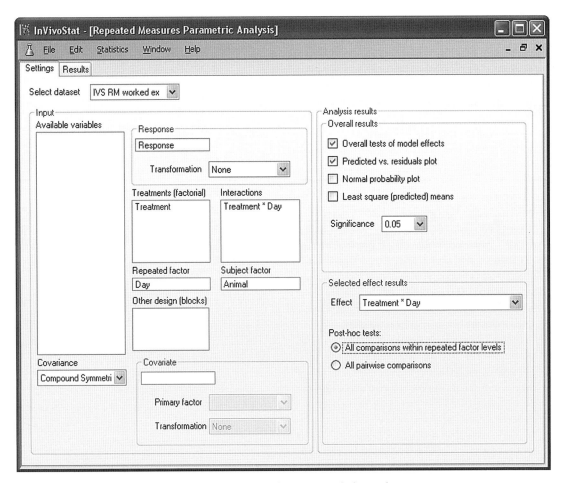

Figure 6.18. Screenshot of the options required for the repeated measures worked example.

analysis approach the researcher can take account of the spatial interrelationships between responses measured on the same animal. It should be noted that this is not the only way to analyse such data; see Crowder and Hand (1990) for other methods and software options available.

InVivoStat does not offer any multiple comparison adjustment procedures in the Repeated Measures Parametric Analysis module. This is for two reasons:

- Within a repeated measures analysis, if an automated procedure is used to calculate the adjusted p-values, then the family of tests that are adjusted for is likely to be larger than is required. For example, it is highly

unlikely that a comparison between the control group on day 1 and a treated group on day 7 will be of practical interest. Unless the researcher can define specifically which comparisons are of interest, then an automated procedure will adjust for all possible pairwise comparisons. This implies that the multiple comparison adjustment will be larger than it needs to be.

- As the observations measured within-animal are related, so will be the p-values for the group mean comparisons. This lack of independence in the tests may not be taken into account by an automated multiple comparison procedure.

Table 6.7. Overall tests of model effects

	Num. df	Den. df	F-value	p-value
Treatment	2	6	448.90	< 0.001
Day	3	18	0.42	0.742
Treatment:Day	6	18	1.35	0.287

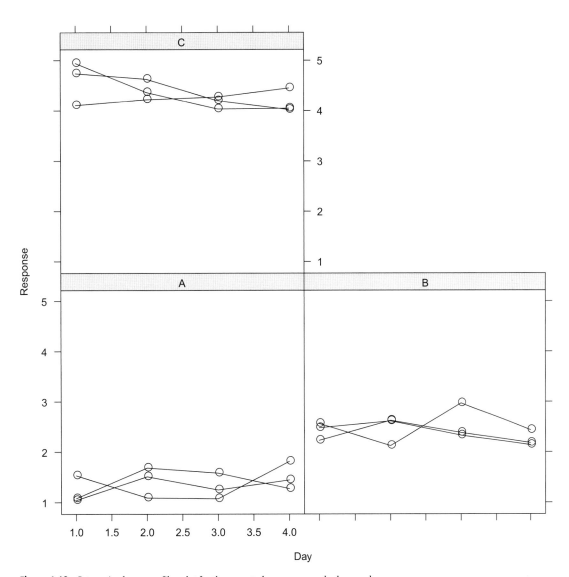

Figure 6.19. Categorised case profiles plot for the repeated measures worked example.

Table 6.8. Pairwise comparisons within the levels of the repeated factor

Comparison	Difference	Lower 95% CI	Upper 95% CI	Std error	p-value
1 : B vs. A	1.209	0.745	1.674	0.221	< 0.001
1 : C vs. A	3.377	2.913	3.841	0.221	< 0.001
2 : B vs. A	1.026	0.562	1.491	0.221	< 0.001
2 : C vs. A	2.975	2.511	3.440	0.221	< 0.001
3 : B vs. A	1.259	0.795	1.724	0.221	< 0.001
3 : C vs. A	2.867	2.402	3.331	0.221	< 0.001
4 : B vs. A	0.743	0.279	1.208	0.221	0.003
4 : C vs. A	2.663	2.199	3.128	0.221	< 0.001
1 : C vs. B	2.168	1.703	2.632	0.221	< 0.001
2 : C vs. B	1.949	1.485	2.413	0.221	< 0.001
3 : C vs. B	1.607	1.143	2.072	0.221	< 0.001
4 : C vs. B	1.920	1.455	2.384	0.221	< 0.001

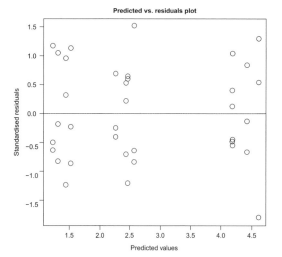

Figure 6.20. Predicted vs. residuals plot for the repeated measures worked example.

For a given Selected effect, InVivoStat will make all pairwise comparisons between the levels of the term corresponding to the Selected effect. The default option is only to make these comparisons within each level of the repeated factor, although there is an option to make comparisons across the levels of the repeated factor by generating all possible pairwise tests.

We recommend either:

- Use the unadjusted p-values themselves, as produced within the Repeated Measures Parametric Analysis module, but only use those that are of interest – the so-called planned comparisons.
- Adjust the p-values generated using the P-Value Adjustment module in InVivoStat (see Section 6.5).

6.5 *P*-Value Adjustment module

Within InVivoStat, the *P*-Value Adjustment module allows the researcher to apply a multiple comparison procedure to a set of unadjusted p-values. Available procedures include Holm, Hochberg, Hommel and Benjamini–Hochberg.

To begin with the researcher generates the unadjusted p-values using one of the other InVivoStat modules or

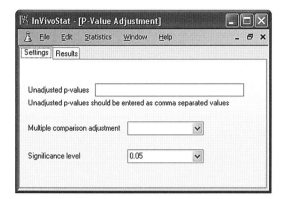

Figure 6.21. Screenshot of the InVivoStat *p*-Value Adjustment module interface.

perhaps another statistical software package. The *p*-values from this family of tests (see Section 5.4.8.2) are then adjusted using the procedure of choice. The size of the adjustment depends on the procedure selected and also the number of tests. The module therefore provides a flexible way of performing a multiple comparison procedure as it makes the requested adjustment based on the correct family of tests. Hence unlike other automated implementations it is not overly conservative as it does not adjust for too many comparisons. The interface is shown in Figure 6.21.

6.5.1 Analysis procedure

The analysis procedure is illustrated in Figure 6.22.

Input selection

1. Entering the *p*-values: The *p*-values are entered in the input box (comma separated and without spaces). The user can enter *p*-values of the form <0.001 and <0.0001 where necessary.

Output selection

2. Defining the procedure: The user then selects a procedure from the drop-down list.
3. Significance level: The user can also choose the significance level, the default being 0.05 or 5%.

Output details

The output contains a table of the adjusted and unadjusted *p*-values. If the user enters a *p*-value of the form <0.001 then the *P*-Value Adjustment module assumes the true *p*-value is 0.0009. This will give a slightly conservative adjusted *p*-value. A warning is given in the output to highlight that this approach has been taken.

6.5.2 Worked example

Consider an example where the researcher has calculated the unadjusted *p*-values as:

0.072, 0.211, <0.001 and 0.049

using the Single Measure Parametric Analysis module. It was decided that an adjustment to these *p*-values was required (to avoid making false positive conclusions) and the Hochberg procedure (at the 5% significance level) was selected. The family of tests to adjust for is therefore of size four. The results are given in Table 6.9.

The unadjusted *p*-value <0.001 was statistically significant at the 5% level, using the Hochberg procedure. However, consider the *p*-value of 0.049. Without adjustment this *p*-value was declared significant at the 5% level as $p < 0.05$. However, following adjustment it was not significant. Perhaps this was originally a false positive result.

Notice that the adjusted *p*-values for the second and third most significant comparisons are the same value. This is because when applying the Hochberg procedure, described in Section 5.4.8.7:

$$p_2' = 0.072 \times 2 = 0.144$$

and

$$p_3' = 0.049 \times 3 = 0.147.$$

Now clearly it is not sensible for the adjusted *p*-values to be in a different order (by size) to the unadjusted *p*-values. When this occurs it is common convention that both adjusted *p*-values are given the same numerical value (to preserve the original order).

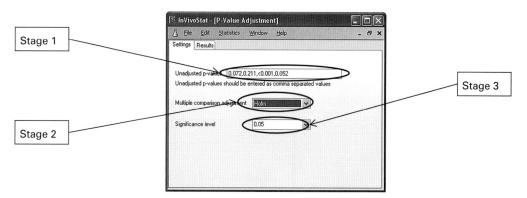

Figure 6.22. Screenshot illustrating the three-stage process for the InVivoStat *P*-Value Adjustment module.

Table 6.9. Unadjusted and adjusted *p*-values for the Hochberg procedure within the *P*-Value Adjustment module

	Unadjusted p-value	Adjusted p-value
1	<0.001	0.004
2	0.049	0.144
3	0.072	0.144
4	0.211	0.211

6.6 Non-Parametric Analysis module

The Non-Parametric Analysis module in InVivoStat is available from the Statistics drop-down menu entitled 'Non-Parametric Analysis'. The interface is given in Figure 6.23.

The Non-Parametric Analysis module performs the Kruskal–Wallis test, the Mann–Whitney test (also known as Wilcoxon rank sum test), Steel's all comparisons back to one test and the Behrens–Fisher all pairwise tests.

6.6.1 Analysis procedure

The analysis procedure is illustrated in Figure 6.24.

Input selection

1. Dataset selection: The analysis begins by selecting a dataset from the drop-down list of available imported datasets.

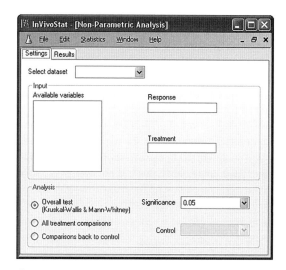

Figure 6.23. Screenshot of the InVivoStat Non-Parametric Analysis module interface.

2. Response and treatment variable selection: The response variable and the treatment factor are then selected from the 'Available variables' list by dragging and dropping the relevant variables into the 'Response' and 'Treatment' boxes.

Output selection

3. Overall comparison: This option produces an overall test of the differences between the treatment factor levels. This is either a Mann–Whitney test, if

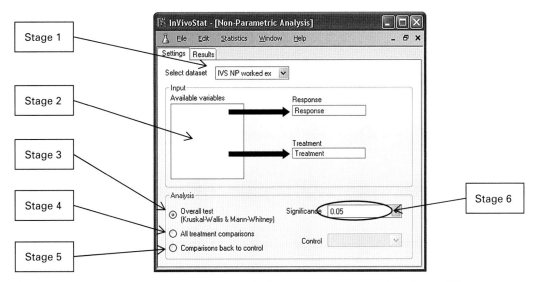

Figure 6.24. Screenshot illustrating the six-stage process for the InVivoStat Non-Parametric Analysis module.

Table 6.10. Summary statistics generated by the Non-Parametric Analysis module within InVivoStat

Group	Minimum	Q1	Median	Q3	Maximum
A	43.000	48.000	53.500	59.500	65.000
B	34.000	39.500	55.000	70.500	76.000
C	3.000	45.000	92.500	277.000	456.000
D	45.000	60.500	155.000	384.000	534.000

there are only two levels of the treatment factor, or a Kruskal–Wallis test otherwise.

4. All treatment comparisons: If this option is selected, then InVivoStat calculates the Behrens–Fisher all pairwise tests along with all pairwise Mann–Whitney tests.

5. Comparisons back to control: If selected, InVivoStat performs Steel's all comparisons back to one test. The user is required to select the control group from a drop-down list.

6. Significance level: The user can also choose the significance level for the tests, the default being 0.05 or 5%.

Output details

1. Summary statistics: InVivoStat produces a table of summary statistics including the median, the inter-quartile range (Q1 and Q3), the minimum observation and the maximum observation. Each row of the table corresponds to one of the levels of the treatment factor.

2. Box-plot: InVivoStat produces a box-plot of the data, as described in Section 5.3.2, categorised by the treatment factor.

3. Overall or pairwise tests: Depending on the option selected, a table of test results is generated. This is

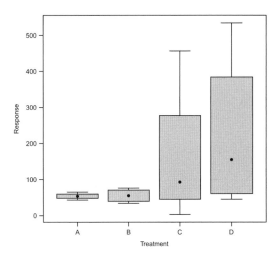

Figure 6.25. Box-plot generated using the InVivoStat Non-Parametric Analysis module.

a Kruskal–Wallis or Mann–Whitney test (depending on the number of levels of the treatment factor), the Behrens–Fisher all pairwise tests and all pairwise Mann–Whitney tests or Steel's all comparisons back to one test.

4. Conclusions: A summary of the conclusions of the analysis is given, at the selected significance level.
5. Description of analysis: A description of the analysis is presented.
6. References: Finally, references for the methods applied in the analysis are given.

6.6.2 Worked example

Consider an experiment involving four treatments (factor Treatment: levels A, B, C and D) administered to four animals per treatment. Due to concerns about the variability of the response, it was decided to analyse the data using the Non-Parametric Analysis module.

Summary data

The output from InVivoStat begins with a table of summary measures, giving an indication of the range of responses within each group. This includes the middle observation (the median), the minimum and maximum observation within each group and also the range

Table 6.11. Table of the overall test (Kruskal–Wallis test) to compare the treatment groups

	Test statistic	Degrees of freedom	p-value
Result	3.68	3	0.298

containing the middle 50% of the data (Q1 to Q3); see Table 6.10.

Box-plot

The values in Table 6.10 are illustrated using a box-plot (see Figure 6.25). The box-plot reveals the response variability is higher in treatment groups C and D.

Overall test

On selecting the Kruskal–Wallis overall comparison option, InVivoStat calculates the Kruskal–Wallis overall test of treatment effects. This test reveals that the overall difference between the treatments was not statistically significant ($p = 0.298$); see Table 6.11. Perhaps this was because the test lacked statistical power due to the small sample size. Performing a parametric analysis, perhaps following a log transformation of the response variable, may have been a more sensitive test.

All pairwise comparisons

We could also make pairwise comparisons between the treatment groups (Mann–Whitney tests) by selecting the 'All treatment comparisons' option. As expected none of the comparisons were statistically significant ($p \geq 0.189$); see Table 6.12.

6.7 Graphics module

The Graphics module allows the user to produce means with SEMs plots, scatterplots, box-plots, histograms and case profiles plots, as described in Section 5.3. The interface is shown in Figure 6.26.

6.7.1 Analysis procedure

The analysis procedure is illustrated in Figure 6.27.

Table 6.12. All pairwise comparison tests (Mann–Whitney tests) to compare the treatment groups

	Gp 1	vs.	Gp 2	p-value
Comparison				
1	A	vs.	B	1.000
2	A	vs.	C	0.312
3	A	vs.	D	0.194
4	B	vs.	C	0.312
5	B	vs.	D	0.189
6	C	vs.	D	0.885

Input selection

1. Dataset selection: The analysis begins by selecting a dataset from the drop-down list of available imported datasets.
2. Variable selection: Graphs are produced by dragging and dropping variables from the 'Available variables' list into the 'X-axis variable' box, the 'Response variable' box, and up to two categorisation factors into the categorisation factor boxes.
3. Response transformation: Once selected, the user can apply a transformation to the response: $\log_{10}$, $\log_e$, square root, rank or arcsine. If the X-axis variable is also numeric, then a transformation can be applied (independently) to this variable.
4. Categorisation format: If categorisation factors are selected, then the categorised plots can be displayed separately or overlaid (with or without a legend).

Output selection

5. The user selects the plots to be produced. Some example plots, and the options required to produce them, are given below.

6.7.2 Example plots

Figures 6.28 to 6.34 illustrate some of the plots that can be created by the Graphics module, alongside the options required to generate them.

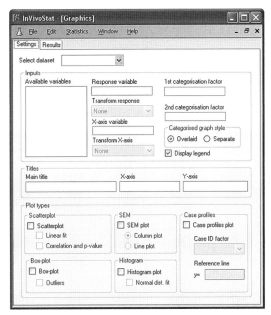

Figure 6.26. Screenshot of the InVivoStat Graphics module interface.

6.8 Power Analysis module

The Power Analysis module in InVivoStat is available from the Statistics drop-down menu entitled 'Power Analysis'. This module allows the user to perform power and sample size calculations to identify how many animals are required in future experiments, as described in Section 3.7.2. The interface is given in Figure 6.35.

6.8.1 Analysis procedure

Input selection

1. Estimating the mean and variance: To perform a power analysis an estimate of the mean and variance of the response is required. There are two ways this information can be entered into the Power Analysis module. The user can manually enter a control mean value and an estimate of the variability (the 'Supplied values'), or let InVivoStat calculate them directly from a dataset (the 'Dataset values').

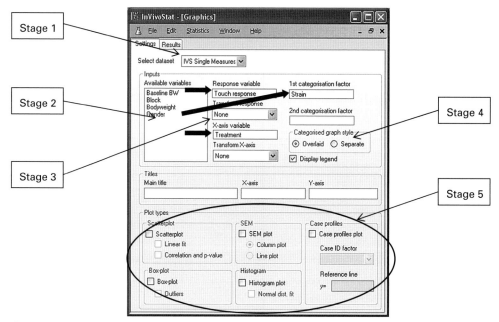

Figure 6.27. Screenshot illustrating the five-stage process for the InVivoStat Graphics module.

Supplied values

If the 'Supplied values' option is selected, then the user can enter an estimate of the mean and variance calculated using another module within InVivoStat or perhaps from another software package (Figure 6.36).

For example, if an ANOVA analysis has been performed (using the Single Measure Parametric Analysis module) then:

$$\text{sample variance} = MS_{\text{Residual}} = \frac{SS_{\text{Residual}}}{DF_{\text{Residual}}}, \qquad (6.1)$$

and

$$\text{sample standard deviation} = \sqrt{\text{sample variance}}. \qquad (6.2)$$

The user could also use other software, such as Excel, to calculate the sample standard deviation and the sample variance. If required, a control group mean (calculated outside the Power Analysis module) can also be entered at this stage.

Dataset values

The user can also let InVivoStat calculate the mean and variance of a response variable. Once the dataset

has been loaded into InVivoStat, then the 'Use variables from the dataset' option should be selected. The response variable is selected by dragging and dropping into the 'Response' box. The user can select a single treatment factor by dragging and dropping the single factor into the 'Treatment factor' box (see Figure 6.37).

The user can select a control group from the drop-down list of treatment factor levels. This is required if the biological differences considered are percentage changes from the control group mean.

2. Selecting the significance level: The user can also choose the significance level for the tests, the default being 0.05 or 5%.

Output selection

3. Plot settings – expected changes: The user will have to decide if the power calculation is performed for a percentage change from control (the 'Percent' option) or an actual change from control (the 'Absolute' option). In each case multiple differences can be entered, each difference separated by a comma.

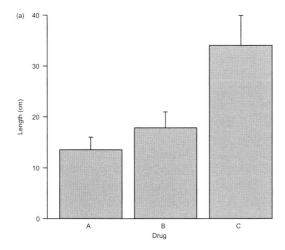

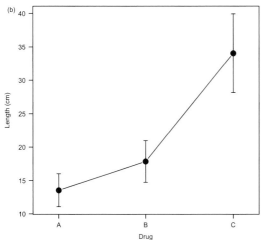

Figure 6.28. Examples of observed means with SEMs plots produced by InVivoStat. (a) Response variable: Length (numerical); *X*-axis variable: Drug (categorical); Plot type: SEM plot; Plot options: Column plot. (b) Response variable: Length (numerical); *X*-axis variable: Drug (categorical); Plot type: SEM plot; Plot options: Line plot.

To select percentage changes, the user must also specify either a control group mean (Supplied values) or a control group (Dataset values).

4. Plot settings – plotting range: The user has various options concerning the ranges of parameters investigated. Power calculations can be performed for a range of sample sizes (recommended). The default

is 6 to 15, although other values may be selected. Alternatively InVivoStat can calculate the range of sample sizes (for the user-defined expected changes) that achieve a desired power. This option can be useful if the purpose of the analysis is to find out how many animals would be required to achieve a target power, given the variability of the data and a certain biologically relevant effect.

5. Graph title: The user can select a title for the power curve plot.

Output details

1. Power curve plot: InVivoStat produces a plot of the power curves, as defined by the user, using the variability estimate.

2. Selected results: InVivoStat produces a text version of selected results from the power analysis.

3. Definitions: This module also provides some information about the statistical terminology used within the Power Analysis module.

4. References: Finally, references for the methods applied in the analysis are given.

6.8.2 Worked example

Assume an experiment was conducted using ten animals per group. The sample mean of the control group was estimated at 12.4 and the variance estimate of the responses was estimated at 3.32. The researcher wished to assess the sample size for future experiments. The size of the biologically relevant effect was thought to be around a 20% to 40% change from the control. The options required are presented in Figure 6.38.

The InVivoStat Power Analysis module was used to assess the sample sizes for 20%, 30% and 40% changes from control. The output from the module revealed that for a 40% change from control, given ten animals per group, the power of the study was around 80%. The power curve plot produced using these options is given in Figure 6.39.

If it was decided that a 20% change from control was biologically relevant, then the power of the study was low (< 50%), even with a sample size greater than 15

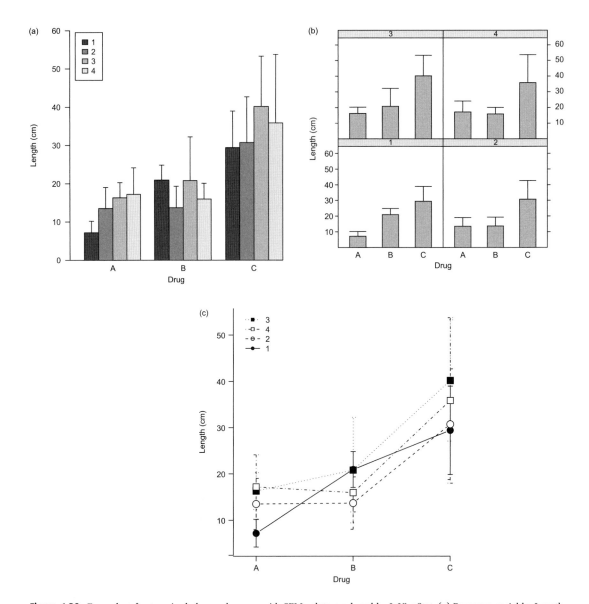

Figure 6.29. Examples of categorised observed means with SEMs plots produced by InVivoStat. (a) Response variable: Length (numerical); *X*-axis variable: Drug (categorical); First category factor: Day (categorical); Category graph option: Overlaid; Plot type: SEM plot; Plot options: Column plot. (b) Response variable: Length (numerical); *X*-axis variable: Drug (categorical); First category factor: Day (categorical); Category graph option: Separate; Plot type: SEM plot; Plot options: Column plot. (c) Response variable: Length (numerical); *X*-axis variable: Drug (categorical); First category factor: Day (categorical); Category graph option: Overlaid; Plot type: SEM plot; Plot options: Line plot.

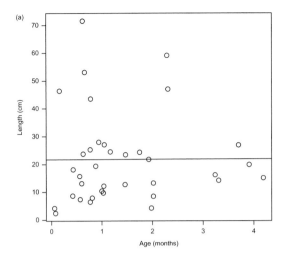

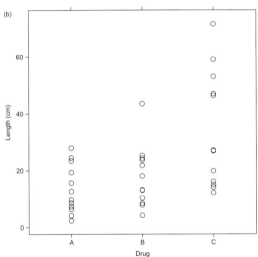

Figure 6.30. Examples of scatterplots produced by InVivoStat. (a) Response variable: Length (numerical); *X*-axis variable: Age (numerical); Plot type: Scatterplot; Plot options: Linear fit. (b) Response variable: Length (numerical); *X*-axis variable: Drug (categorical); Plot type: Scatterplot.

animals per group. This indicated that the researcher should try to find ways to reduce the variability, perhaps by using a blocking factor in the experimental design and analysis. If the variability cannot be reduced then the sample size would need to be increased, perhaps to unacceptably large numbers. The researcher could also try to increase the window of opportunity using a large

factorial design or ultimately choose a different animal model.

6.9 Unpaired *t*-test Analysis module

The Unpaired *t*-test Analysis module within InVivoStat is a tool for performing the unpaired *t*-test under the assumption of equal or unequal variances across the two groups. It is available within the Additional Analyses sub-menu of the Statistics drop-down menu. The interface is given in Figure 6.40.

6.9.1 Analysis procedure

The analysis procedure is illustrated in Figure 6.41.

Input selection

1. Dataset selection: The analysis begins by selecting a dataset from the drop-down list of available imported datasets.
2. Response and treatment variable selection: The response variable is dragged and dropped from the 'Available variables' list onto the 'Response' box and the treatment factor variable onto the 'Treatment' box. The treatment factor must consist of two levels.
3. Response transformation: Once selected, the user has the option of applying a transformation to the response: $\log_{10}$, $\log_e$, square root, rank or arcsine. Note if the variability is different between the two groups then we can perform the analysis under the assumption of unequal between-group variances, rather than perform a transformation.

Output selection

4. Equal variance case: If this option is selected, the unpaired *t*-test is performed using a single pooled estimate of the variability.
5. Unequal variance case: If this option is selected, the unpaired *t*-test is performed under the assumption that the variability is different across the two groups. This test is known as Welch's *t*-test.

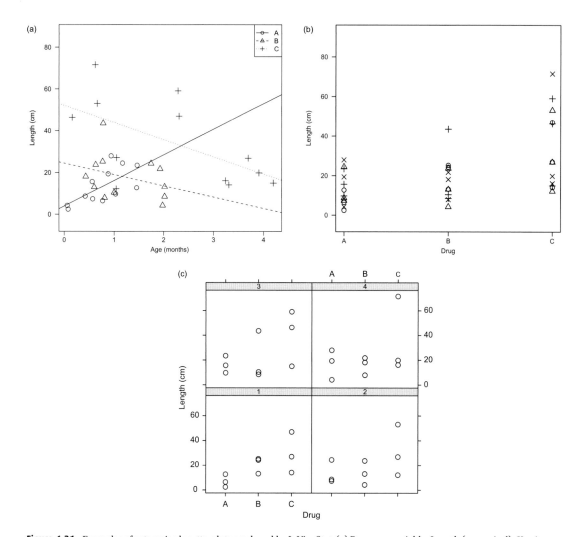

Figure 6.31. Examples of categorised scatterplots produced by InVivoStat. (a) Response variable: Length (numerical); X-axis variable: Age (numerical); First category factor: Drug; Category graph option: Overlaid; Plot type: Scatterplot; Plot options: Linear fit. (b) Response variable: Length (numerical); X-axis variable: Drug (categorical); First category factor: Day; Category graph option: Overlaid; Plot type: Scatterplot. (c) Response variable: Length (numerical); X-axis variable: Drug (categorical); First category factor: Day; Category graph option: Separate; Plot type: Scatterplot.

6. Predicted vs. residuals plot: This plot allows the user to check the homogeneity of variance assumption of the parametric analysis (applicable if equal variances are assumed).
7. Normal probability plot: This plot allows the user to check the normality assumption of the parametric t-test analysis.

8. Significance: The user can also choose the significance level for the test, the default being 0.05 or 5%.

Output details

1. Response: This text contains information about the response selected for analysis.

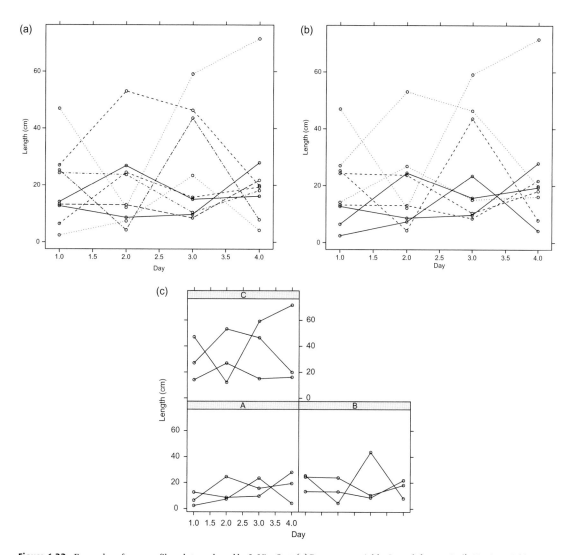

Figure 6.32. Examples of case profiles plot produced by InVivoStat. (a) Response variable: Length (numerical); *X*-axis variable: Day (continuous); Plot type: Case profiles plot; Case ID factor: Animal. (b) Response variable: Length (numerical); *X*-axis variable: Day (continuous); First category factor: Drug; Category graph option: Overlaid; Plot type: Case profiles plot; Plot options: Display legend deselected; Case ID factor: Animal. (c) Response variable: Length (numerical); *X*-axis variable: Day (continuous); First category factor: Drug; Category graph option: Separate; Plot type: Case profiles plot; Case ID factor: Animal.

2. Scatterplot of the data: This plot of the data allows the user to see if there are any outliers in the dataset.

3. Unpaired *t*-test assuming equal variances: If selected, this table contains the results of the unpaired *t*-test (assuming equal variances). Also

given is a table of the least square (predicted) means with confidence intervals.

4. Unpaired *t*-test assuming unequal variances: If selected, this table contains the results of the unpaired *t*-test (assuming unequal variances). Also

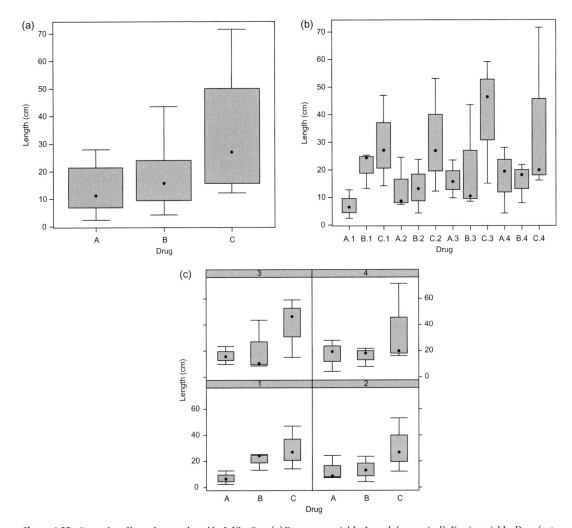

Figure 6.33. Examples of box-plots produced by InVivoStat. (a) Response variable: Length (numerical); *X*-axis variable: Drug (categorical); Plot type: Box-plot. (b) Response variable: Length (numerical); *X*-axis variable: Drug (categorical); First category factor: Day (categorical); Category graph option: Overlaid; Plot type: Box-plot. (c) Response variable: Length (numerical); *X*-axis variable: Drug (categorical); First category factor: Day (categorical); Category graph option: Separate; Plot type: Box-plot.

given is a table of the least square (predicted) means with confidence intervals.

5. Diagnostic plots: If requested InVivoStat produces the predicted vs. residuals plot and the normal probability plot. The residuals plotted on the predicted vs. residuals plot are the externally Studentised residuals as these can provide a test for outliers. Any observation with an externally Studentised residual greater (or less than) three could be considered an outlier.

6. References: Finally, references for the methods applied in the analysis are given.

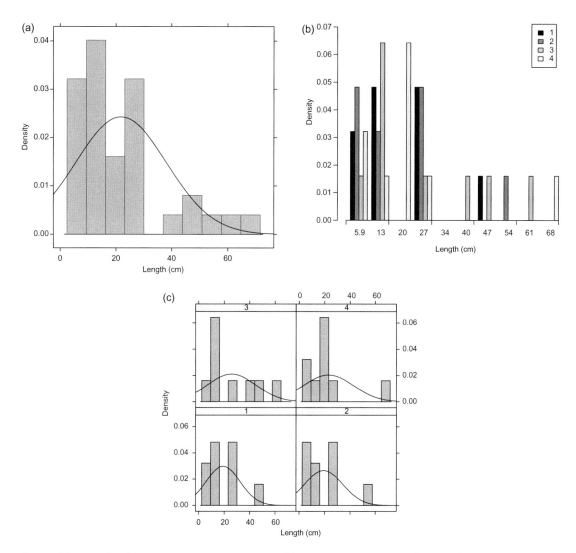

Figure 6.34. Examples of histograms produced by InVivoStat. (a) Response variable: Length (numerical); Plot type: Histogram; Plot options: Normal distribution fit. (b) Response variable: Length (numerical); First category factor: Drug (categorical); Category graph option: Overlaid; Plot type: Histogram. (c) Response variable: Length (numerical); First category factor: Drug (categorical); Category graph option: Separate; Plot type: Histogram; Plot options: Normal distribution fit.

6.9.2 Worked example

Consider an experiment that involved a treatment (factor Treatment, levels: A and B) with 12 animals per group. Each animal was administered either treatment A or B. A scatterplot of the data revealed a clear treatment effect; the variability appeared to be similar across the two groups (see Figure 6.42).

The unpaired *t*-test assuming equal variances revealed a significant treatment effect (see Table 6.13).

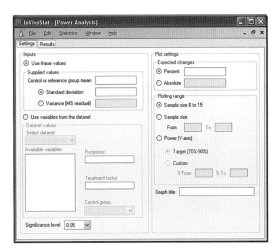

Figure 6.35. Screenshot of the InVivoStat Power Analysis module interface.

As the spread of responses was similar across the two treatment groups, the results of Welch's *t*-test, assuming unequal variances, were similar to the test performed assuming equal variances (see Table 6.14).

6.10 Paired *t*-test/within-subject Analysis module

The Paired *t*-test/within-subject Analysis module in InVivoStat is a tool for performing paired *t*-tests and, more generally, within-subject analyses where more than two treatments are administered to each of the animals. It is available within the Additional Analyses sub-menu of the Statistics drop-down menu. It fits models that consist of a single repeated factor and optionally other design (blocking) factors and a single covariate. This module can be used to analyse data generated using dose-escalation designs (see Section 3.8.2). Note if the experimental design also includes between-animal factors of interest, then the Repeated Measures Parametric Analysis module should be used instead.

This module performs a paired *t*-test when the repeated (treatment) factor consists of two levels. For the case where the number of levels of the repeated

(treatment) factor is greater than two, the module performs a within-subject repeated measures analysis. In both cases InVivoStat uses a repeated measures mixed-model analysis approach. If any individual animal is missing an observation, then the remaining observation(s) for that animal will be included in the analysis. The interface is shown in Figure 6.43.

6.10.1 Analysis procedure

The analysis procedure is illustrated in Figure 6.44.

Input selection

1. Dataset selection: The analysis begins by selecting a dataset from the drop-down list of available imported datasets.
2. Response, treatment and subject variables: The user can select the variables to include in the analysis by dragging and dropping them from the 'Available variables' list into the 'Response', 'Treatment factor', 'Other design (blocks)', 'Covariate' and 'Subject factor' boxes.
3. Response transformation: Once selected, the user has the option of applying a transformation to the response: $\log_{10}$, $\log_e$, square root, rank or arcsine. If selected the covariate will be transformed using the same transformation as the response, although this can be changed manually if required.
4. Covariance structure: Finally the user can select a covariance structure to account for the spatial interrelationships between the within-subject observations. The default option is the compound symmetric structure (all observations within-subject are equally correlated). Other options include autoregressive (recommended if the repeated factor is time-related and the time points are equally spaced) or unstructured (recommended if the sample sizes are not too small).

Output selection

5. Overall tests of statistical model effects: This option produces overall tests of the significance of the terms present in the statistical model.

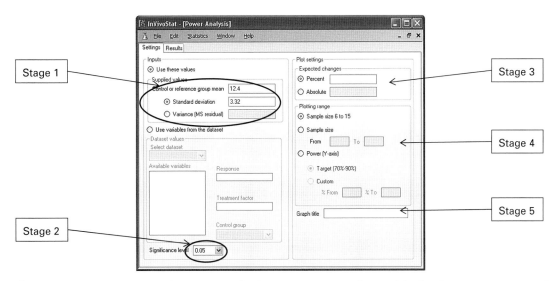

Figure 6.36. Screenshot illustrating the input options for the InVivoStat Power Analysis module when the user enters a mean and standard deviation manually. The significance level is set at the default (5%).

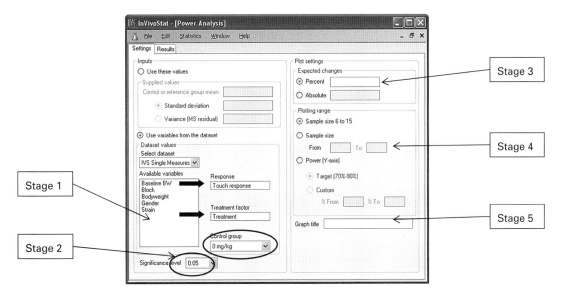

Figure 6.37. Screenshot illustrating the input options for the InVivoStat Power Analysis module when the module is required to calculate the mean and variance estimates from a dataset. The user selects the response variable , the treatment variable (optional), the control group (optional) and the significance level (default 5%).

6. Predicted vs. residuals plot: This plot allows the user to check the homogeneity of variance assumption of the parametric analysis, when required.

7. Normal probability plot: This plot allows the user to check the normality assumption of the parametric analysis.

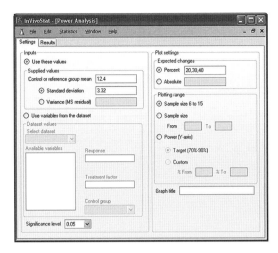

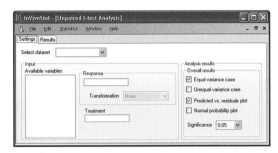

Figure 6.40. Screenshot of the InVivoStat Unpaired *t*-test Analysis module interface.

Figure 6.38. Options required by the InVivoStat Power Analysis module with sample mean 12.4, standard deviation 3.23 with power curves for 20%, 30% and 40% change from control.

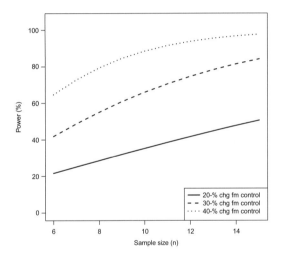

Figure 6.39. Power curves created by the InVivoStat Power Analysis module with sample mean 12.4, standard deviation 3.23 with power curves for 20%, 30% and 40% change from control.

8. Least square (predicted) means: The module produces a plot of the least square (predicted) means (with confidence intervals) of the levels of the repeated factor.

9. Significance level: The user can also choose the significance level for the tests, the default being 0.05 or 5%.

Output details

1. Response, covariance structure and covariate: InVivoStat identifies the response being analysed, the covariance structure used and also the covariate (if one is selected). This section also describes any transformations that have been applied.

2. Case profiles plot of the data: InVivoStat produces a case profiles plot of the data (see the Graphics module in Section 6.7).

3. Categorised scatterplot of the data: When fitting a covariate in a statistical analysis, certain assumptions are made. This plot allows the user to assess these assumptions. A list of the assumptions is shown below the plot and also advice on how the plot should be used to assess them.

4. Overall tests of model effects table: The ANOVA-style table contains overall tests of the significance of the repeated factor and the covariate, if selected. Below the table any statistically significant results are described.

5. Diagnostic plots: If requested InVivoStat produces the predicted vs. residuals plot and the normal probability plot. The residuals plotted on the predicted vs. residuals plot are the standardised residuals as these can provide a test for outliers. Any observation with a standardised residual greater (or less than) three could be considered an outlier.

6. Plot of the least square (predicted) means: InVivoStat produces a plot and table of the predicted means of the repeated factor. Also included on the plot are confidence intervals around the predicted means.

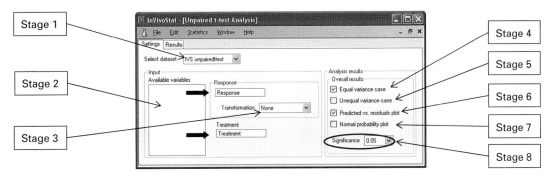

Figure 6.41. Screenshot illustrating the eight-stage process for the InVivoStat Unpaired *t*-test Analysis module.

Table 6.13. Unpaired *t*-test (assuming equal variance)

	t-statistic	Degrees of Freedom	p-value
Equal variance unpaired t-test	-10.124	22	< 0.001

Table 6.14. Unpaired *t*-test (assuming unequal variance)

	t-statistic	Degrees of Freedom	p-value
Unequal variance unpaired t-test	-10.124	21.90	< 0.001

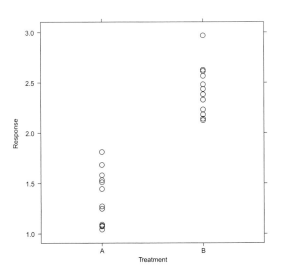

Figure 6.42. Scatterplot of the data, produced by the InVivoStat Unpaired *t*-test Analysis module.

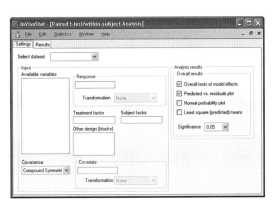

Figure 6.43. Screenshot of the InVivoStat Paired *t*-test/within-subject Analysis module interface.

7. Pairwise comparisons on the least square (predicted) means: InVivoStat produces a table of all pairwise comparisons of the predicted means of the repeated

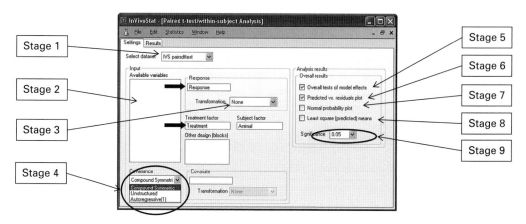

Figure 6.44. Screenshot illustrating the nine-stage process for the InVivoStat Paired *t*-test/within-subject Analysis module.

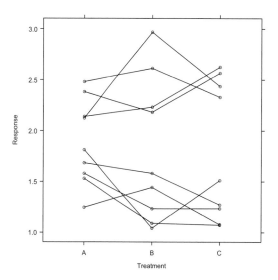

Figure 6.45. Case profiles plot produced by the Paired *t*-test/within-subject Analysis module.

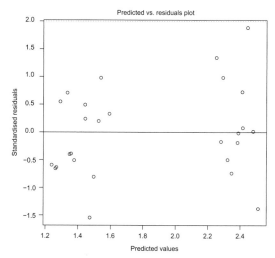

Figure 6.46. Predicted vs. residuals plot produced by the Paired *t*-test/within-subject Analysis module.

Table 6.15. Overall test between the three treatment means

	Num. df	Den. df	F-value	p-value
Treatment	2	16	0.28	0.762

factor. As well as the size of the difference between the means and the confidence intervals, InVivoStat also provides *p*-values to assess the significance of these differences. A list of statistically significant comparisons is given below the table.

8. References: Finally, references for the methods applied in the analysis are given.

6.10.2 Worked example

Consider an experiment where animals were administered three treatments (factor Treatment, levels: A, B and C) in a non-random order. The data were analysed using the Paired *t*-test/within-subject Analysis module. A case profiles plot (Figure 6.45) revealed little evidence of a treatment effect, although there appeared to be two

Table 6.16. All pairwise comparisons, without adjustment for multiplicity

Comparison	Difference	Lower 95% CI	Upper 95% CI	Std error	p-value
B vs. A	−0.066	−0.345	0.212	0.131	0.620
C vs. A	−0.095	−0.374	0.183	0.131	0.479
C vs. B	−0.029	−0.307	0.250	0.131	0.830

sub-populations in the data that could mask any real effect.

There was no overall treatment effect ($F_{(2,16)} = 0.28$, $p = 0.762$); see Table 6.15. The predicted vs. residuals plot indicated there was some evidence of a need to transform the data (Figure 6.46). However, for the purposes of illustration we shall not consider this further. None of the pairwise comparisons were statistically significant, although investigating the cause of the two sub-populations may be of more interest than testing the differences between the three treatments (see Table 6.16).

6.11 Dose-Response Analysis module

The Dose-Response Analysis module in InVivoStat is available from the Statistics drop-down menu entitled 'Dose-Response Analysis'. This module allows the user to fit four-parameter logistic curves to the data, as described in Section 3.6.1. It also has additional functionality for the analysis of data generated from quantitative research assays. Finally other non-linear curves can be fitted using the 'User defined equation' option. The interface is given in Figure 6.47.

6.11.1 Technical details on curve fitting

When modelling the dose-response relationship using a non-linear curve, the researcher must first select the type of curve to fit to the data. For example, the type of curve could be logistic, exponential or quadratic. The choice should reflect either:

- The relationship observed in the data. This can be obtained from a scatterplot of the data.

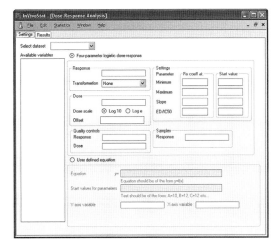

Figure 6.47. Screenshot of the InVivoStat Dose-Response Analysis module interface.

- The theoretical relationship based on known biological mechanisms. For example, if we know the responses increase exponentially as we increase the dose of the compound, then it is sensible to try to fit an exponential curve to the data.

Once the type of curve has been selected, then the actual curve fitted to the data will depend on the numerical value of the parameters that define the curve. For example, you may decide to fit a four-parameter logistic curve to your data, but the actual curve will depend on the numerical values of the four parameters that define the curve.

The Dose-Response Analysis module uses the *nls* algorithm in R to determine the non-linear (weighted) least squares estimates of the parameters that define the fitted curve. The non-linear (weighted) least squares algorithm works iteratively to generate a solution. The process involves a series of stages:

1. To begin with the type of non-linear curve to fit to the data has to be selected by the user.
2. Once the type has been selected, a curve is superimposed on the data using a set of arbitrary *start values* for the parameters that define the curve. The start values can either be generated automatically by InVivoStat or chosen by the user.
3. The *nls* algorithm will then search for a new set of parameters that define a curve that is a better fit to the data (i.e. the residuals from the model fit are smaller). Usually the algorithm goes through a series of stages (iteratively) slowly improving the fit of the curve to the data until no improvements are possible. InVivoStat uses the Gauss–Newton algorithm to search intelligently for curves that are a better fit to the data.

6.11.2 Fitting logistic curves to data

The Dose-Response Analysis module can be used to fit logistic curves to data that have been generated, for example, using a dose-response design (as described in Section 3.6.1). The logistic equation employed by InVivoStat is:

$$\text{Response} = D + \frac{(A - D)}{\left(1 + \left(10^{\log_{10}(Dose) - C}\right)^{B}\right)} \tag{6.3}$$

where A is the maximum, D is the minimum, C is the log D_{50} (an estimate of the dose that causes a 50% increase (or decrease) in response on the log scale) and B is the Hill slope. Note the definitions of A and D are interchangeable, depending on the sign of the Hill slope parameter B.

Within the Dose-Response Analysis module the user has several options when fitting a logistic curve:

Select the start values Sometimes the algorithm does not converge or converges to an obviously incorrect solution (when using the default start values). For example, if the underlying relationship between response and dose is masked by the response variability or if the type of curve chosen is not an appropriate

one. The user can select a set of start values so that the initial curve is already a good fit to the data.

Fix some of the parameters Sometimes the user may wish to fix some of the parameters. In particular, the minimum and/or the maximum of the curve can sometimes be fixed due to practical constraints.

Choose an offset for the dose axis As discussed above in Section 3.6.3, it is not possible to include a zero (control) group if the doses are transformed onto the log scale. By default InVivoStat will add a small offset onto the individual doses to allow the zero (control) dose to be included in the analysis. This default offset is either:

(lowest non-zero dose)/10   (for analyses on the $\log_{10}$ scale)
(lowest non-zero dose)/e (for analyses on the $\log_e$ scale)

If the user wishes to apply a different offset, then this should be carried out prior to importing the dataset into InVivoStat. Once imported this offset will need to be defined within the Dose-Response Analysis module so that the correct back-transformed D_{50} estimates can be calculated.

6.11.3 Analysis of quantitative assays

The Dose-Response Analysis module can be used to analyse results generated from quantitative assays where the underlying response/concentration relationship is logistic. The analysis involves a series of stages:

Standard curve calibration

The analysis begins by estimating the standard curve using responses generated from known concentrations of the analyte. In the Dose-Response Analysis module it is assumed that the standard curve is an example of a logistic curve. This stage of the process follows the approach discussed in the previous section.

Quality controls

Quality control (QC) samples may also be included in the assay to assess the reliability of the standard curve.

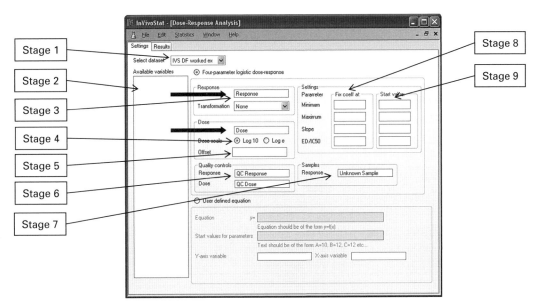

Figure 6.48. Screenshot illustrating the nine-stage process when using the InVivoStat Dose-Response Analysis module.

They are independent samples of known nominal concentration and are not used to calibrate the standard curve. QC responses (usually assessed in triplicate at each known concentration) are individually back-calculated onto the standard curve and then the triplicates for each concentration are averaged (on the log scale). These mean QC estimates (on the log scale) are then back-transformed onto the original scale to allow comparison between the nominal and the predicted QC concentrations.

It is also standard practice to use predefined assay-dependent acceptance criteria, based on the summary statistics of the estimated QC concentrations, to decide if the assay is fit for purpose. Some of these calculations can be performed within the Dose-Response Analysis module. Acceptance criteria calculated by InVivoStat include the percentage relative error:

$$\%RE = 100 \times \frac{\left(\text{Predicted concentration} - \text{Nominal concentration}\right)}{\text{Nominal concentration}} \quad (6.4)$$

and the percentage coefficient of variation:

$$\%CV = \frac{100 \times \text{PSD}}{\text{Predicted concentration}} \quad (6.5)$$

where $\text{PSD} = \sqrt{10^{2\bar{\mu}} \times 10^{s^2} \left(10^{s^2} - 1\right)}$ is the standard deviation of the predicted concentration mean (also known as the geometric standard deviation), $\bar{\mu}$ is the estimate of the predicted concentration on the log scale and s^2 is the associated variance estimate also on the log scale.

Unknown sample assessment

Assuming the assay passes the acceptance criteria on the QC samples, the unknown sample results are back-calculated onto the standard curve to estimate the concentration of the unknown samples.

6.11.4 Analysis procedure

The analysis procedure is illustrated in Figure 6.48. Stages 1 to 5, 8 and 9 are required when fitting a logistic curve to data. Stages 6 and 7 are required when analysing quantitative assays.

Table 6.17. Dataset in the format required for the analysis of a quantitative assay using the Dose-Response Analysis module

Standard response	Standard concentration	Unknown sample response	QC response	QC concentration
0.99	0	2.14	8.25	0.08
0.71	0	6.82	7.41	0.08
1.25	0	4.01	8.11	0.08
1.60	0.001	2.63	6.40	0.03
0.44	0.001	6.27	9.10	0.03
1.25	0.001	7.25	8.30	0.03
3.54	0.01	9.75	4.31	0.01
3.42	0.01	2.88	4.56	0.01
5.29	0.01	10.24	3.61	0.01
7.70	0.1	0.47		
8.88	0.1	0.28		
10.20	0.1			
9.93	1			

Input dataset

The dataset consists of variables that define the response and the corresponding dose or concentration. In quantitative assays these correspond to the response and the known concentration of the standards. There may also be variables in the dataset containing the unknown sample responses, the QC responses and the corresponding QC concentrations. An example is given in Table 6.17.

Input selection

1. Dataset selection: The analysis begins by selecting a dataset from the drop-down list of available imported datasets.
2. Selecting the response and dose/concentration variables: The user selects the response and dose/concentration variables by dragging and dropping variables from the 'Available variables' list into the relevant boxes.
3. Response transformation: Once selected, the user has the option of applying a transformation to the response variable: $\log_{10}$, $\log_e$, square root, rank or arcsine.
4. Dose scale: Doses and concentrations are usually selected so that they are equally spaced on an increasing logarithmic scale, for example 0.01, 0.1, 1 and 10 mg/kg. The user can select the log scale that

will be used to transform the dose variable (either $\log_{10}$ or $\log_e$) by selecting the correct 'Dose scale' option.

5. Defining the offset: As discussed in Section 3.6.3.3, InVivoStat adds an offset onto all the dose variable values prior to log transformation to allow the zero (control) group to be included on the log dose scale. However, if the user wishes to apply a different offset to the dose variable, then this should be added to the dose variable prior to importing the dataset into InVivoStat. The offset must then be defined in the 'Offset' box to: (1) inform InVivoStat that an offset has already been added and the addition of the default offset is not required and (2) allow InVivoStat to back-calculate the X_{50} estimate onto the original scale correctly.

6. Selecting the quality controls: The user can select QCs to assess the reliability of the estimate of the standard curve. The QC response and QC concentration variables are selected by dragging and dropping into the relevant boxes. Both a QC response and QC concentration variable are required for the QC assessment to proceed. Any user-defined transformation applied to the response variable will also be applied to the QC response variable. It is also assumed that any offset that has been manually added to the

concentration variable has also been applied to the QC concentration variable.

7. Selecting the unknown samples: The variable containing the unknown samples (that need to be back-calculated onto the standard curve) can be selected by dragging and dropping the variable into the 'Samples' box. Any transformation applied to the response variable will also be applied to the variable containing the unknown samples.

8. Fixing the logistic curve parameters: The user has the option to fix some of the parameters (by populating the 'Fix coeff. at' boxes). This allows greater flexibility in the choice of logistic curve that can be fitted to the data. It is common practice to fix the plateaux of the curve, for example the minimum plateau is fixed at 0% and/or the maximum plateau is fixed at 100%.

9. Selecting the start values: As discussed above the non-linear (weighted) least squares algorithm requires a set of start values for the parameters for the iteration process. The default choice of start values for the unknown parameters (calculated within the module) should be sufficient for the process to fit a curve to the data, especially if the analysis involves calibrating a standard curve. However, in certain cases the user may need to use specific start values by populating the 'Start value' boxes with start values that are close to the final parameters.

Output details

The output from the module may include:

1. A description of the analysis performed.
2. A scatterplot of the response variable vs. the dose/concentration variable.
3. A scatterplot of the response variable vs. the dose/concentration variable, including the fitted curve. Also included on the plot are any QC samples.
4. A table of curve parameter estimates.
5. A table of the back-transformed X_{50} estimate along with 95% confidence intervals.
6. A table of the back-calculated QC samples with %RE and %CV acceptance criteria.
7. A table of the predicted back-calculated unknown sample concentrations.

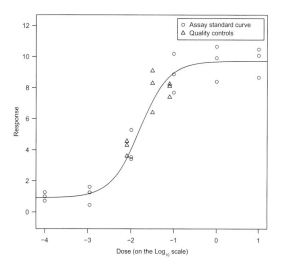

Figure 6.49. Scatterplot of the response vs. concentration (on the $\log_{10}$ scale) for the standards and the QC samples with the best-fit logistic curve.

6.11.5 Worked example: a biological assay

An assay was conducted to estimate the amount of compound absorbed into the rat bloodstream. A standard curve for the assay was composed using known standards and this curve was used to back-calculate the concentration of the compound in the unknown samples collected from the rat.

Responses were measured in triplicate at five concentrations of the standard (0.001, 0.01, 0.1, 1 and 10 mg/kg) and control (0 mg/kg). Using these responses a standard curve for the assay was estimated. Three quality control samples (with a known concentration of 0.01, 0.03 and 0.08 mg/kg), each assayed in triplicate, were tested to assess the reliability of the standard curve. The acceptance criteria were set at 20% for both the %RE and %CV (in other words the estimated %RE and %CV need to be less than 20% for the assay to be deemed valid). Also included in the dataset were a number of unknown samples.

A scatterplot of the data, including the predicted standard curve, revealed a reasonable fit to the data (see Figure 6.49). The QC samples, however, appeared to question the validity of the standard curve. For example, the 0.01 mg/kg QC had a relative error of 30.13%

Table 6.18. Summary statistics of the quality controls

True QC mean	Back-calculated QC mean	Std dev of back-calculated QC mean	No. of back-calculated QCs	Relative error (%)	Coefficient of variation (%)
0.008	0.010	0.001	3	30.13	12.90
0.032	0.055	0.036	3	72.41	66.60
0.079	0.047	0.007	3	-41.10	15.99

and a coefficient of variation of 12.90%. The first of these values was greater than 20%, and hence the assay failed the predefined acceptance criteria. The other QC samples are even more questionable with a %RE of 72% and 41% (see Table 6.18).

If the QC samples had passed the predefined acceptance criteria then the researcher could have considered the back-calculated unknown sample concentrations (see Table 6.19). Note some of the back-calculated concentrations were not computed. They are denoted by 'NaN'. This was because they were outside the estimated minimum/maximum range of the standard curve.

6.11.6 User-defined equation option

Rather than fit a logistic curve to the data, the user has the option of entering a different equation in the 'User defined equation' boxes (see Figure 6.50). The equation should be entered in the form:

$$y = f(x) \tag{6.6}$$

Every unknown parameter in the equation has to have a corresponding start parameter. This is entered in the 'Start values for parameters' box and should be entered as a comma separated list of the form:

$$A = 1, B = 1, C = 1$$

The user must also define the response (Y-axis) variable and the X-axis variable by dragging and dropping variables into the relevant boxes.

The output includes a table of unknown parameter estimates (that define the user-defined non-linear curve) and a plot of the observations with the predicted curve fitted to the data. If InVivoStat fails to generate any output then this may be because:

Table 6.19. Back-calculated unknown samples

Sample ID	Sample response	Back-calculated response
1	2.1418	0.004
2	6.8183	0.028
3	4.0096	0.010
4	2.6323	0.005
5	6.2721	0.022
6	7.2454	0.033
7	9.7476	NaN
8	2.8806	0.006
9	10.2398	NaN
10	0.4717	NaN
11	0.2760	NaN

- The start values for the unknown parameters are not sufficiently close to the true curve parameter estimates. Try different start values.
- The type of curve selected by the user does not explain the relationship between the response and the X-axis variable. Perhaps an alternative type of curve is more appropriate. Use the Graphics module to produce a scatterplot of the data to investigate which type of non-linear curve is appropriate.

6.12 Chi-squared Test and Fisher's Exact Test module

The Chi-squared Test and Fisher's Exact Test module within InVivoStat is a tool for analysing proportions, as discussed in Section 5.5.2. It is available within the

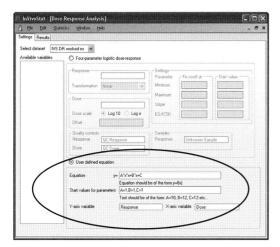

Figure 6.50. Screenshot of the options required for the user-defined equation within the InVivoStat Dose-Response Analysis module.

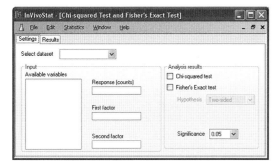

Figure 6.51. Screenshot of the InVivoStat Chi-squared Test and Fisher's Exact Test module interface.

Additional Analyses sub-menu of the Statistics drop-down menu. This module performs a one-sided chi-squared test and a one- or two-sided Fisher's exact test. The interface is given in Figure 6.51.

6.12.1 Analysis procedure

Input dataset

The dataset for this module can be created in the format of a contingency table, where the individual animals are grouped into categories. An example is given

Table 6.20. Contingency table for an experiment involving two treatments where the animals were categorised by the severity of their condition

Treatment	Condition	Count
vehicle	mild	5
vehicle	moderate	3
vehicle	severe	2
drug	mild	2
drug	moderate	4
drug	severe	4

in Table 6.20. In this experiment there were ten animals per group. The condition of each animal was defined as mild, moderate or severe, depending on the disease severity. Alternatively the dataset for this experiment can consist of one row per animal (see Table 6.21). Note this format requires the inclusion of a 'Count' variable consisting of all ones. Either format can be analysed by the InVivoStat Chi-squared Test and Fisher's Exact Test module. The analysis procedure is illustrated in Figure 6.52.

Input selection

1. Dataset selection: The analysis begins by selecting a dataset from the drop-down list of available imported datasets.
2. Variable selection: The (count) response variable is dragged and dropped from the 'Available variables' list onto the 'Response (counts)' box. The two variables that define the experimental groups and the response categories are then dragged and dropped onto the 'First factor' and 'Second factor' boxes (it is not important which variable is assigned to which box).

Output selection

The user has several choices for the analysis.
3. Chi-squared test: Select this option to perform the chi-squared test of association.
4. Fisher's exact test: Select this option to perform the Fisher's exact test of association.

Table 6.21. Individual animal data for an experiment involving two treatments where the animals were categorised by the severity of their condition

Treatment (individual)	Condition (individual)	Count (individual)	Animal
vehicle	mild	1	1
vehicle	mild	1	2
vehicle	mild	1	3
vehicle	mild	1	4
vehicle	mild	1	5
vehicle	moderate	1	6
vehicle	moderate	1	7
vehicle	moderate	1	8
vehicle	severe	1	9
vehicle	severe	1	10
drug	mild	1	11
drug	mild	1	12
drug	moderate	1	13
drug	moderate	1	14
drug	moderate	1	15
drug	moderate	1	16
drug	severe	1	17
drug	severe	1	18
drug	severe	1	19
drug	severe	1	20

5. Hypothesis: This option allows the user to perform either a one-sided or two-sided Fisher's exact test when the response consists of two categories and there are only two experimental groups in the experimental design.
6. Significance: The user can also choose the significance level for the tests, the default being 0.05 or 5%.

Output details

1. Response: This text contains information about the response variable and the variables used to categorise the responses.
2. Contingency table of counts: This table contains a summary of the observed counts, categorised by the two variables that define the experimental groups and response categories.
3. Table of expected counts: This table contains the counts that you would expect to see, given the row and column totals in the table, if the null hypothesis

of no association between the response categories and the experimental groups is true.
4. Chi-squared test: If selected, this table contains the chi-squared test result.
5. Fisher's exact test: If selected, this table contains the Fisher's exact test result.
6. References: Finally, references for the methods applied in the analysis are given.

6.12.2 Worked example

Consider the experiment described above that involved a Treatment factor (factor Treatment, levels: drug and vehicle) with ten animals per group. For each animal the disease state was defined as being mild, moderate or severe. The total number of animals in each category is given in the contingency table of counts (Table 6.22).

Under the assumption that there were no treatment-related effects, and given the total number of animals in

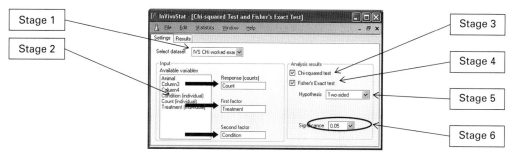

Figure 6.52. Screenshot illustrating the six-stage process for the InVivoStat Chi-squared Test and Fisher's Exact Test module.

Table 6.22. Contingency table of counts

	mild	moderate	severe
drug	2	4	4
vehicle	5	3	2

each of the three categories (7, 7 and 6 for mild, moderate and severe, respectively) you would expect to see 3.5 animals in each treatment group classified as mild, 3.5 in each group classified as moderate and 3 in each group classified as severe. This is displayed in the table of expected results (Table 6.23).

The chi-squared test compares the expected results to the observed results, as described in Section 5.5.2.2. This test was not significant at the 5% significance level $(\chi_{(2)} = 2.1, p = 0.351)$, see Table 6.24, indicating that the proportion of animals in each of the disease states was similar across the drug-treated and control groups.

However, as the numbers of animals in some of the categories were less than five, the above chi-squared test is not a reliable test. The preferred test in this situation is Fisher's exact test. The two-sided Fisher's exact test (Table 6.25) was not statistically significant $(p = 0.536)$, confirming that there were no treatment-related effects in this experiment.

6.13 R-Runner module

InVivoStat is based on the free-to-use R language (R Development Core Team, 2012). If the user has existing programs written in R, then these can be run within

the R-Runner module. This allows access to functionality available within R that is not implemented within the InVivoStat core modules. The interface is given in Figure 6.53.

User-defined R programs can be written in the R script window, or existing code loaded into InVivoStat using the 'Load' button (and similarly R programs can be saved using the 'Save' button). Information about how to use this module, and how to set up the output so that it is displayed in the Results tab, is given within the default R script window.

The benefits of using the R-Runner module to run existing R code is that the output is available in HTML format, programs can be shared (and run) by others who may not be familiar with R and also that variables need not be hard coded but can be dragged and dropped into the variable boxes, thus allowing more flexibility when programming in R.

6.14 Nested Design Analysis module

The Nested Design Analysis module is a power analysis tool that allows the user to assess the effect of varying the levels of replication of the multiple random factors within a higher-order nested design. It is an implementation of the methods described in Section 3.7.3.5.

The Nested Design Analysis module assumes that treatments (or other fixed factors of interest) will be tested against the between-animal variability. This is the random factor at the top of the nested design's hierarchical structure (Random factor 1 on the interface, see Figure 6.54). In the power analyses conducted

Table 6.23. Expected results

	mild	moderate	severe	Column totals
drug	3.50	3.50	3.00	10
vehicle	3.50	3.50	3.00	10
Row totals	7	7	6	20

Table 6.24. Chi-squared test result

	Test statistic	Degrees of freedom	p-value
Result	2.10	2	0.351

Table 6.25. Fisher's exact test result

	p-value
Result	0.536

within this module it is this source of variability that is used as the variance estimate.

The user can enter any number of fixed factors but can only enter up to four nested random factors. If there are more than four nested random factors in the experimental design, then the results should be averaged up to the fourth-level random factor. Experimental designs that involve crossed random factors, rather than simply nested random factors, are beyond the scope of this module. The interface is given in Figure 6.54.

For each random factor the user can investigate the effect of varying the replication of the levels of the nested random factors on the statistical power of the statistical tests. To achieve this, the replication of the levels of each of the nested random factors *within the levels of the factor that nests it* needs to be defined. For example, if there are eight animals per group and three samples per animal then the user may wish to investigate changing the number of samples per animal from the original three to two or four. It is these numbers (three and four) that are entered into the Nested Design Analysis module and not the total number of samples in the experiment.

6.14.1 Analysis procedure

Setting up the dataset

The dataset required by the Nested Design Analysis module needs to be created in a specific format. The responses are written down in a single variable within

the dataset alongside a variable for each of the fixed and random factors.

The random factor variables should be set up so that each level of a random factor in the dataset has a unique practical meaning. So if, for each of the random factors, two rows in the dataset are assigned the same factor label, then the corresponding responses share the same level of the random factor in the experiment itself.

Example 3.36 (continued): Assessing joint pain using applied pressure

Consider Example 3.36, a study that consists of two treatments (factor Treatment, levels: control and FCA), eight rats per treatment group (factor Animal, levels: 1 to 16) and three trials per animal (factor Trial, levels: 1 to 48). We assume that the first trial for animal 2 is not related in any way to the first trial in animal 1, so it is numbered trial 4 (the first three trials are for animal 1). The first 15 rows of the dataset are given in Table 6.26.

In the dataset required for this module, there should be a variable within the dataset that indexes the individual observations (Trial in this case). It is numbered 1 up to n, where n is the total number of observations measured. The analysis procedure is illustrated in Figure 6.55.

Input selection

1. Dataset selection: The analysis begins by selecting a dataset from the drop-down list of available imported datasets.
2. Variable selection: The user selects (by dragging and dropping) the response into the 'Response' box, the fixed factors into the 'Treatment (factorial)' box and the random factors into the 'Random factor'

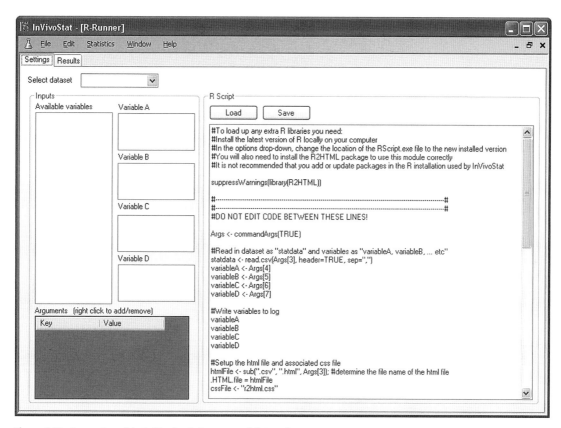

Figure 6.53. Screenshot of the InVivoStat R-Runner module interface.

boxes. Be careful when defining the random factors as the order that the random factors are added to the 'Random factor' boxes is important. Within the Nested Design Analysis module interface 'Random factor 1' is the random factor that resides at the top of the hierarchical nested design structure, the random factor below this is 'Random factor 2' and so on. In many cases it follows that the Animal random factor will be defined as Random factor 1.

The user can also select blocking factors and a covariate to include in the statistical model.

3. Response transformation: Once selected, the user has the option of applying a transformation to the response: $\log_{10}$, $\log_e$, square root, rank or arcsine. If selected the covariate will be transformed using the same transformation as the response, although this can be manually changed if required.

4. Significance level: The user can also choose the significance level for the tests, the default being 0.05 or 5%.

Output selection

5. Replication of random factors: The user can now investigate varying the replication of the levels of the random factors by entering (using a comma separated list) a series of integers corresponding to different levels of replication of the nested random factors. As mentioned above, these numbers correspond to the level of replication of the factor within each level of the factor that nests it. It is recommended that values are selected that are close to the replication actually used in the actual experiment.

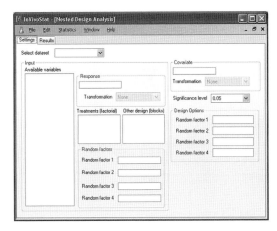

Figure 6.54. Screenshot of the InVivoStat Nested Design Analysis module interface.

Output details

InVivoStat will now calculate an estimate of the between-animal variability for experimental designs based on the replication of the levels of the random factors defined by the user; see Section 3.7.3.5 for more details. For each random factor we vary the replication of the levels of the factor while keeping the replication of the other random factors at a level that is equal to the average replication in the original design (rounded to a whole number). For each level of replication (i.e. each proposed experimental design) a new estimate of the between-animal variability is calculated. InVivoStat then produces a separate power curve corresponding to each of these experimental designs.

The power curve plots produced are different from those created in the Power Analysis module described above, although they do share many similarities. For example, in both modules the Y-axis corresponds to the statistical power. The X-axis in the Nested Design Analysis module plots corresponds to the size of effect (rather than sample size, as is the case in the plots generated by the Power Analysis module) and the different lines on the graph correspond to different designs, i.e. different levels of replication of the random factors. The X-axis range selected by InVivoStat is not necessarily a biologically meaningful range of effects. The range is

Table 6.26. First 15 rows of a dataset showing how to label the levels of the factors of a nested design

Response	Treatment	Animal	Trial
6.19	control	1	1
5.44	control	1	2
4.06	control	1	3
4.19	control	2	4
22.98	control	2	5
18.02	control	2	6
15.26	control	3	7
25.43	control	3	8
21.39	control	3	9
16.32	control	4	10
13.12	control	4	11
22.08	control	4	12
19.67	FCA	5	13
38.94	FCA	5	14
23.02	FCA	5	15
...	...	...	...

merely selected to highlight the differences between the statistical powers of the various experimental designs. The purpose of the power curve plots in the Nested Design Analysis module is to allow the user to compare the competing designs, rather than make any decisions about the power of individual treatment comparisons.

The output includes:

1. Response variable: InVivoStat identifies the response being analysed and also the covariate (if one is selected). This section also describes any transformations that have been applied to the response.

2. Table of estimated variance components: This table contains the estimated variance components of the random factors (see Section 3.7.3.3). These estimates are used when assessing the effect of varying the replication of the levels of the random factors in the experimental design.

3. Table of average replication in the original design: When assessing the effect of varying the replication of the random factors in the experimental design, the replication of the other factors is held constant at the average level. This table informs the user at what replication level the other factors will be held.

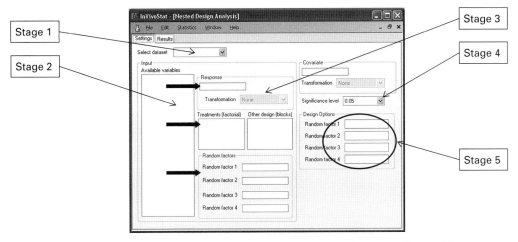

Figure 6.55. Screenshot illustrating the five-stage process for the InVivoStat Nested Design Analysis module.

4. Power curve plot of the original design: The Nested Design Analysis module provides the user with a graphical display of the power of an experimental design where the replications of the levels of the random factors are as defined in the previous table. This power curve will effectively be an approximate power curve of the original design.

5. Power curve plots for alternative designs: The module now provides a series of graphical plots of the power curves. These plots are defined by the different replications of the levels of the random factors, as defined by the user.

6.14.2 Worked example

Consider Example 3.36 described above. In the analysis Treatment was the only fixed factor, Animal was Random factor 1 and Trial was Random factor 2. The replication of the random factors investigated was 6 to 10 (for Animal) and 1 to 6 (for Trial within Animal). These options are presented in Figure 6.56. The output from this analysis, including the power curve plots produced and the conclusions drawn from the analysis, is discussed in Section 3.7.3.5.

6.15 Survival Analysis module

The Survival Analysis module within InVivoStat is a tool for analysing censored data. As discussed in Section 5.5.3, censored data occurs when an animal's actual response cannot be measured but it is known to be beyond a certain censored value. For example, in the hotplate test there is a 30-second limit to how long an animal's paw can be placed on the hotplate. If an animal does not withdraw its paw within this time then the test is discontinued and the response recorded is the censored value of 30 seconds.

The Survival Analysis module is available within the Additional Analyses sub-menu of the Statistics drop-down menu. This module produces a plot of the Kaplan–Meier survival curves and performs a log-rank test to compare the experimental groups. The interface is given in Figure 6.57.

6.15.1 Analysis procedure

Input dataset

This module requires a dataset that consists of three variables. This includes the response variable to be analysed (usually time to event or time of censored observation), a variable identifying the experimental group and a censorship variable. The censorship variable contains either 0 or 1 values, where 0 corresponds to a censored observation. Each experimental unit (usually animal) is one row of the dataset. An example is given in Table 6.27, where censorship occurred on days 2 and 3 in the treatment group. The analysis procedure is illustrated in Figure 6.58.

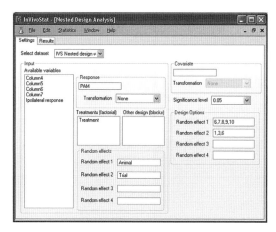

Figure 6.56. Screenshot of the options required by the InVivoStat Nested Design Analysis module for Example 3.36.

Table 6.27. Example of the first ten rows of the dataset required for the Survival Analysis module.

Group	Day	Censor
control	4	0
control	4	0
control	4	0
control	4	0
control	4	0
control	4	0
control	4	0
treatment	2	1
treatment	3	1
treatment	4	0
...	...	...

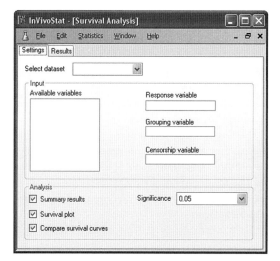

Figure 6.57. Screenshot of the InVivoStat Survival Analysis module interface.

Input selection

1. Dataset selection: The analysis begins by select-ing a dataset from the drop-down list of available imported datasets.
2. Variable selection: The response variable is dragged and dropped from the 'Available variables' list onto the 'Response variable' box. The variable that defines the experimental groups is dragged and dropped onto the 'Grouping variable' box and the censorship variable is dragged and dropped onto the 'Censorship variable' box.

Output selection

The user has several choices for the analysis.
3. Summary results: Select this option to generate summary statistics of the dataset, including the total number of records, the start size of each group, the number of recorded events (that are not censored), the median response and a 95% confidence interval around the median.
4. Survival plot: This option produces the Kaplan–Meier survival plot.
5. Compare survival curves: This option allows the user to perform a log-rank test to compare the sur-vival rates across groups.
6. Significance: The user can also choose the signifi-cance level for the tests, the default being 0.05 or 5%.

Output details

1. Response: This text contains information about the response, grouping and censorship variables.
2. Summary results: If selected, this table contains a summary of the results, categorised by the grouping variable.

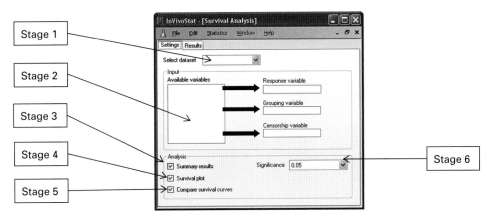

Figure 6.58. Screenshot illustrating the six-stage process when using the InVivoStat Survival Analysis module.

Table 6.28. Summary results

Group	Records	n	Start size	Events	Median	Lower 95% CI	Upper 95% CI
05% ligation	10	10	10	0			
10% ligation	10	10	10	1			
20% ligation	10	10	10	4		2	
25% ligation	10	10	10	8	2	1	2
30% ligation	10	10	10	9	2	1	3
35% ligation	10	10	10	10	2	1	2

3. Comparing survival curves: If selected, this table contains the results of the log-rank test.
4. Kaplan–Meier survival plot: If selected, the Kaplan–Meier survival plot is produced.
5. References: Finally, references for the methods applied in the analysis are given.

6.15.2 Worked example

Consider Example 5.29, described in Section 5.5.3, consisting of six treatment groups (corresponding to between 5% and 35% ligation) with ten animals per group. The summary results are given in Table 6.28. There were ten animals in each group at the start of the study and the number of deaths per group ranged between zero and ten in an apparently dose-related way. It was only possible to calculate confidence intervals for some of the treatment group due to the sparsity of data.

The log-rank test results are presented in Table 6.29. The chi-squared test statistic (37.34) and the associated p-value ($p < 0.001$) indicate there is almost certainly a difference in survival rates across the groups. The Kaplan–Meier survival plot for this analysis is presented above in Section 5.5.3.1.

Table 6.29. Log-rank test results

Group	N	Observed	Expected	(O-E)^2/E	(O-E)^2/V	Chi-sq	p-value
05% ligation	10	0	6.70	6.70	10.92	37.34	< 0.001
10% ligation	10	1	6.25	4.41	7.02		
20% ligation	10	4	5.94	0.63	0.99		
25% ligation	10	8	4.27	3.27	4.93		
30% ligation	10	9	4.77	3.75	5.71		
35% ligation	10	10	4.08	8.61	13.18		

7

Conclusion

In this text we have aimed to show the reader how the use of experimental design and statistics can help the researcher gather the most information from each animal experiment while using as few animals as possible. Returning to the statement of Russell and Burch (1959, p. 111):

Every time any particle of statistical method is properly used, fewer animals are employed than would otherwise have been necessary.

We hope that this text has convinced the reader that there is much merit in this statement.

The book has been aimed at any researcher performing animal experiments. Some of the subject matter can be applied by scientists without the help of a professional statistician. We have also used this platform to introduce the reader to some of the more complicated examples of experimental design and statistical analysis, examples of which are commonly found in real-life experiments. Hopefully we have given a flavour of these methods and encouraged the reader to either try them out for themselves or seek professional help to get started. Remember, as explained in Gaines Das (2004), sometimes it is the collaboration between the biologist and the statistician at all stages of the experimental process that leads to a successful experiment.

The emphasis in the text has been experimental designs. We feel that the scientist can, using rules based on common sense, construct complicated yet useful experimental designs without resorting to the mathematical theory underpinning the designs. Once a design is selected then the choice of statistical analysis should be relatively straightforward and has, in our experience, led to reliable conclusions being drawn.

If the reader applies the principles outlined in this text during their research, then it should be possible to achieve valid scientific results while using as few animals as possible. We end this book with a few summary thoughts that the researcher should always consider.

Experimental design

1. Don't ignore the variability at the expense of the signal.
2. Use blocking factors to reduce the variability and remove bias from the signal.
3. Use factorial designs to gain a better understanding of how the experimental factors are interrelated.
4. Make sure you use enough animals to obtain reliable results. There is no point running experiments that generate tests that do not have sufficient statistical power to reject the null hypothesis.
5. Be aware of pseudo-replication.
6. Choose continuous responses where possible.
7. Always perform a power analysis to confirm appropriate sample sizes in future studies.
8. Use nested designs to identify suitable within-animal replication.
9. Identify the experimental units.
10. Consider using dose-escalation techniques rather than testing doses of compounds relative to the control.

Randomisation

11. Use blinding and randomisation to avoid all forms of bias.

Statistical analysis

12. Limit the standard t-test to situations where it is valid, i.e. a single treatment group against a control, and not when multiple treatments are being compared or other factors are likely to be important, e.g. sex of animal or initial body weight.
13. Graph the data, preferably the raw data.
14. Use estimation procedures (the difference between treatments and confidence intervals) rather than relying on hypothesis tests and p-values.
15. Transform the data if necessary to satisfy the assumptions of the analysis.
16. Use all of the information recorded for the animals using covariates or linear predictors.
17. If the levels of a factor are not involved in the randomisation (for example Time in a repeated measures or Dose in a dose-escalation design) then use repeated measures techniques to analyse the data.

Reporting results

18. When reporting results say how many non-significant results were found.
19. Always report an estimate of the variability alongside the results.
20. Have the confidence always to question the design and analysis strategies used by your peers.

There will always be concerns about the conclusions drawn from animal experiments. With sample sizes limited by ethical considerations, biological variability and questions about the applicability of the animal models to human disease, there are many challenges. However, the choice of a good experimental design and statistical analysis can improve the power of the experiment to detect the important differences. Good experimental design and an appropriate statistical analysis technique can, if applied correctly, improve the quality of animal research.

Glossary

Term	Definition
A priori	Relating to prior knowledge
Arithmetic mean for group i	$\left(x_{1i} + x_{2i} + \ldots + x_{n,i}\right)/\, n_i$
Continuous distribution	Data presented as numbers that can take any numerical value, e.g. body weight, time to event
Correlation	Measure of the linear relationship between two variables
Covariance	A measure of the degree to which two variables vary together
Covariate	A measure of a feature of the subject, e.g. body weight, which may explain some of the variability in the posttreatment results and is unaffected by the treatment being applied in the experiment. Usually a pretreatment measure
Degrees of freedom	A measure of the number of independent pieces of information available to estimate the parameters in the statistical analysis, usually the number of factor levels minus 1
Factor	A variable controlled by the researcher that can be used to quantify a source of variability in the experiment. For example, the Treatment factor is a variable that is part of the experimental design and quantifies the treatment effects
False negative	The incorrect acceptance of the null hypothesis when it is false
False positive	The incorrect rejection of the null hypothesis when it is true
FDR	False discovery rate – the chance of making at least one false positive conclusion in a statistical analysis
F-value	The test used in the ANOVA table. It is a signal-to-noise ratio, that is the size of the effect vs. underlying variability
FWE	Family-wise error rate – the proportion of false positives in a statistical analysis
Geometric mean for group i	$\left(x_{1i} \times x_{2i} \times \ldots \times x_{n,i}\right)^{1/n_i}$
Homogeneity of variance	We assume the variability is the same in all experimental groups (ANOVA uses an average variability)
Independence	One experimental observation should not be influenced by, or related to, any other
Level	The set of levels a factor can take. For example control, low, medium, high dose are levels of the Treatment factor
Linear predictor	A measure taken on each animal, e.g. terminal body weight, which is related in a linear fashion to the experimental response. Unlike covariates, linear predictors may be influenced by the treatments. It may be of interest to see how the linear predictors are related, or correlated, with the response using a regression analysis
Mean	Sum of a series of values divided by the number of values measured
Median	The middle or central value of a set of values
Mixed-model	A statistical analysis approach that contains both fixed and random factors. Used in the analysis of complex analyses and repeated measures analyses

Term	Definition
Mode	Most frequently occurring value of a set of values
Multiple comparison procedure	A process that involves an adjustment, usually applied to p-values and confidence intervals, to maintain a specified risk of finding a false positive result
n_i	Sample size for the ith group
Noise	Variation in a sample
Non-parametric	Statistics that do not rely on certain assumptions about the distribution of the measurements (for example the assumption that the data are normally distributed)
Normal distribution (Gaussian)	Hypothetical frequency distribution with special characteristics (bell shaped, symmetrical and with a central tendency)
Normally distributed	The distribution of the residuals of the measurements (if plotted as a histogram say) follows a normal or Gaussian (bell-shaped) curve
One-way ANOVA	ANalysis Of VAriance. Used when you have only one factor in the experiment
Parametric	When the measured responses from a population are assumed to fit to a normal distribution
Parametric test	Statistical test that relies on the assumption that the population of animal responses is normally distributed
Population	Set of potential animals that we wish to make predictions about
Post hoc	Examining the data after the experiment has finished
p-value	Probability of obtaining a result at least as extreme as a given data point, assuming the null hypothesis is true
Random sample	A sample chosen by an unpredictable method to ensure that every member of the population has an equal chance of being selected
Residual	The observed value minus the predicted value
Response	A quantity measured by the researcher that reflects an animal's response to the experimental intervention. Responses can be continuous, discrete, ordinal, nominal or binary
Sphericity	One of the assumptions that can be made when performing a repeated measures analysis. It is the assumption that the variances of the differences between pairs of treatment group means are the same
Standard deviation (SD)	A measure of the variation of the observations from their predicted means: $SD = \sqrt{Variance}$
Standard error of the mean (SEM)	The standard deviation of the ith sample mean: $SEM = \sqrt{Variance} / n_i$
Statistical significance	A result that is unlikely to have occurred by chance
Transformation	Mathematical operation required before the statistical analysis if the data are not normally distributed or the within-group variances are different. A log or square root transformation of the response is most common
t-test	The t-test assesses whether two group means are *statistically* different from each other. This test is appropriate whenever you have a study with only two groups
Two-way ANOVA	Used when you have two factors and wish to investigate how they interact with each other
Type I error	False positive determination – rejecting the null hypothesis when the null hypothesis is actually true
Type II error	False negative determination – failing to reject the null hypothesis when the alternative hypothesis is actually true
Variable	A column of the dataset corresponding to a single experimental design factor or a set of measurements
Variance	A measure of the underlying variability of the response, once all known factors have been accounted for. Variance equals the standard deviation squared
$x_{1i}, ..., x_{ni}$	n responses for the ith group

References

Afsarinejad, K. (1983). Balanced repeated measurements designs. *Biometrika*, 70(1), 199–204.

Anderson, V. L. and McLean, R. A. (1974). *Design of Experiments*. Marcel Dekker Inc.: New York.

Andreasen, J. T., Henningsen, K., Bate, S. T., Christiansen, S. and Wiborg, O. (2011). Nicotine reverses anhedonic-like response and cognitive impairment in the rat chronic mild stress model of depression: comparison with sertraline. *Journal of Psychopharmacology*, 25(8), 1134–41.

Armitage, P., Berry, G. and Matthews, J. N. S. (2002). *Statistical Methods in Medical Research*, 4th edition. Wiley-Blackwell: Malden, MA.

Aylott, M., Bate, S. T., Collins, S., Jarvis, P. and Saul, J. (2011). Review of the statistical analysis of the dog telemetry study. *Pharmaceutical Statistics*, 10(3), 236–49.

Bailey, R. A. (2008). *Design of Comparative Experiments*. Cambridge University Press: Cambridge, UK.

Bartlett, M. S. (1937). Properties of sufficiency and statistical tests. *Proceedings of the Royal Statistical Society Series A – Mathematical and Physical Sciences*, 160(901), 268–82.

Barton, N. J., Strickland, I. T., Bond, S. M., *et al.* (2007). Pressure application measurement (PAM): a novel behavioural technique for measuring hypersensitivity in a rat model of joint pain. *Journal of Neuroscience Methods*, 163(1), 67–75.

Bate, S. T. and Boxall, J. (2008). The construction of multi-factor crossover designs in animal husbandry studies. *Pharmaceutical Statistics*, 7(3), 179–94.

Bate, S. T. and Jones, B. (2008). A review of uniform cross-over designs. *Journal of Statistical Planning and Inference*, 138(2), 336–51.

Belluzzi, J. D., Lee, A. G., Oliff, H. S. and Leslie, F. M. (2004). Age-dependent effects of nicotine on locomotor activity and conditioned place preference in rats. *Psychopharmacology*, 174, 389–95.

Benjamini, Y. and Hochberg, Y. (1995). Controlling the false discovery rate: a practical and powerful approach to multiple testing. *Journal of the Royal Statistical Society Series B*, 57, 289–300.

Bennett, C. M., Wolford, G. L. and Miller, M. B. (2009). The principled control of false positives in neuroimaging. *Social Cognitive and Affective Neuroscience*, 4(4), 417–22.

Bianchi, M. and Baulieu, E. E. (2012). 3β-methoxy-pregnenolone (MAP4343) as an innovative therapeutic approach for depressive disorders. *Proceedings of the National Academy of Sciences*, 109(5), 1713–18.

Biggers, J. D., Baskar, J. F. and Torchiana, D. F. (1981). Reduction of fertility of mice by the intrauterine injection of prostaglandin antagonists. *Journal of Reproduction and Fertility*, 63, 365–72.

Bison, S., Carboni, L., Arban, R., *et al.* (2009). Differential behavioral, physiological, and hormonal sensitivity to LPS challenge in rats. *International Journal of Interferon, Cytokine and Mediator Research*, 1, 1–13.

Blakesley, R. E., Mazumdar, S., Dew, M. A., *et al.* (2009). Comparisons of methods for multiple hypothesis testing in neuropsychological research. *Neuropsychology*, 23(2), 255–64.

Bonferroni, C. E. (1936). Teoria statistica delle classi e calcolo delle probabilita. *Pubblicazioni del R Istituto Superiore di Scienze Economiche e Commerciali di Firenze*, 8, 3–62.

Box, G. E. P. (1953). Non-normality and tests on variance. *Biometrika*, 40(3/4), 318–35.

Boxall, J., Heath, S., Bate, S. and Brautigam, J. (2004). Modern concepts of socialisation for dogs: implications for their behaviour, welfare and use in scientific procedures. *ATLA. Alternatives to Laboratory Animals*, 32, 81–93.

Brammer, R. J. (2003). Modelling covariance structure in ascending dose studies of isolated tissues and organs. *Pharmaceutical Statistics*, 2(2), 103–12.

Bright, J., Aylott, M., Bate, S., *et al.* (2011). Recommendations on the statistical analysis of the Comet assay. *Pharmaceutical Statistics*, 10(6), 485–93.

Brooks, K. J., Bunce, K. T., Hasse, M. V., *et al.* (2005). MRI quantification *in vivo* of corticosteroid induced thymus involution in mice: correlation with *ex vivo* measurements. *Steroids*, 70(4), 267–72.

Brown, M. B. and Forsythe, A. B. (1974). Robust tests for equality of variances. *Journal of the American Statistical Society*, 69(346), 364–7.

Burden, R. L. and Faires, J. D. (2011). *Numerical Analysis*, 9th edition. Brooks/Cole Publishing: Pacific Grove, CA.

Button, K. S., Ioannidis, J. P., Mokrysz, C., *et al.* (2013). Power failure: why small sample size undermines the reliability of neuroscience. *Nature Reviews Neuroscience*, 14, 365–76.

Chaves, A. A., Keller, W. J., O'Sullivan, S., *et al.* (2006). Cardiovascular monkey telemetry: sensitivity to detect QT interval prolongation. *Journal of Pharmacological and Toxicological Methods*, 54(2), 150–8.

Clark, R. A., Shoaib, M., Hewitt, K. N., Stanford, S. C. and Bate, S. T. (2012). A comparison of InVivoStat with other statistical software packages for analysis of data generated from animal experiments. *Journal of Psychopharmacology*, 26(8), 1136–42.

Clarke, G. M. and Kempson, R. E. (1997). *Introduction to the Design and Analysis of Experiments*. Arnold: London.

Cochran, W. G. and Cox, G. M. (1957). *Experimental Designs*, 2nd edition. Wiley & Sons, Inc.: New York, London.

Cohen, J. (1988). *Statistical Power Analysis for the Behavioural Sciences*, 2nd edition. Lawrence Erlbaum Associates: Hillsdale, NJ.

Crowder, M. J. and Hand, D. J. (1990). *Analysis of Repeated Measures*. Chapman and Hall/CRC: London.

Cumming, G., Fidler, F. and Vaux, D. L. (2007). Error bars in experimental biology. *The Journal of Cell Biology*, 177(1), 7–11.

Curran-Everett, D. (2000). Multiple comparisons: philosophies and illustrations. *American Journal of Physiology – Regulatory, Integrative and Comparative Physiology*, 279(1), R1–8.

Curtin, L. I., Grakowsky, J. A., Suarez, M., *et al.* (2009). Evaluation of buprenorphine in a postoperative pain model in rats. *Comparative Medicine*, 59(1), 60–71.

Downie, D., Antipatis, C., Delday, M. I., Maltin, C. A. and Sneddon, A. A. (2005). Moderate maternal vitamin A deficiency alters myogenic regulatory protein expression and perinatal organ growth in the rat. *American Journal of Physiology – Regulatory, Integrative and Comparative Physiology*, 288(1), 73–9.

Dudchenko, P. A., Wood, E. R. and Eichenbaum, H. (2000). Neurotoxic hippocampal lesions have no effect on odor span and little effect on odor recognition memory but produce significant impairments on spatial span, recognition, and alteration. *The Journal of Neuroscience*, 20(8), 2964–77.

Duncan, D. B. (1955). Multiple range and multiple F tests. *Biometrics*, 11(1), 1–42.

Dunnett, C. W. (1955). A multiple comparison procedure for comparing several treatments with a control. *Journal of the American Statistical Association*, 50(272), 1096–121.

Dunnett, C. W. (1964). New tables for multiple comparisons with a control. *Biometrics*, 20(3), 482–91.

Elashoff, J. D. (1981). Down with multiple t-tests! *Gastroenterology*, 80, 615–20.

Festing, M. F. W. (1994). Reduction of animal use: experimental design and quality of experiments. *Laboratory Animals*, 28(3), 212–21.

Festing, M. F. W. (2003a). Principles: the need for better experimental design. *Trends in Pharmacological Sciences*, 24(7), 341-5.

Festing, M. F. W. (2003b). We should be designing better experiments. *Veterinary Anaesthesia and Analgesia*, 30, 58-60.

Festing, M. F. W. and Altman, D. G. (2002). Guidelines for the design and statistical analysis of experiments using laboratory animals. *ILAR Journal*, 43(4), 244-58.

Festing, M. F. W., Diamanti, P. and Turton, J. A. (2001). Strain differences in haematological response to chloroamphenicol succinate in mice: implications for toxicological research. *Food and Chemical Toxicology*, 39(4), 375-83.

Festing, M. F. W., Overend, P., Gaines Das, R., Cortina-Borja, M. and Berdoy, M. (2002). *The Design of Animal Experiments: Reducing the Use of Animals in Research through Better Experimental Design*. Royal Society of Medicine Press: London.

Field, A. (1998). A bluffer's guide to... sphericity. *The British Psychological Society: Mathematical, Statistical & Computing Section Newsletter*, 6, 13-22.

Findlay, J. W. A. and Dillard, R. F. (2007). Appropriate calibration curve fitting in ligand binding assays. *The AAPS Journal*, 9(2), E260-7.

Ford, D. J. (1977). Effect of autoclaving and physical structure of diets on their utilization by mice. *Laboratory Animals*, 11(4), 235-9.

Gaines Das, R. (2004). 'Statistics' is not a sausage machine: a statistician's viewpoint and some comments on experimental design. *ATLA. Alternatives to Laboratory Animals*, 32(2), 5-8.

Gaines Das, R., Fry, D., Preziosi, R. and Hudson, M. (2009). Planning for reduction. *ATLA. Alternatives to Laboratory Animals*, 37(1), 27-32.

Giesbrecht, F. G. and Gumpertz, M. L. (2004). *Planning, Construction, and Statistical Analysis of Comparative Experiments*. Wiley & Sons, Inc.: Hoboken, NJ.

Godolphin, J. D. (2004). Simple pilot procedures for the avoidance of disconnected experimental designs. *Journal of the Royal Statistical Society Series C (Applied Statistics)*, 53(1), 133-47.

Gore, K. H. and Stanley, P. J. (2005). An illustration that statistical design mitigates environmental variation and ensures unambiguous study conclusions. *Animal Welfare*, 14(4), 361-5.

Grayson, B., Idris, N. F. and Neill, J. C. (2007). Atypical antipsychotics attenuate a sub-chronic PCP-induced cognitive deficit in the novel object recognition task in the rat. *Behavioural Brain Research*, 184(1), 31-8.

Green, C. R., Ham, K. N. and Tange, J. D. (1969). Kidney lesions induced in rats by p-aminophenol. *British Medical Journal*, 18(1), 162-4.

Harris, R. B. S., Zhou, J., Youngblood, B. D., *et al.* (1998). Effect of repeated stress on body weight and body composition of rats fed low- and high-fat diets. *American Journal of Physiology – Regulatory, Integrative and Comparative Physiology*, 275(6), R1928-38.

Hatcher, P. D., Brown, V. J., Tait, D. S., *et al.* (2005). 5-HT6 receptor antagonists improve performance in an attentional set shifting task in rats. *Psychopharmacology*, 181(2), 253-9.

Hedenqvist, P., Roughan, J. V., Antunes, L., Orr, H. and Flecknell, P. A. (2001). Induction of anaesthesia with desflurane and isoflurane in the rabbit. *Laboratory Animals*, 35(2), 172-9.

Hille, C., Bate, S., Davis, J. and Gonzalez, M. I. (2008). 5-HT4 receptor agonism in the five-choice serial reaction time task. *Behavioural Brain Research*, 195(1), 180-6.

Hochberg, Y. (1988). A sharper Bonferroni procedure for multiple tests of significance. *Biometrika*, 75(4), 800-3.

Hoenig, J. M. and Heisey, D. M. (2001). The abuse of power: the pervasive fallacy of power calculations for data analysis. *The American Statistician*, 55(1), 19-24.

Holland, B. S. and Copenhaver, M. D. (1988). Improved Bonferroni-type multiple testing procedures. *Psychological Bulletin*, 104(1), 145-9.

Holm, S. (1979). A simple sequentially rejective multiple test procedure. *Scandinavian Journal of Statistics*, 6, 65-70.

Holson, R. R., Freshwater, L., Maurissen, J. P. J., Moser, V. C. and Phang, W. (2008). Statistical issues and techniques appropriate for developmental neurotoxicity testing: a report from the ILSI Research Foundation/Risk Science Institute expert working group on neurodevelopmental endpoints. *Neurotoxicology and Teratology*, 30(4), 326-48.

Hommel, G. (1988). A stagewise rejective multiple test procedure based on a modified Bonferroni test. *Biometrika*, 75(2), 383-6.

Hsu, J. (1996). *Multiple Comparisons: Theory and Methods*. Chapman and Hall/CRC: London.

Hulshoff, J. E. G, Van Dijk, K., van der Waerden, J. P. C. M., *et al.* (1996). Evaluation of plasma-spray and magnetron-sputter Ca-P-coated implants: an *in vivo* experiment using rabbits. *Journal of Biomedical Materials Research*, 31(3), 329-37.

Ingram-Ross, J. L., Curran, A. K., Miyamoto, M., *et al.* (2012). Cardiorespiratory safety evaluation in non-human primates. *Journal of Pharmacological and Toxicological Methods*, 66, 114-24.

Jones, B. and Kenward, M. G. (2003). *Design and Analysis of Cross-Over Trials*. Chapman and Hall/CRC: London.

Kalinichev, M., Bate, S. T. and Jones, D. N. C. (2009). Models of aspects of schizophrenia: behavioral sensitization induced by subchronic phencyclidine administration. *Current Protocols in Pharmacology*, 45, 5.54.1–13.

Karp, N. A., Segonds-Pichon, A., Gerdin, A. K. B., Ramirez-Solis, R. and White, J. K. (2012). The fallacy of ratio correction to address confounding factors. *Laboratory Animals*, 46(3), 245–52.

Keuls, M. (1952). The use of the 'studentized range' in connection with an analysis of variance. *Euphytica*, 1(2), 112–22.

Kilkenny, C., Brown, W. J., Cuthill, I. C., Emerson, M. and Altman, D. G. (2010). Improving bioscience research: the ARRIVE guidelines for reporting animal research. *PLoS Biol*, 8(6), e1000412.

Kilkenny, C., Parsons, N., Kadyszewski, E., *et al.* (2009). Survey of the quality of experimental design, statistical analysis and reporting of research using animals. *PLoS One*, 4(11), e7824.

Kleinbaum, D. G. and Klein, M. (2005). *Survival Analysis: A Self-Learning Text*, 2nd edition. Springer: New York.

Kolmogorov, A. N. (1933). Sulla determinazione empirica di una legge di distribuzione. *Giornale dell'Istituto Italiano degli Attuari*, 4(1), 83–91.

Kramer, C. Y. (1956). Extension of multiple range tests to group means with unequal numbers of replications. *Biometrics*, 12(3), 307–10.

Kuentz, M., Rothlisberger, D. and Richter, W. (2003). Design of experiment (DoE) methods maximize information from a minimal number of animals in special cases of preclinical bioavailability testing. *Pharmaceutical Development and Technology*, 8(4), 453–8.

Kwan, K. Y., Allchorne, A. J., Vollrath, M. A., *et al.* (2006). TRPA1 contributes to cold, mechanical, and chemical nociception but is not essential for hair-cell transduction. *Neuron*, 50, 277–89.

Lazic, S. E. (2010). The problem of pseudoreplication in neuroscientific studies: is it affecting your analysis? *BMC Neuroscience*, 11(1), 5.

Lehmann, E. L. (1999). *Elements of Large-Sample Theory*. Springer: New York.

Levene, H. (1960). Robust tests for equality of variances. In *Contributions to Probability and Statistics: Essays in Honor of Harold Hotelling*, editors Olkin, I., Ghurye, S. G., Hoeffding, W., Madow, W. G. and Mann, H. B. 278–292. Stanford University Press: Stanford, CA.

Liao, J. J. Z. and Liu, R. (2009). Re-parameterization of five-parameter logistic function. *Journal of Chemometrics*, 23(5), 248–53.

Ludbrook, J. (1998). Multiple comparison procedures updated. *Clinical and Experimental Pharmacology and Physiology*, 25(12), 1032–7.

Macleod, M. R., Fisher, M., O'Collins, V., *et al.* (2009). Reprint: good laboratory practice: preventing introduction of bias at the bench. *Journal of Cerebral Blood Flow and Metabolism*, 29, 2213.

Maheswaran, S., Barjat, H., Rueckert, D., *et al.* (2009). Longitudinal regional brain volume changes quantified in normal aging and Alzheimer's APP × PS1 mice using MRI. *Brain Research*, 1270, 19–32.

Manser, C. E., Broom, D. M., Overend, P. and Morris, T. H. (1998). Investigations into the preferences of laboratory rats for nest-boxes and nesting materials. *Laboratory Animals*, 32(1), 23–35.

Mathew, G., Watson, D. I., Rofe, A. M., *et al.* (1996). Wound metastases following laparoscopic and open surgery for abdominal cancer in a rat model. *British Journal of Surgery*, 83(8), 1087–90.

Mauchly, J. W. (1940). Test for sphericity of a normal *n*-variate distribution. *Annals of Mathematical Statistics*, 11(2), 204–9.

McCance, I. (1995). Assessment of statistical procedures used in papers in the Australian Veterinary Journal. *Australian Veterinary Journal*, 72(9), 322–8.

McQuade, R., Creton, D. and Stanford, S. C. (1999). Effect of novel environmental stimuli on rat behaviour and central noradrenaline function measured by *in vivo* microdialysis. *Psychopharmacology*, 145(4), 393–400.

Mead, R. (1988). *The Design of Experiments: Statistical Principles for Practical Applications*. Cambridge University Press: Cambridge.

Mead, R., Curnow, R. N. and Hasted, A. M. (2003). *Statistical Methods in Agriculture and Experimental Biology*, 3rd edition. Chapman and Hall/CRC: London.

Miller, R. G. (1981). *Simultaneous Statistical Inference*, 2nd edition. Springer-Verlag: New York.

Milliken, G. A. and Johnson, D. E. (2002). *Analysis of Messy Data Volume III: Analysis of Covariance*. Chapman & Hall/CRC: New York.

Miyazaki, H., Watanabe, H., Kitayama, T., *et al.* (2005). QT PRODACT: sensitivity and specificity of the canine telemetry assay for detecting drug-induced QT interval prolongation. *Journal of Pharmacological Sciences*, 99, 523–9.

Montgomery, D. C. (1997). *Design and Analysis of Experiments*, 4th edition. Wiley: New York.

Morris, T. R. (1999). *Experimental Design and Analysis in Animal Sciences*. CABI Publishing: Wallingford, UK.

Murphy, N., Bruckdorfer, K. R., Grimsditch, D. C., *et al.* (2003). Temporal relationships between circulating levels of CC and CXC chemokines and developing atherosclerosis in Apolipoprotein E*3 Leiden mice. *Arteriosclerosis, Thrombosis, and Vascular Biology*, 23, 1615–20.

Nakagawa, S. (2004). A farewell to Bonferroni: the problems of low statistical power and publication bias. *Behavioral Ecology*, 15(6), 1044–5.

Nesnow, S., Mass, M. J., Ross, J. A., *et al.* (1998). Lung tumourigenic interactions in strain A/J mice of five environmental polycyclic aromatic hydrocarbons. *Environmental Health Perspectives*, 106(Suppl 6), 1337–46.

Newman, D. (1939). The distribution of range in samples from a normal population, expressed in terms of an independent estimate of standard deviation. *Biometrika*, 31(1/2), 20–30.

Nieuwenhuis, S., Forstmann, B. U. and Wagenmakers, E. J. (2011). Erroneous analyses of interactions in neuroscience: a problem of significance. *Nature Neuroscience*, 14(9), 1105–7.

Onyango, E. M. and Adeola, O. (2011). Dietary cholecalciferol lowers the maximal activity of intestinal mucosa phytase in ducklings fed low-phosphorus diets. *Canadian Journal of Animal Science*, 91(3), 399–404.

Parkin, S. L., Pritchett, J. P., Grimsditch, D. C., *et al.* (2004). Circulating levels of the chemokines JE and KC in female C3H apolipoprotein-E-deficient and C57BL apolipoprotein-E-deficient mice as potential markers of atherosclerosis development. *Biochemical Society Transactions*, 32(1), 128–30.

Patel, S. R., Murphy, K. G., Thompson, E. L., *et al.* (2008). Pyroglutamylated RFamide peptide 43 stimulates the hypothalamic-pituitary-gonadal axis via gonadotropin-releasing hormone in rats. *Endocrinology*, 149(9), 4747–54.

Pinheiro, J., Bates, D., DebRoy, S. and Sarkar, D. (2008). The R Development Core Team. nlme: linear and nonlinear mixed effects models. R package version 3.1–93. R Foundation for Statistical Computing, Vienna, Austria. www.R-project.org.

Plackett, R. L. and Burman, J. P. (1946). The design of optimal multifactorial experiments. *Biometrika*, 33(4), 305–25.

Pugh, P. L., Richardson, J. C., Bate, S. T., Upton, N. and Sunter, D. (2007). Non-cognitive behaviours in an APP/PS1 transgenic model of Alzheimer's disease. *Behavioural Brain Research*, 178(1), 18–28.

R Development Core Team (2012). *R: A language and environment for statistical computing*. R Foundation for Statistical Computing, Vienna, Austria. ISBN 3-900051-07-0, www.R-project.org.

Rooke, E. D. M., Vesterinen, H. M., Sena, E. S., Egan, K. J. and Macleod, M. R. (2011). Dopamine agonists in animal models of Parkinson's disease: A systematic review and meta-analysis. *Parkinsonism and Related Disorders*, 17(5), 313–20.

Rosnow, R. L. and Rosenthal, R. (1989). Statistical procedures and the justification of knowledge in psychological science. *American Psychologist*, 44(10), 1276–84.

Rumble, R., Saville, M., Simmons, L., *et al.* (2005). The preference of the common marmoset for nest boxes made from three different materials – wood, plastic, metal. *Animal Technology and Welfare*, 4(3), 185–7.

Russell, W. M. S. and Burch, R. L. (1959). *The Principles of Humane Experimental Technique*. Methuen & Co. Ltd: London.

Ruxton, G. G. and Colegrave, N. (2006). *Experimental Design for the Life Sciences*. Oxford University Press: Oxford.

Scheffé, H. (1953). A method for judging all contrasts in the analysis of variance. *Biometrika*, 40(1–2), 87–110.

Schleiss, M. R., Anderson, J. L. and McGregor, A. (2006). Cyclic cidofovir (cHPMPC) prevents congenital cytomegalovirus infection in a guinea pig model. *Virology Journal*, 3, 9.

Seacat, A. M., Thomford, P. J., Hansen, K. J., *et al.* (2002). Subchronic toxicity studies on perfluorooctanesulfonate potassium salt in cynomolgus monkeys. *Toxicological Sciences*, 68(1), 249–64.

Semela, D., Piguet, A. C., Kolev, M., *et al.* (2007). Vascular remodeling and antitumoral effects of mTOR inhibition in a rat model of hepatocellular carcinoma. *Journal of Hepatology*, 46(5), 840–8.

Sena, E. S., van der Worp, H. B., Bath, P. M. W., Howells, D. W. and Macleod, M. R. (2010). Publication bias in reports of animal stroke studies leads to major overstatement of efficacy. *PLoS Biol*, 8(3), e1000344.

Shaffer, J. P. (1995). Multiple hypothesis testing. *Annual Review of Psychology*, 46, 561–84.

Shapiro, S. S. and Wilk, M. B. (1965). An analysis of variance test for normality (complete samples). *Biometrika*, 52(3–4), 591–9.

Shaw, R. (2004). Reduction in laboratory animal use by factorial design. *Alternatives to Laboratory Animals: ATLA*, 32(2), 49–51.

Shaw, R., Festing, M. F. W., Peers, I. and Furlong, L. (2002). Use of factorial designs to optimize animal experiments and reduce animal use. *ILAR Journal*, 43(4), 223–32.

Shoaib, M., Sidhpura, N. and Shafait, S. (2003). Investigating the actions of bupropion on dependence-related effects of nicotine in rats. *Psychopharmacology* 165, 404–12.

Shirley, E. A. C. (1977). The analysis of organ weight data. *Toxicology*, 8, 13–22.

Šidák, Z. (1967). Rectangular confidence regions for the means of multivariate normal distributions. *Journal of the American Statistical Association*, 62(318), 626–33.

Singleton, K. D. and Wischmeyer, P. E. (2003). Distance of cecum ligated influences mortality, tumor necrosis factor-alpha and interleukin-6 expression following cecal ligation and puncture in the rat. *European Surgical Research*, 35(6), 486–91.

Sjödin, L., Visser, S. and Al-Saffar, A. (2011). Using pharmacokinetic modeling to determine the effect of drug and food on gastrointestinal transit in dogs. *Journal of Pharmacological and Toxicological Methods*, 64(1), 42–52.

Skene, S. S. and Kenward, M. G. (2010). The analysis of very small samples of repeated measurements I: an adjusted sandwich estimator. *Statistics in Medicine*, 29(27), 2825–37.

Slob, W. (2002). Dose-response modeling of continuous endpoints. *Toxicological Sciences*, 66(2), 298–312.

Slotten, H. A., Kalinichev, M., Hagan, J. J., Marsden, C. A. and Fone, K. C. F. (2006). Long-lasting changes in behavioural and neuroendocrine indices in the rat following neonatal maternal separation: gender-dependent effects. *Brain Research*, 1097(1), 123–32.

Smirnov, N. V. (1939). Estimation of deviation between empirical distribution functions in two independent samples. *Bulletin Moscow University*, 2(2), 3–16.

Smith, P. F. (2012). A note on the advantages of using linear mixed model analysis with maximal likelihood estimation over repeated measures ANOVAs in psychopharmacology: comment on Clark *et al.* (2012). *Journal of Psychopharmacology*, 26(12), 1605–7.

Smith, C. C., Adkins, D. J., Martin, E. A. and O'Donovan, M. R. (2008). Recommendations for design of the rat comet assay. *Mutagenesis*, 23(3), 233–40.

Snedecor, G. W. and Cochran, W. G. (1989). *Statistical Methods*, 8th edition. Iowa State University Press: Ames, IA.

Stufken, J. (1996). Optimal crossover designs. In *Handbook of Statistics 13: Design and Analysis of Experiments*, editors Ghosh, S. and Rao, C. R. 63–90. North-Holland: Amsterdam.

Tallarida, R. J. (2000). *Drug Synergism and Dose-Effect Data Analysis*. Chapman and Hall/CRC Press: Boca Raton, FL.

Tallarida, R. J. and Jacob, L. S. (1979). *The Dose-Response Relation in Pharmacology*. Springer-Verlag: New York.

Teng, Y. D., Lavik, E. B., Qu, X., *et al.* (2002). Functional recovery following traumatic spinal cord injury mediated by a unique polymer scaffold seeded with neural stem cells. *Proceedings of the National Academy of Sciences*, 99(5), 3024–9.

Toothaker, L. E. (1993). *Multiple Comparison Procedures*. No. 89. SAGE Publications Inc.: London, UK.

Torrallardona, D., Conde, M. R., Badiola, I., Polo, J. and Brufau, J. (2003). Effect of fishmeal replacement with spray-dried animal plasma and colistin on intestinal structure, intestinal microbiology, and performance of weanling pigs challenged with *Escherichia coli* K99. *Journal of Animal Science*, 81(5), 1220–6.

Tufte, E. R. (1983). *The Visual Display of Quantitative Information*. Graphics Press: Cheshire, CT.

Tukey, J. W. (1953). *The Problem of Multiple Comparisons*. Unpublished Notes, Princeton University.

van der Worp, H. B., Howells, D. W., Sena, E. S., *et al.* (2010). Can animal models of disease reliably inform human studies? *PLoS Medicine*, 7(3), e1000245.

Vesterinen, H. M., Sena, E. S., ffrench-Constant, C., *et al.* (2010). Improving the translational hit of experimental treatments in multiple sclerosis. *Multiple Sclerosis*, 16(9), 1044–55.

Wiklund, S. J. and Agurell, E. (2003). Aspects of design and statistical analysis in the Comet assay. *Mutagenesis*, 18(2), 167–75.

Williams, E. J. (1949). Experimental designs balanced for the estimation of residual effects of treatments. *Australian Journal of Scientific Research Series A*, 2, 149–68.

Wolfram, S., Raederstorff, D., Preller, M., *et al.* (2006). Epigallocatechin gallate supplementation alleviates diabetes in rodents. *The Journal of Nutrition*, 136, 2512–18.

Woolley, M. L., Pemberton, D. J., Bate, S., Corti, C. and Jones, D. N. C. (2008). The mGlu2 but not the mGlu3 receptor mediates the actions of the mGluR2/3 agonist, LY379268, in mouse models predictive of antipsychotic activity. *Psychopharmacology*, 196(3), 431–40.

Index